Public Awareness of Food Products, Preferences and Practices

Public Awareness of Food Products, Preferences and Practices

Editors

F. Xavier Medina
Francesc Fusté-Forné
Nela Filimon

MDPI • Basel • Beijing • Wuhan • Barcelona • Belgrade • Manchester • Tokyo • Cluj • Tianjin

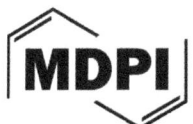

Editors

F. Xavier Medina
Faculty of Health Sciences
Universitat Oberta de
Catalunya
Barcelona
Spain

Francesc Fusté-Forné
Department of Business,
Faculty of Business and
Economic Sciences
University of Girona
Girona
Spain

Nela Filimon
Department of Business,
Faculty of Business and
Economic Sciences
University of Girona
Girona
Spain

Editorial Office
MDPI
St. Alban-Anlage 66
4052 Basel, Switzerland

This is a reprint of articles from the Special Issue published online in the open access journal *International Journal of Environmental Research and Public Health* (ISSN 1660-4601) (available at: www.mdpi.com/journal/ijerph/special_issues/Public_Awareness_Food).

For citation purposes, cite each article independently as indicated on the article page online and as indicated below:

LastName, A.A.; LastName, B.B.; LastName, C.C. Article Title. *Journal Name* **Year**, *Volume Number*, Page Range.

ISBN 978-3-0365-8545-1 (Hbk)
ISBN 978-3-0365-8544-4 (PDF)

© 2023 by the authors. Articles in this book are Open Access and distributed under the Creative Commons Attribution (CC BY) license, which allows users to download, copy and build upon published articles, as long as the author and publisher are properly credited, which ensures maximum dissemination and a wider impact of our publications.

The book as a whole is distributed by MDPI under the terms and conditions of the Creative Commons license CC BY-NC-ND.

Contents

About the Editors vii

Preface to "Public Awareness of Food Products, Preferences and Practices" ix

F. Xavier Medina, Francesc Fusté-Forné and Nela Filimon
Public Awareness of Food Products, Preferences and Practices: Old Challenges and New Insights
Reprinted from: *Int. J. Environ. Res. Public Health* **2023**, *20*, 5691, doi:10.3390/ijerph20095691 . . . 1

Claudia Valli, Marilina Santero, Anna Prokop-Dorner, Victoria Howatt, Bradley C. Johnston and Joanna Zajac et al.
Health Related Values and Preferences Regarding Meat Intake: A Cross-Sectional Mixed-Methods Study
Reprinted from: *Int. J. Environ. Res. Public Health* **2021**, *18*, 11585, doi:10.3390/ijerph182111585 . 5

Renata Nestorowicz, Ewa Jerzyk and Anna Rogala
In the Labyrinth of Dietary Patterns and Well-Being—When Eating Healthy Is Not Enough to Be Well
Reprinted from: *Int. J. Environ. Res. Public Health* **2022**, *19*, 1259, doi:10.3390/ijerph19031259 . . . 23

Carolin V. Zorell
Central Persons in Sustainable (Food) Consumption
Reprinted from: *Int. J. Environ. Res. Public Health* **2022**, *19*, 3139, doi:10.3390/ijerph19053139 . . . 39

Muhammad Zeeshan Zafar, Xiangjiao Shi, Hailan Yang, Jaffar Abbas and Jiakui Chen
The Impact of Interpretive Packaged Food Labels on Consumer Purchase Intention: The Comparative Analysis of Efficacy and Inefficiency of Food Labels
Reprinted from: *Int. J. Environ. Res. Public Health* **2022**, *19*, 15098, doi:10.3390/ijerph192215098 . 57

Yezheng Li, Pinyi Yao, Syuhaily Osman, Norzalina Zainudin and Mohamad Fazli Sabri
A Thematic Review on Using Food Delivery Services during the Pandemic: Insights for the Post-COVID-19 Era
Reprinted from: *Int. J. Environ. Res. Public Health* **2022**, *19*, 15267, doi:10.3390/ijerph192215267 . 73

Carmen Cipriano-Crespo, Francesc-Xavier Medina and Lorenzo Mariano-Juárez
Culinary Solitude in the Diet of People with Functional Diversity
Reprinted from: *Int. J. Environ. Res. Public Health* **2022**, *19*, 3624, doi:10.3390/ijerph19063624 . . . 95

Cecilia Díaz-Méndez, Sonia Otero-Estévez and Sandra Sánchez-Sánchez
Are Spanish Surveys Ready to Detect the Social Factors of Obesity?
Reprinted from: *Int. J. Environ. Res. Public Health* **2022**, *19*, 11156, doi:10.3390/ijerph191811156 . 109

Araceli Muñoz, Cristina Larrea-Killinger, Andrés Fontalba-Navas and Miguel Company-Morales
Categorizations of Trust and Distrust in the Classifications and Social Representations of Food among Pregnant and Breastfeeding Women in Spain—Applying the Cultural Domains' Pile Sort Technique
Reprinted from: *Int. J. Environ. Res. Public Health* **2023**, *20*, 4195, doi:10.3390/ijerph20054195 . . . 119

Josep M. Sole-Sedeno, Ester Miralpeix, Maria-Dolors Muns, Cristina Rodriguez-Cosmen, Berta Fabrego and Nadwa Kanjou et al.
Protein Supplementation in a Prehabilitation Program in Patients Undergoing Surgery for Endometrial Cancer
Reprinted from: *Int. J. Environ. Res. Public Health* **2023**, *20*, 5502, doi:10.3390/ijerph20085502 . . . 137

Agnieszka Dudziak and Anna Kocira
Preference-Based Determinants of Consumer Choice on the Polish Organic Food Market
Reprinted from: *Int. J. Environ. Res. Public Health* **2022**, *19*, 10895, doi:10.3390/ijerph191710895 . **145**

Magdalena Raftowicz
Prospects for the Development of the Demand for Carp in Poland among Young Consumers
Reprinted from: *Int. J. Environ. Res. Public Health* **2022**, *19*, 3831, doi:10.3390/ijerph19073831 . . . **163**

Marta Ros-Baró, Patricia Casas-Agustench, Diana Alícia Díaz-Rizzolo, Laura Batlle-Bayer, Ferran Adrià-Acosta and Alícia Aguilar-Martínez et al.
Edible Insect Consumption for Human and Planetary Health: A Systematic Review
Reprinted from: *Int. J. Environ. Res. Public Health* **2022**, *19*, 11653, doi:10.3390/ijerph191811653 . **181**

Marta Ros-Baró, Violeida Sánchez-Socarrás, Maria Santos-Pagès, Anna Bach-Faig and Alicia Aguilar-Martínez
Consumers' Acceptability and Perception of Edible Insects as an Emerging Protein Source
Reprinted from: *Int. J. Environ. Res. Public Health* **2022**, *19*, 15756, doi:10.3390/ijerph192315756 . **211**

Mª Genoveva Dancausa Millán and Mª Genoveva Millán Vázquez de la Torre
Quality Food Products as a Tourist Attraction in the Province of Córdoba (Spain)
Reprinted from: *Int. J. Environ. Res. Public Health* **2022**, *19*, 12754, doi:10.3390/ijerph191912754 . **225**

Mian Yang, Wenjie Fan, Jian Qiu, Sining Zhang and Jinting Li
The Evaluation of Rural Outdoor Dining Environment from Consumer Perspective
Reprinted from: *Int. J. Environ. Res. Public Health* **2022**, *19*, 13767, doi:10.3390/ijerph192113767 . **249**

About the Editors

F. Xavier Medina

F. Xavier Medina holds a PhD in Social Anthropology by the University of Barcelona, and is a full professor (Anthropology of Food), Department of Food, Nutrition and Physical Activity, Faculty of Health Sciences, Universitat Oberta de Catalunya / Open University of Catalonia, in Barcelona (Spain). He is the Director of the UNESCO Chair on Food, Culture and Development, and World President of the International Commission on the Anthropology of Food and Nutrition (ICAF). He is also the principal investigator (PI) of the FoodLab, a multi-disciplinary group carrying out research into food, nutrition, society and health.

Francesc Fusté-Forné

Francesc Fusté-Forné holds a PhD in Tourism by the University of Girona and a PhD in Communication (Ramon Llull University), and is a lecturer at the Department of Business, Faculty of Business and Economic Sciences, Universitat de Girona (Spain). He is also a researcher at the Multidisciplinary Laboratory of Tourism Research, member of the Institute of Tourism Studies (INSETUR) and the Director of the Chair of Maritime Studies at the University of Girona.

Nela Filimon

Nela Filimon holds a PhD in Economics from the Universitat Autònoma de Barcelona, and is a Serra Húnter associate professor at the Department of Business, Faculty of Business and Economic Sciences, Universitat de Girona (Spain).

Preface to "Public Awareness of Food Products, Preferences and Practices"

This reprint is the result of a Special Issue that took place in the International Journal of Environmental Research and Public Health (IJERPH) during 2022-2023. The general topic of the reprint discusses the different uses, protection and promotion of food, always from a broad perspective, through 15 innovative research papers, from both qualitative and quantitative methodological approaches.

This subject is relevant for various reasons: on the one hand, because of its interdisciplinarity; on the other hand, due to the multiplicity of topics and approaches. But, in any case, all of them focus on food, as a complex aspect of human life, which affects all people at all ages and at all times of life.

The articles published in this reprint reproduce the format and order in which they were published in the original Special Issue. Their joint publication, however, provides an overview that is useful and relevant for people interested in these issues. Issues, by the way, that have not yet received enough attention from interdisciplinary and open perspectives. This reprint tries, albeit insufficiently, to fill a part of this void.

F. Xavier Medina, Francesc Fusté-Forné, and Nela Filimon
Editors

Editorial

Public Awareness of Food Products, Preferences and Practices: Old Challenges and New Insights

F. Xavier Medina [1,*], Francesc Fusté-Forné [2] and Nela Filimon [2]

1. Unesco Chair on Food, Culture and Development, Department of Food and Nutrition, Faculty of Health Sciences, Universitat Oberta de Catalunya (UOC), Rambla del Poblenou, 156, 08035 Barcelona, Spain
2. Department of Business, Faculty of Business and Economic Sciences, Edifici Econòmiques, c/ de la Universitat de Girona, 10, Campus Montilivi, University of Girona, 17003 Girona, Spain; francesc.fusteforne@udg.edu (F.F.-F.); nela.filimon@udg.edu (N.F.)
* Correspondence: fxmedina@uoc.edu

Food is not only a source of nutrition for humans; it also encompasses social, cultural, and psychological dynamics. Understanding of food products, preferences, and practices provides us with knowledge of historical, cultural and contemporary uses [1]. In addition, food and drink act as both identifiers and attractions of regions around the world. In this regard, there are a great variety of actors, cultures, and practices within the food value chain. This Special Issue on 'Public Awareness of Food Products, Preferences and Practices' discusses the protection and promotion of food, from a broad perspective, through 15 innovative research papers and systematic reviews, from both qualitative and quantitative methodological approaches.

In the first paper published in this Special Issue, Valli et al. [2] analyze the influence of people's values and preferences on daily food choices in relation to unprocessed and processed red meat. Based on a cross-sectional mixed-methods study, they revealed that the majority of their sample was unwilling to stop, and even to reduce, their red meat consumption; this line of thinking is driven by the familial and social context of meat consumption, and by health- and non-health-related concerns about meat consumption. In a similar manner, Nestorowicz et al. [3] studied the relationship between food consumption and wellbeing, and how the diet influences levels of wellbeing. Drawing on a quantitative approach, they determined that the consumption of organic food and following a regimen such as a vegan, low-salt, or low-sugar diet results in higher levels of wellbeing; this conclusion was not only based on health, but also on pleasure and the social dimension of food.

Zorell [4] highlighted the role of influencers on individuals' consumption decisions. Informed by a quantitative analysis, their paper shows that social media is a primary source of information about food, along with families and schools, and that this source may also lead to environmentally friendlier food consumption. Zafar et al. [5] analyzed the impact of food labels on consumers' attitudes and intentions towards healthy and nutritional foods. Based on a quantitative study, their results show that food labels and their format not only influence consumers' attitudes, but also their purchasing decisions. The study by Li et al. [6] focuses on food delivery services as an example of online-to-offline (O2O) commerce. The authors develop a literature review and reveal current research and industry trends.

In addition, Cipriano-Crespo et al. [7] present a qualitative ethnographic study identifying how the feeding process of people with functional diversity results in different eating situations. Their results show that influences on eating situations are mainly driven by three themes: social ghettoization and culinary loneliness; stigma, shame, feeling like a burden, and loneliness; and exclusion or self-exclusion at the dining table. Additionally, Díaz-Méndez et al. [8] analyzed the social factors that contribute to obesity as a public health problem. Based on the case of Spain, they reveal that while official statistics include socio-demographic variables, health and social variables, always understood from a social perspective, could allow the provision of more tangible support for halting obesity [9].

Muñoz et al. [10] focused on the role of food in pregnant and breastfeeding women, and its influence on both their own health and the health of their child. The paper analyzes discourses and practices in relation to the dietary intake of the participants, and shows the role of trust and mistrust in relation to food products, foods' origins, and modes of production. Additionally, in the context of dietary intake, but specifically of nutritional interventions in surgery patients from a hospital perspective, Sole-Sedeno et al. [11] explored the impact of protein supplementation in a prehabilitation program in endometrial cancer patients undergoing laparoscopic surgery.

In the context of Poland as a particular example in Europe, Raftowicz [12] analyzed the situation of the country's carp fishing economy. The paper alerts readers to the stagnation of a centuries-old tradition, and explains the challenges facing the development of the market because of a decrease in carp consumption by young adult consumers. On the other hand, Dudziak and Kocira [13] focused their research on the development of the organic food market. They study the barriers related to the availability of organic food and also the lack of awareness of consumers. Based on a quantitative design, the paper analyzes the determinants affecting people's choices of organic food, these determinants being price and product labeling.

Ros-Baró et al. [14] carried out a systematic review aiming to examine the role of edible insect consumption in health outcomes, alongside its environmental impact. They reveal that edible insects are an alternative protein source that can improve human and animal nutrition, and improve the health of the planet. Later, Ros-Baró et al. [15] analyzed the factors involved in consumer acceptability of insect consumption in the Mediterranean area in a more applied way. Their quantitative study demonstrated that neophobia, social norms, familiarity, experiences of consumption, and knowledge of benefits are crucial to spread information and therefore increase insect consumption.

Dancausa Millán and Millán Vázquez de la Torre [16] analyzed the relationships between food and tourism based on quality foods endorsed by protected designations of origin (PDOs). They focused on olive oil, wine and ham. Drawing from the perspectives of gastronomic tourists, they propose strategies to deseasonalize tourism through food.

Finally, in the context of the relationship between food and tourism, Yang et al. [17] focused on the rural catering industry. They also analyzed the perspectives of consumers through social media data. Their results show that agricultural resources, safety, and a hygienic environment are important factors in the competitiveness of rural restaurants, and explain the differences between three different groups of clientele (regular customers, customers with children, and elderly customers).

This Special Issue on 'Public Awareness of Food Products, Preferences and Practices' discusses the conception, protection, and promotion of food from a broad perspective, analyzing food-based experiences, consumption, food cultures, social behavior related to food, and healthy and sustainable food practices. All these papers came from original and innovative international research and case studies that show food, from all perspectives, as it is: a necessary fact that straddles the biological and the social, with strong implications for our daily life. They also invite researchers and decision-makers in the field to look into future lines of research, which will span various different areas, such as artificial intelligence, advances in measuring food carbon footprint, demographic and climate change, the preservation of biodiversity, and other factors that could affect individuals' food preferences, lifestyle, health, and wellbeing.

Author Contributions: Conceptualization, F.F.-F., F.X.M. and N.F.; validation, F.F.-F., F.X.M. and N.F.; writing—original draft preparation, F.F.-F.; writing—review and editing, F.X.M. and N.F.; visualization, F.F.-F., F.X.M. and N.F.; supervision, F.X.M.; project administration, F.F.-F., F.X.M. and N.F. N.F. is Serra Húnter Fellow. All authors have read and agreed to the published version of the manuscript.

Conflicts of Interest: The authors declare no conflict of interest.

References

1. Medina, F.X. Food Culture: Anthropology of Food and Nutrition. In *Encyclopedia of Food Security and Sustainability*; Ferranti, P., Berry, E., Anderson, J.R., Eds.; Elsevier: Oxford, UK, 2019; Volume 2.
2. Valli, C.; Santero, M.; Prokop-Dorner, A.; Howatt, V.; Johnston, B.C.; Zajac, J.; Han, M.-A.; Pereira, A.; Kenji Nampo, F.; Guyatt, G.H.; et al. Health Related Values and Preferences Regarding Meat Intake: A Cross-Sectional Mixed-Methods Study. *Int. J. Environ. Res. Public Health* **2021**, *18*, 11585. [CrossRef] [PubMed]
3. Nestorowicz, R.; Jerzyk, E.; Rogala, A. In the Labyrinth of Dietary Patterns and Well-Being—When Eating Healthy Is Not Enough to Be Well. *Int. J. Environ. Res. Public Health* **2022**, *19*, 1259. [CrossRef] [PubMed]
4. Zorell, C.V. Central Persons in Sustainable (Food) Consumption. *Int. J. Environ. Res. Public Health* **2022**, *19*, 3139. [CrossRef] [PubMed]
5. Zafar, M.Z.; Shi, X.; Yang, H.; Abbas, J.; Chen, J. The Impact of Interpretive Packaged Food Labels on Consumer Purchase Intention: The Comparative Analysis of Efficacy and Inefficiency of Food Labels. *Int. J. Environ. Res. Public Health* **2022**, *19*, 15098. [CrossRef] [PubMed]
6. Li, Y.; Yao, P.; Osman, S.; Zainudin, N.; Sabri, M.F. A Thematic Review on Using Food Delivery Services during the Pandemic: Insights for the Post-COVID-19 Era. *Int. J. Environ. Res. Public Health* **2022**, *19*, 15267. [CrossRef]
7. Cipriano-Crespo, C.; Medina, F.X.; Mariano-Juárez, L. Culinary Solitude in the Diet of People with Functional Diversity. *Int. J. Environ. Res. Public Health* **2022**, *19*, 3624. [CrossRef] [PubMed]
8. Díaz-Méndez, C.; Otero-Estévez, S.; Sánchez-Sánchez, S. Are Spanish Surveys Ready to Detect the Social Factors of Obesity? *Int. J. Environ. Res. Public Health* **2022**, *19*, 11156. [CrossRef]
9. Medina, F.X.; Solé-Sedeno, J.M.; Bach-Faig, A.; Aguilar-Martínez, A. Obesity, Mediterranean Diet, and Public Health: A Vision of Obesity in the Mediterranean Context from a Sociocultural Perspective. *Int. J. Environ. Res. Public Health* **2021**, *18*, 3715. [CrossRef] [PubMed]
10. Muñoz, A.; Larrea-Killinger, C.; Fontalba-Navas, A.; Company-Morales, M. Categorizations of Trust and Distrust in the Classifications and Social Representations of Food among Pregnant and Breastfeeding Women in Spain—Applying the Cultural Domains' Pile Sort Technique. *Int. J. Environ. Res. Public Health* **2023**, *20*, 4195. [CrossRef] [PubMed]
11. Sole-Sedeno, J.M.; Miralpeix, E.; Muns, M.-D.; Rodriguez-Cosmen, C.; Fabrego, B.; Kanjou, N.; Medina, F.-X.; Mancebo, G. Protein Supplementation in a Prehabilitation Program in Patients Undergoing Surgery for Endometrial Cancer. *Int. J. Environ. Res. Public Health* **2023**, *20*, 5502. [CrossRef] [PubMed]
12. Raftowicz, M. Prospects for the Development of the Demand for Carp in Poland among Young Consumers. *Int. J. Environ. Res. Public Health* **2022**, *19*, 3831. [CrossRef] [PubMed]
13. Dudziak, A.; Kocira, A. Preference-Based Determinants of Consumer Choice on the Polish Organic Food Market. *Int. J. Environ. Res. Public Health* **2022**, *19*, 10895. [CrossRef] [PubMed]
14. Ros-Baró, M.; Casas-Agustench, P.; Díaz-Rizzolo, D.A.; Batlle-Bayer, L.; Adrià-Acosta, F.; Aguilar-Martínez, A.; Medina, F.-X.; Pujolà, M.; Bach-Faig, A. Edible Insect Consumption for Human and Planetary Health: A Systematic Review. *Int. J. Environ. Res. Public Health* **2022**, *19*, 11653. [CrossRef] [PubMed]
15. Ros-Baró, M.; Sánchez-Socarrás, V.; Santos-Pagès, M.; Bach-Faig, A.; Aguilar-Martínez, A. Consumers' Acceptability and Perception of Edible Insects as an Emerging Protein Source. *Int. J. Environ. Res. Public Health* **2022**, *19*, 15756. [CrossRef] [PubMed]
16. Dancausa Millán, M.G.; Millán Vázquez de la Torre, M.G. Quality Food Products as a Tourist Attraction in the Province of Córdoba (Spain). *Int. J. Environ. Res. Public Health* **2022**, *19*, 12754. [CrossRef] [PubMed]
17. Yang, M.; Fan, W.; Qiu, J.; Zhang, S.; Li, J. The Evaluation of Rural Outdoor Dining Environment from Consumer Perspective. *Int. J. Environ. Res. Public Health* **2022**, *19*, 13767. [CrossRef] [PubMed]

Disclaimer/Publisher's Note: The statements, opinions and data contained in all publications are solely those of the individual author(s) and contributor(s) and not of MDPI and/or the editor(s). MDPI and/or the editor(s) disclaim responsibility for any injury to people or property resulting from any ideas, methods, instructions or products referred to in the content.

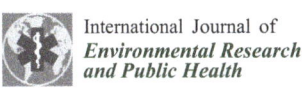

Article

Health Related Values and Preferences Regarding Meat Intake: A Cross-Sectional Mixed-Methods Study

Claudia Valli [1,2,*], Marilina Santero [1,2], Anna Prokop-Dorner [3], Victoria Howatt [4,5], Bradley C. Johnston [6,7], Joanna Zajac [8], Mi-Ah Han [9], Ana Pereira [10,11], Fernando Kenji Nampo [12], Gordon H. Guyatt [13], Malgorzata M. Bala [8], Pablo Alonso-Coello [2,14] and Montserrat Rabassa [2]

1. Department of Paediatrics, Obstetrics, Gynaecology and Preventive Medicine, Universidad Autónoma de Barcelona, 08193 Barcelona, Spain; marilinasantero@gmail.com
2. Iberoamerican Cochrane Centre, Biomedical Research Institute San Pau (IIB Sant Pau), 08025 Barcelona, Spain; PAlonso@santpau.cat (P.A.-C.); mrabassa.cochrane@gmail.com (M.R.)
3. Department of Medical Sociology, Chair of Epidemiology and Preventive Medicine, Jagiellonian University Medical College, 31-034 Krakow, Poland; anna.prokop@uj.edu.pl
4. Faculty of Medicine, Dalhousie University, Halifax, NS B3H 4R2, Canada; vhowatt@dal.ca
5. Department of Community Health and Epidemiology, Dalhousie University, Halifax, NS B3H 4R2, Canada
6. Department Epidemiology and Biostatistics, School of Public Health, Texas A&M University, College Station, TX 77843, USA; bjohnston@dal.ca
7. Department of Nutrition, Texas A&M University, College Station, TX 77843, USA
8. Department of Hygiene and Dietetics, Chair Department of Epidemiology and Preventive Medicine, Jagiellonian University Medical College, 31-034 Krakow, Poland; joanna.faustyna.zajac@gmail.com (J.Z.); malgorzata.1.bala@uj.edu.pl (M.M.B.)
9. College of Medicine, Chosun University, Gwangju 61452, Korea; mahan@chosun.ac.kr
10. Servicio Madrileño de Salud (SERMAS), 28008 Madrid, Spain; pereiraiglesiasana@gmail.com
11. Sociedad Madrileña de Medicina de Familia Comunitaria (SoMaMFyC), 28004 Madrid, Spain
12. Evidence-Based Public Health Research Group, Latin-American Institute of Life and Nature Sciences, Federal University of Latin-American Integration, Foz do Iguassu 85866-000, PR, Brazil; fernando.nampo@unila.edu.br
13. Department of Medicine, McMaster University, Hamilton, ON L8N 3Z5, Canada; guyatt@mcmaster.ca
14. CIBER de Epidemiología y Salud Pública (CIBERESP), 28029 Madrid, Spain
* Correspondence: cvalli@santpau.cat or claudia.valli89@gmail.com

Abstract: Background. In addition to social and environmental determinants, people's values and preferences determine daily food choices. This study evaluated adults' values and preferences regarding unprocessed red meat (URM) and processed meat (PM) and their willingness to change their consumption in the face of possible undesirable health consequences. Methods. A cross-sectional mixed-methods study including a quantitative assessment through an online survey, a qualitative inquiry through semi-structured interviews, and a follow-up assessment through a telephone survey. We performed descriptive statistics, logistic regressions, and thematic analysis. Results. Of 304 participants, over 75% were unwilling to stop their consumption of either URM or PM, and of those unwilling to stop, over 80% were also unwilling to reduce. Men were less likely to stop meat intake than women (odds ratios < 0.4). From the semi-structured interviews, we identified three main themes: the social and/or family context of meat consumption, health- and non-health-related concerns about meat, and uncertainty of the evidence. At three months, 63% of participants reported no changes in meat intake. Conclusions. When informed about the cancer incidence and mortality risks of meat consumption, most respondents would not reduce their intake. Public health and clinical nutrition guidelines should ensure that their recommendations are consistent with population values and preferences.

Keywords: health; values and preferences; red meat; processed meat; cross-sectional study; mixed methods; explanatory sequential; survey

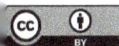

1. Introduction

Many believe that people's dietary choices have important consequences for their health. All individuals face the daily choice regarding what to eat, and in what quantity [1]. People's food choices, in addition to social and environmental determinants, may depend on their beliefs regarding health effects, their beliefs about the environmental effects of their diet, the pleasure they take in eating, their social and cultural milieu and the relative importance they place on these issues.

When developing guidance for public dietary behaviour, respect for individual autonomy requires understanding the health-outcome-related values and preferences that are linked to diet among members of the public. Most dietary guidelines have, however, not only failed to conduct systematic reviews (SRs) of people's values and preferences, but have also neglected this issue when making their recommendations [2,3].

With regard to meat, given the association between unprocessed red meat (URM) and processed meat (PM) consumption and adverse health outcomes (cancer and cardiovascular events) [4], dietary guidelines have generally recommended limiting meat intake [5–7]. In developing a guideline regarding meat consumption, our group undertook a SR that addressed relevant health-related values and preferences. We found that reasons for meat consumption varied and that people's willingness to change their meat consumption is generally low [8], but because researchers had never undertaken the most relevant studies to inform the question, the evidence was only low quality.

We therefore developed and conducted a cross-sectional explanatory sequential mixed-methods study in order to evaluate adults' values and preferences regarding URM and PM intake and their willingness to change their intake in the face of possible undesirable health consequences based on the dose–response meta-analysis SR of meat and cancer risk [9]. Unprocessed red meat was defined as mammalian meat (e.g., beef, pork, lamb), and processed meat was defined as white or red meat that was preserved by smoking, curing, salting, or by the addition of preservatives (e.g., hot dogs, charcuterie, sausage, ham, and cold cut deli meats). One serving corresponded to 120 g for unprocessed red meat, and 50 g for processed meat [10].

2. Methods

2.1. Study Design and Setting

This cross-sectional explanatory sequential mixed-methods study included a quantitative assessment through an online survey, a qualitative inquiry through semi-structured interviews, and a follow-up assessment through a telephone survey. Our team conducted the study in Spain between November 2020 and March 2021, based on a previously published study protocol where further details on the methods are provided [11]. The report follows STROBE guidelines [12].

This work constitutes one part of NutriRECS (Nutritional Recommendations; www.nutrirecs.com, accessed on 26 November 2020), an initiative that aims, by following a rigorous and transparent approach based on the methods promoted by the National Academy of Medicine, Guideline International Network and GRADE, and that includes the incorporation of values and preferences of the public [13], in order to develop trustworthy nutritional recommendations.

2.2. Study Population

People learned about this study thorough the Cochrane website and Twitter, where we published all of the information related to the study, eligibility criteria, contact information of the researcher carrying out the study, and the related link to access the online survey. People who were interested in participating completed the online consent form and accessed the survey. Respondents included adults between 18 and 80 years of age who currently consume URM and/or PM. We excluded adults who had active cancer and those who had suffered a major cardiovascular event such as: stroke, angina, myocardial infarction, heart failure, symptomatic peripheral arterial disease, as well as pregnant women and those unwilling or unable to provide informed consent.

2.3. Questionnaire and Study Procedures

The questionnaire was first developed and reviewed by experts on the topic in order to ensure the validity of the included items in the questionnaire; secondly, we pilot-tested it in English in a convenience sample of participants [14]. On the basis of the pilot study, our team modified the questionnaire, performed a translation into Spanish—one researcher translated the survey that was reviewed and a second researcher confirmed it—and finally, we developed an online version that we tested on 34 Spanish participants to establish clarity and understanding. Based on the findings of the pre-testing, we refined the survey to improve face and content validity. See Supplementary Materials for the Spanish version of the online survey.

The questionnaire addressed the participants' demographic characteristics, their medical history and meat consumption beliefs and behaviours, and it also included a direct-choice exercise. This exercise presented scenarios that were tailored to each individual's weekly meat consumption and included, based on a prior SR and dose–response meta-analysis, the best estimates of the risk reduction of overall lifetime cancer incidences and cancer mortality that is associated with a decrease in URM and/or PM consumption [9]. In order to keep the presentation understandable and assimilable, we decided to focus only on cancer and thus, we omitted the possible cardiovascular effects. The scenarios also presented the corresponding certainty of the evidence for the potential risk reductions. The questionnaire was tailored to participants' individual meat consumption (i.e., after they had stated their mean consumption, subsequent questions referred to those prior responses) and participants' willingness to change their meat intake (those unwilling to change responded to additional questions regarding whether higher quality evidence or a larger effect would change their willingness).

Participants first considered the cancer-incidence scenario and expressed their willingness to "stop" their URM and PM intake using a 7-point Likert-scale with 1 (meaning definitely unwilling) and 7 (meaning definitely willing) (Question 1). If participants were unwilling to stop (≤ 4 of the Likert-scale), they were asked, using a 7-point Likert-scale question (Question a), if they would stop their intake if the certainty of the evidence was higher. If they were still unwilling to stop (≤ 4 of the Likert-scale), we asked them, using a multiple-choice question (Question b), if they were willing to stop if the evidence showed a larger risk reduction. If, after the above questions, participants were still unwilling to stop, we presented them with an additional 7-point Likert-scale question about their willingness to "reduce" their intake (Question 2). Similar to what was reported above, participants unwilling to reduce their intake (≤ 4 of the Likert-scale), were presented with the questions about the certainty of the evidence (Question a) and, if still unwilling, the magnitude of the risk (Question b). If participants were also unwilling to reduce their intake (≤ 4 of the Likert-scale), they were finally presented with a question about whether they were instead willing to increase their meat consumption using a 7-point Likert-scale question (Question 3). This logic of questions was applied for both types of meat and for both the cancer-incidence and cancer-mortality scenarios (Figure 1).

Two additional questions invited respondents to participate in a semi-structured interview and a follow-up assessment at 3 months. If the respondents had agreed to participate in the semi-structured interviews, then we arranged a meeting (through a secured Skype/Zoom call or by telephone) in which we reviewed and discussed their answers from the online survey and asked additional questions addressing their motives to change or continue with their current URM and/or PM consumption. At 3 months after the online survey, we conducted follow-up interviews via email and/or phone and asked the participants who had agreed to be contacted if they had made any changes in their meat consumption.

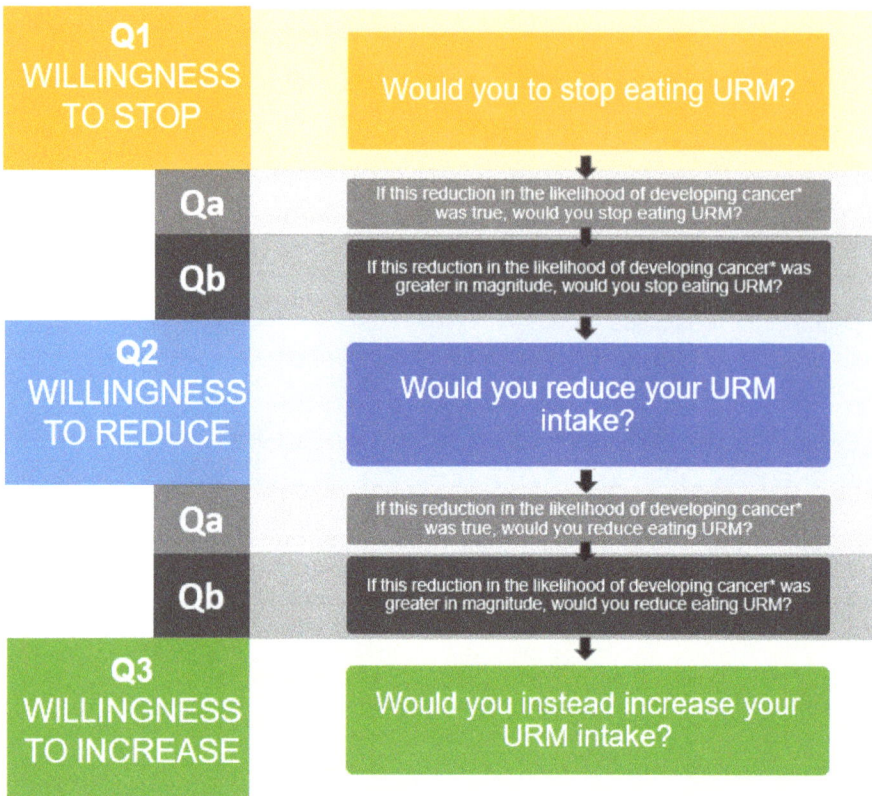

Figure 1. Questions framework for the direct-choice cancer-incidence exercise for unprocessed red meat. Abbreviations: URM = unprocessed red meat; Q1 = Question 1; Q2 = question2; Q3 = Question3; Qa = Question a; Qb = Question b. Q1–Q2–Q3: Willingness to stop, reduce and increase meat intake was based on a 7-point Likert-scale with 1 (meaning definitely not) and 7 (meaning definitely yes). Qa: Willingness to stop and reduce meat intake with higher certainty was based on a 7-point Likert-scale with 1 (meaning definitely not) and 7 (meaning definitely yes). Qb: Willingness to stop and reduce processed meat consumption with a larger risk reduction was formulated as a multiple-choice question. This logic of questions was applied for both types of meat and for both cancer-incidence and cancer-mortality scenarios. * For the mortality scenarios "developing cancer" was changed into "dying from cancer".

2.4. Data Synthesis and Analysis

2.4.1. Quantitative Analysis

All statistical analyses were performed using RStudio (version 1.2.5033) [15]. Data were checked for normal distribution using the Kolmogorov–Smirnov test. An independent samples t-test (normal distribution) or a Mann–Whitney U test (non-normal distribution) was used to assess the differences between the two groups. For categorical variables, differences between groups were analyzed by the chi-square test. Missing values were excluded from the analysis.

We described the participants' demographic and medical history information as well as their meat consumption behaviours using mean ± standard deviation or as median and inter-quartile-range (IQR) and number (percentage). Because the data were not normally distributed, we presented the participants' willingness to stop, reduce and increase meat consumption in the face of undesirable cancer as medians and IQRs.

We performed a separate logistic regression analysis for each dependent variable in order to explore the determinants of the participants' willingness to change meat consumption in the direct-choice scenarios. The dependent variables were the choice (unwilling versus willing) to stop and reduce eating URM and/or PM in the face of cancer-incidence risks as well as cancer-mortality risks. The team identified the independent variables of sex, age, level of education, occupational status and religious belief a priori as known potential confounders and they were included in each statistical model. Linear regression was not performed as planned in the protocol because the assumption of linearity was violated.

We calculated the number and percentage of participants who had made any changes in their meat consumption at the follow-up after three months.

2.4.2. Qualitative Analysis

After collecting the data and transcribing the semi-structured interviews, we conducted an iterative, thematic analysis, using constant comparison within and across the transcripts of the study's participants by following a six-step approach (i.e., familiarisation with the data, generating initial codes, searching for themes, reviewing the themes, defining and naming the themes and producing the final report) [16].

2.4.3. Integrating Qualitative and Quantitative Analyses

We conducted a sequential analysis of the quantitative and qualitative components of the data. We analysed each dataset separately and then, at the end of the study, listed the findings from each component of our study and drew meta-inferences. Findings of interest from both data sets were compared and contrasted for convergence (whether findings from each data set agree), complementarity (whether findings offer complementary information on the same issue), dissonance (appear to contradict each other) and "silence" (a particular finding could only be explored in one data set) [17]. The integrated data were presented using a joint display [18], which presents each theme from the qualitative analyses according to the proportion that was obtained from the relevant online survey questions.

3. Results

3.1. Online Survey

3.1.1. Participants' Characteristics

Of the 304 individuals who participated in our study, typical respondents were women around 40 years old with a university degree (85%), employed (81%), and having at least one comorbidity (74%) (Table 1).

Table 1. Participants' sociodemographic and medical history.

	Overall (n = 304)
Sex, n (%)	
Women	189 (62.0)
Men	115 (38.0)
Age, years	
Mean (SD)	39.8 (10.7)
Median (Q1, Q3)	38.0 (32.0, 46.0)
Education level, n (%)	
Primary education	3 (1.0)
Secondary education	14 (4.6)
Professional education	24 (7.9)
University education	259 (85.2)
No studies	1 (0.3)
Employment status, n (%)	
Employed	247 (81.2)
Unemployed	34 (11.2)

Table 1. Cont.

	Overall (n = 304)
Student	20 (6.6)
Marital status, n (%)	
Married	94 (30.9)
Common-law couple	5 (1.6)
Living with my partner or family	87 (28.6)
Separated	2 (0.7)
Divorced	12 (3.9)
Widow/widower	1 (0.3)
Single	100 (32.9)
Children, n (%)	
One child	42 (13.8)
Two children	62 (20.4)
Three or more children	14 (4.6)
None	183 (60.2)
Religion, n (%)	
Catholicism	62 (20.4)
Other	9 (3.0)
None	230 (75.7)
Physical activity intensity [¥], n (%)	
Low	82 (27.0)
Moderate	139 (45.7)
High	80 (26.3)
Weight, kg	
Mean (SD)	69.9 (14.5)
Median (Q1, Q3)	68.0 (59.8, 79.0)
Height, m	
Mean (SD)	1.70 (0.1)
Median (Q1, Q3)	1.70 (1.6, 1.8)
BMI	
Mean (SD)	24.3 (4.1)
Median (Q1, Q3)	23.6 (21.5, 26.2)
Comorbidities, n (%)	
Hormonal system disorders	14 (4.6)
Digestive diseases	12 (3.9)
Musculoskeletal disorders	8 (2.6)
Other	41 (13.5)
None	226 (74.3)
Family history of cancer, n (%)	
Yes	198 (65.1)
No	73 (24.0)
I don't know	30 (9.9)

Abbreviations: SD = standard deviation; Q1 = Quartile 1; Q3 = Quartile 3, kg = kilograms; m = meters; BMI = body mass index. [¥] Physical activity (PA) intensity was categorized as follows: participants who reported doing PA every day were categorized in the "high" category; who reported doing PA at least once a week was categorized in the "moderate" one and the rest of participants were categorized in the "low" category.

3.1.2. Participants' Meat Consumption Behaviour

Many participants reported consuming less than three servings of meat per week (76% of URM and 57% of PM), 24% of participants consumed three or more servings of URM and 43% of PM. Figure 2 presents the meat-consumption frequency behaviour. The type of URM most frequently consumed was beef or veal (76.0%) and, for PM, Serrano ham or shoulder ham (71.4%) (See Supplementary Materials: Figures S1 and S2). The three main reasons for meat consumption among the participants included flavour, cost and availability, and were similar for URM and PM (See Supplementary Materials: Table S1).

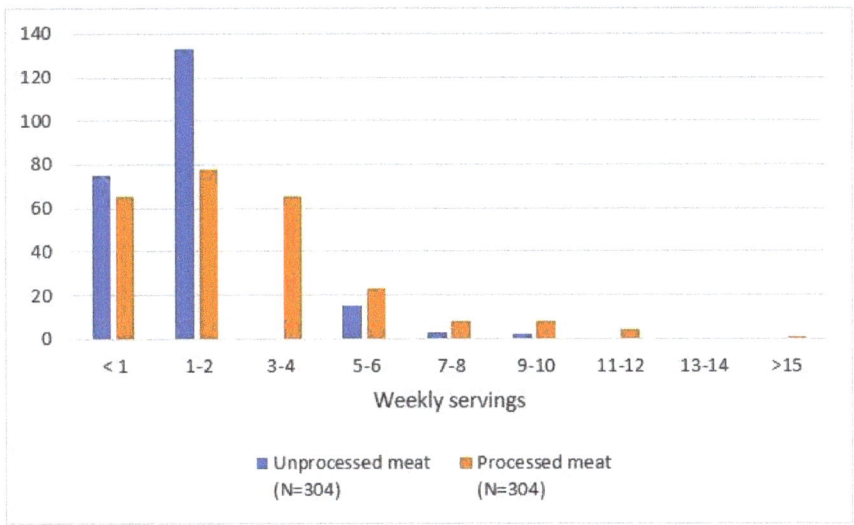

Figure 2. Meat consumption frequency behavior.

With regard to URM consumption, 27.3% had previously reduced consumption for health; for PM, the same was true of 38.2% of participants, whereas 38.5% reported to have reduced their intake of meat in general for other non-health-related reasons. Among the eight different non-health-related reasons participants could choose from, animal welfare and environmental concerns were the most frequently reported (Table 2).

Table 2. Participants' meat reduction in the past.

Past reduction due to health reasons	
Unprocessed red meat	
N	283
No, n (%)	200 (65.8)
Yes, n (%)	83 (27.3)
Processed meat	
N	283
No, n (%)	167 (54.9)
Yes, n (%)	116 (38.2)
Past reduction due to other reasons	
Meat in general	
N	282
No, n (%)	165 (54.3)
Yes, n (%)	117 (38.5)
Other reasons, n (%)	
Animal welfare	62 (20.4)
Environmental concerns	67 (22.0)
Family preferences	15 (4.9)
Social context	7 (2.3)
Availability/accessibility	5 (1.6)
Flavour	21 (6.9)
Cost	14 (4.6)
Other	31 (10.2)

Unprocessed red meat was defined as mammalian meat (e.g., beef, pork, lamb), and processed meat was defined as white or red meat that was preserved by smoking, curing, salting, or by the addition of preservatives (e.g., hot dogs, charcuterie, sausage, ham, and cold cut deli meats). One serving corresponded to 120 g for unprocessed red meat and 50 g for processed meat.

3.1.3. Willingness to Change Meat Consumption (Questions 1, 2 and 3)

The majority of participants were unwilling to introduce any changes to their URM and PM consumption in the face of the associated reductions in overall cancer-incidence and cancer-mortality risks. Most respondents were unwilling to stop their intake (URM: 78.6%; PM: 77.9%); of those unwilling to stop, most were also unwilling to reduce (URM: 81.1%; PM: 91.5%) their intake when presented with the cancer-incidence scenario; likewise, most participants were unwilling to stop (URM: 75.4%; PM: 76.4%), and of those unwilling to stop, to reduce (URM: 85.7%; PM: 80%) when presented with the mortality scenario. Similarly, none of the participants were willing to increase their URM and/or PM intake. Table 3 presents the participants' willingness to stop, and if unwilling to stop, to reduce, and if unwilling to reduce, to increase URM and PM consumption in the face of cancer-incidence and cancer-mortality risks.

Table 3. Willingness to change meat consumption in the face of cancer-incidence and cancer-mortality risks.

	URM	PM
Willingness to stop—Question 1		
Cancer Incidence		
N	126	163
Willing, n (%)	27 (21.4)	36 (22.1)
Unwilling, n (%)	99 (78.6)	127 (77.9)
Median	3.0	3.0
Q1, Q3	(1.0, 4.0)	(2.0, 4.0)
Cancer Mortality		
N	118	157
Willing, n (%)	29 (24.6)	37 (23.6)
Unwilling, n (%)	89 (75.4)	120 (76.4)
Median	3.0	3.0
Q1, Q3	(1.0, 4.0)	(2.0, 4.0)
Willingness to stop with higher certainty—Question a		
Cancer Incidence		
N	94	120
Willing, n (%)	25 (26.6)	43 (35.8)
Unwilling, n (%)	69 (73.4)	77 (64.2)
Median	3.0	3.0
Q1, Q3	(2.0, 5.0)	(2.0, 5.0)
Cancer Mortality		
N	84	106
Willing, n (%)	16 (19.0)	31 (29.2)
Unwilling, n (%)	68 (81.0)	75 (70.8)
Median	3.0	3.0
Q1, Q3	(1.0, 4.0)	(2.0, 5.0)

Table 3. *Cont.*

	URM	PM
Willingness to stop with a larger risk reduction—Question b		
Cancer Incidence		
N	68	50
Unwilling, n (%)	21 (31.0)	17 (34.0)
Willing, n (%)	25 (37.0)	19 (38.0)
Neither unwilling nor willing, n (%)	22 (32.0)	14 (28.0)
Cancer Mortality		
N	67	74
Unwilling, n (%)	21 (31.0)	17 (23.0)
Willing, n (%)	28 (42.0)	41 (55.0)
Neither unwilling nor willing, n (%)	18 (27.0)	16 (22.0)
Willingness to reduce—Question 2		
Cancer Incidence		
N	37	47
Willing, n (%)	7 (18.9)	4 (8.5)
Unwilling, n (%)	30 (81.1)	43 (91.5)
Median	3.0	2.0
Q1, Q3	(1.0, 4.0)	(1.0, 3.0)
Cancer Mortality		
N	35	30
Willing, n (%)	5 (14.3)	6 (20.0)
Unwilling, n (%)	30 (85.7)	24 (80.0)
Median	3.0	3.0
Q1, Q3	(1.0, 4.0)	(2.0, 4.0)
Willingness to reduce with higher certainty—Question a		
Cancer Incidence		
N	30	39
Willing, n (%)	2 (6.7)	4 (10.3)
Unwilling, n (%)	28 (93.3)	35 (89.7)
Median	3.0	3.0
Q1, Q3	(1.0, 4.0)	(2.0, 4.0)
Cancer Mortality		
N	29	22
Willing, n (%)	2 (6.9)	3 (13.6)
Unwilling, n (%)	27 (93.1)	19 (86.4)
Median	2.0	3.0
Q1, Q3	(1.0, 4.0)	(1.3, 4.0)
Willingness to reduce with a larger risk reduction—Question b		
Cancer Incidence		
N	27	20
Unwilling, n (%)	12 (44.0)	10 (50.0)
Willing, n (%)	15 (56.0)	10 (50.0)
Neither unwilling nor willing, n (%)	0 (0)	0 (0)
Cancer Mortality		
N	26	20
Unwilling, n (%)	12 (46.0)	10 (50.0)
Willing, n (%)	14 (54.0)	10 (50.0)
Neither unwilling nor willing, n (%)	0 (0)	0 (0)

Table 3. Cont.

	URM	PM
Willingness to increase—Question 3		
Cancer Incidence		
N	22	25
Willing, n (%)	0	0 (0.0)
Unwilling, n (%)	22 (100.0)	25 (100.0)
Median	1.0	1.0
Q1, Q3	(1.0, 2.0)	(1.0, 2.0)
Cancer Mortality		
N	13	13
Willing, n (%)	0 (0.0)	0 (0.0)
Unwilling, n (%)	13 (100.0)	13 (100.0)
Median	1.0	1.0
Q1, Q3	(1.0, 1.0)	(1.0, 4.0)

Abbreviations: URM = unprocessed red meat, PM = processed meat, Q1 = Quartile 1; Q3 = Quartile 3. Question 1,2,3: Willingness to stop and reduce meat intake was based on a 7-point Likert-scale with 1 (meaning definitely not) and 7 (meaning definitely yes). Question a: Willingness to stop and reduce meat intake with higher certainty was based on a 7-point Likert-scale with 1 (meaning definitely not) and 7 (meaning definitely yes). Question b: Willingness to stop and reduce unprocessed red meat consumption with a larger risk reduction was formulated as a multiple-choice question. Unwilling =≤4 of the Likert-scale, Willing =≥ 5 of the Likert-scale. The sample size (N) varied across the Willingness and cancer scenarios and type of meat because the questionnaire was tailored according to the participants' responses.

3.1.4. Willingness to Change Meat Consumption with Higher Certainty (Questions a)

The availability of higher-certainty evidence affected the participants' willingness to change their consumption in a minority of respondents who were unwilling to stop or reduce in response to the initial evidence presentation: 26.6% participants were willing to stop and 6.7% were willing to reduce their URM intake when they were presented with the cancer-incidence scenario. Similarly, with the cancer-mortality scenario, 19.0% were willing to sop and 6.9% were willing to reduce their intake. For PM, 35.8% of participants were willing to stop and 10.3% to reduce their intake when presented with the cancer-incidence scenario; similarly, for the cancer-mortality scenario, 29.2% were willing to stop and 13.6% to reduce. Table 3 presents the participants' willingness to stop and reduce URM and PC consumption in the face of cancer-incidence and cancer-mortality risks with higher certainty.

3.1.5. Willingness to Change Meat Consumption with a Larger Risk Reduction (Questions b)

The availability of a hypothetically larger reduction in cancer risk affected the willingness to change the meat consumption of some participants who were unwilling to stop or reduce in response to higher-certainty evidence: 37.0% participants reported to be willing to stop and 56.0% to reduce their URM intake when presented with the cancer-incidence scenario. Similarly, with the cancer-mortality scenario, 42.0% participants reported to be willing to stop and 54.0% to reduce their URM intake. For PM, 38.0% of participants were willing to stop and 50.0% to reduce their PM intake when presented with the cancer-incidence scenario, whereas in the cancer-mortality scenario, 55.0% of participants reported to be willing to stop and 53.0% to reduce their PM intake. Table 3 presents the participants' willingness to stop and reduce URM and PC consumption in the face of cancer-incidence and cancer-mortality risks with a larger risk reduction.

3.1.6. Predictors of Willingness to Change Meat Consumption

In the logistic regression analysis, gender appeared to be the only significant predictor of willingness to stop PM consumption in the cancer-incidence scenario (OR: 0.40; 95% CI: 0.15–0.93) and URM consumption in the cancer-mortality scenario (OR: 0.34; 95% CI:

0.11–0.88), with men being less willing to stop compared to women. Men also appeared to be less willing to stop eating PM (OR: 0.43; 95% CI: 0.18–0.96) and URM (OR: 0.27; 95% CI: 0.08–0.74) if the certainty was higher when presented with the cancer-incidence and cancer-mortality scenarios, respectively. Age, level of education, occupational status and religious belief did not appear to be significant predictors for any other dependent variables of willingness.

3.2. Semi-Structured Interviews

3.2.1. Participants' Characteristics

Of the 304 participants, seven agreed to participate in the semi-structured interviews; there were four men and three women, with a mean age of 38.6 years (SD = 5.0). All participants (100%) reported having a university degree, being employed, and six (86%) reported not having any comorbidity. Table S2 (See Supplementary Materials) presents the participants' sociodemographic and medical history.

3.2.2. Participants' Meat Consumption Behaviour

Participants' meat consumption varied. Three participants consumed between 3 and 4 servings of PM per week, one participant consumed between 11 and 12 servings per week and three participants declared consuming less than one serving per week. Regarding URM, three participants declared to consume less than one serving per week, two declared consuming between 1 and 2 servings per week and two consumed between 3 and 4 servings per week (See Supplementary Materials: Figure S3).

When asked if they had reduced their meat consumption in the past for health reasons and/or for other reasons, three participants declared having reduced both their URM and PM intake in the past due to health reasons, two participants reported having reduced their intake for animal welfare and environmental concerns and one participant reported cost as the main reason for having reduced his consumption. From the survey, none of the participants reported to be willing to stop or reduce their meat intake in the future.

3.2.3. Meat Consumption Preferences

We have identified three main themes reflecting the participants' preferences: (1) Social and/or family context of meat consumption, (2) Health- and non-health-related concerns about meat, and (3) Uncertainty of the evidence. Here we present some quotations from research participants.

Social and/or Family Context Meat Consumption

Two participants did not consider themselves regular meat eaters and reported eating meat mainly in social contexts.

"I'm not vegetarian and not vegan either, but if it was for me, I wouldn't choose meat as part of my daily meals. But once in a while if I go out with friends, I do eat it. I haven't eaten meat on a regular basis for a year now" (Female participant, 33 years old)

"I have not eaten meat on a regular basis for many years now. I consume meat especially for social occasions" (Male participant, 41 years old)

One participant reported consuming meat for its nutritional properties and mainly in social contexts.

"I have not completely stopped eating meat, as I consider it necessary to have certain nutritional values such as iron or vitamin B12. In addition, due to my origin one of my favourite foods is Iberian ham. On the other hand, the meat that I usually consume is of high quality and does not usually come from large farms. Even, for tradition, I consume game meat when I return to the family home" (Male participant, 32 years old)

One participant reported consuming meat mainly for the health and nutritional needs of her family.

"If it was for me, I would follow a more vegetarian diet, but I have to adapt to the needs of my children and family" (Female participant, 39 years old)

Health- and Non-Health-Related Concerns about Meat

Two participants reported health as the main reason for having reduced their meat intake in the past.

"In 2015 when I became a mother, I started to look for information about nutrition and get more information about what was healthy to take care of me and my son, that is when I decided to reduce my meat consumption" (Female participant, 39 years old)

"I had this idea that meat was high in fat and more expensive. So, I started to reduce my meat consumption, especially red meat, and in the end, I was eating mostly chicken. Gradually, I started to remove all types of meat from my daily meals" (Female participant, 33 years old)

Two participants highlighted other aspects that should be of concern when consuming meat. Animal welfare and/or environmental concerns were stated as important aspects to be considered when consuming meat.

"In recent years, there has been a lot of investigative journalism about the situation of large-scale animal farms and the deplorable conditions in which they are raised. In addition, livestock farming is directly related to greenhouse gas emissions and the deforestation of huge regions to grow pasture and feed for livestock. Livestock farming is one of the human activities that generates the most CO_2 emissions" (Male participant, 32 years old)

"From what I have read, too much meat can lead to diseases but on the other hand I am concerned about the sustainability aspects related to its consumption. This doesn't mean I don't eat meat, but I don't buy processed meat. I do eat beef sometimes and when I buy it, I go to the butcher so that I can choose the type of meat, the cut, and make sure of the origin" (Male participant, 41 years old)

Uncertainty of the Evidence

Three participants reported that the certainty of the evidence was not sufficiently convincing to cause changes in their meat consumption.

"I have no proof, nor enough evidence to think that I should reduce my consumption. If the evidence said that there was a real and significant reduction, I would reduce my consumption." (Male participant, 39 years old).

"I like meat, and it is for sure a barrier to reduce or quit its consumption, especially when the evidence is unclear." (Male participant, 47 years old).

"As far as I can see, the evidence is not valid enough to completely stop eating meat." (Female participant, 39 years old).

3.3. Integrated Data

In Table 4, the data from the quantitative (online survey) and qualitative (semi-structured interviews) analyses are integrated and presented in a joint display, which allows a deeper understanding of the participants' values and preferences around meat consumption. The quotes from the transcripts that most clearly represent the participants' views have been included in the right column. Table 4 will be interpreted in the discussion.

3.4. Follow-Up Assessment at 3 Months

The same seven participants who participated in the semi-structured interviews completed the follow-up assessment, with the addition of one woman participant; four men and four women with a mean age of 39.3 years (SD = 5.0) participated. Five participants (63%, three men and two women) reported not having made any changes in their URM and PM consumption, two participants (25%, one man and one woman) reported having increased their meat intake—one participant for URM and the other for PM—and finally, one woman participant (12%) reported having reduced the intake of PM.

Table 4. Joint display of integrated data from qualitative and quantitative data sets.

Qualitative Data		Quantitative Data		
Semi-Structured Interview Themes	Online Survey Questions	Online Survey Results	Representative Quotes	Interpretation
Social and/or family context meat consumption	What are the most important factors that favour your consumption of red meat and processed meat? Select all that apply *	Social context was selected as a factor favouring unprocessed red meat and processed meat consumption by 52% and 40% of participants respectively.	"I consume meat especially social occasions"	Participants reported that social gatherings influenced their meat consumption.
		Family preference was selected as a factor favouring unprocessed red meat and processed meat consumption by 50% and 33% of participants respectively.	"I have to adapt to the needs of my children and family"	Participants reported that family preference influenced their meat consumption.
		Tradition was selected as a factor favouring unprocessed red meat and processed meat consumption by 57% and 33% of participants respectively.	"Even, for tradition, I consume game meat when I return to the family home"	Participants reported that tradition influenced their meat consumption
Health- and non-health-related concerns about meat	What are the most important factors that favour your consumption of unprocessed red meat? Select all that apply *	Health was selected by 41% of participants as a factor favouring unprocessed red meat consumption.	"I consider red meat necessary to have certain nutritional values such as iron or vitamin B12"	Participants highlighted the nutritional value of unprocessed red meat as a reason for consuming it.
	In the past, have you cut back on red and/or processed meat for non-health reasons?	Environmental concerns were selected by 22% of participants. The second highest selected reason as a non-health-related reason for having reduced meat consumption in the past.	"Livestock farming is one of the human activities that generates the most CO_2 emissions"	Non-health-related reasons such as environmental concerns play an important role in people's meat consumption habits.
Uncertainty of the evidence	What are the most important factors that favour your consumption of unprocessed red meat and processed meat? Select all that apply *	Taste was selected as a factor favouring unprocessed red meat and processed meat consumption by 79% and 49% of participants respectevely. The most selected factor.	"I like meat, and it is for sure a barrier to reduce or quit its consumption, especially when the evidence is unclear"	Taste was one of the most voted factors for consuming meat, and this could explain why in the face of uncertain evidence, participants were unwilling to stop and/or reduce their intake.

* 11 factors were provided to choose from, see Table S1 in the Supplementary Materials.

4. Discussion

4.1. Main Findings

In this cross-sectional explanatory sequential mixed-methods study that included more than 300 adults in Spain, we found that, in the face of the available evidence regarding cancer-incidence and cancer-mortality risk reductions they would achieve, most people were unwilling to reduce their meat intake. Men were appreciably less willing to reduce meat consumption than were women. In the semi-structured interviews, participants reported consuming meat in social contexts and/or in response to family preferences. Health proved to be one important factor in favour of consuming meat and other aspects such as environmental concerns emerged as important considerations. Three of seven participants reported that the evidence was too uncertain for them to make changes in their current consumption. Overall, quantitative and qualitative findings were in agreement.

The included participants can be considered as infrequent meat eaters since the majority consumed between 1 and 2 servings of meat per week versus the estimated average consumption of three servings of meat per week [19]. This could explain why people who already had a low meat consumption were not willing to further decrease their meat intake. In fact, during the semi-structured interviews, some participants did not consider themselves as regular meat eaters and reported consuming meat occasionally, mainly in social contexts or because of tradition and/or family preferences. The participants' unwillingness to reduce or increase consumption suggests that participants were satisfied with their meat consumption habits and did not feel the need to make any changes; as emerged during the interviews, people felt that they were already consuming a healthy amount of meat that did not need to be changed.

4.2. Our Results in the Context of Previous Research

Our results are similar to the findings from a previous mixed-methods systematic review that was conducted by our team [8]. In this review, we showed that most omnivores were unwilling to change their meat intake. More recent studies also show a low willingness to change meat consumption [14,20,21]. Both our review and further studies also showed that men were more attached to meat consumption, and less willing to change their intake. In addition, although our results showed that participants were unwilling to reduce their meat in the face of cancer risks, many had reduced their intake in the past for other aspects, such as environmental concerns and animal welfare reasons. These aspects, which emerged during the interviews, are similar to the conclusions of a recent systematic review that found that environmental motives were already appealing to significant proportions of Western meat-eaters, who were adopting certain meat-curtailment strategies such as meat-free days [22].

4.3. Strengths and Limitations

Our study has several strengths. It is the first study, to our knowledge, that has comprehensively and explicitly evaluated people's health-related values and preferences, and their willingness to change meat consumption when informed of the potential adverse cancer risk and the uncertainty around this evidence. The information that patients received was based on a recent rigorous dose–response meta-analysis [9]. We developed and published a protocol reporting this study's methodology [13]. We followed an explanatory mixed-methods approach to the collection of both quantitative and qualitative evidence that enhanced the interpretability of our results. We used health states to ensure a similar understanding among participants of the presented outcomes.

Our study also has some limitations. Most of the included participants had a university degree and consumed less than three servings per week, which was the average meat intake in Spain [19]; therefore, our results might not be representative for the rest of the Spanish population. Although we provided information about the associated reductions in cancer risk in different formats, we did not check for understanding. We also only presented data on cancer risk and did not present other health risks, such as cardiovascular effects, in order not to overburden the participants. In addition, while the semi-structured interviews and follow-up assessment findings were collected from a small proportion and convenience sample of participants (only 7 and 8 participants agreed to participate, respectively); however, their sociodemographic characteristics and their meat consumption behaviours were very similar to the rest of study's participants. The response rate for the survey questions on willingness varied. The less willing they were to change meat consumption, the more questions a participant had to answer (see study procedures).

4.4. Implications for Practice and Research

This study will be informative in the development of both public health and clinical nutritional recommendations regarding meat consumption. For example, given that people are unlikely to modify their meat consumption on the basis of small and uncertain health benefits, panels would be more likely to make conditional rather than strong recommendations for the reduction of meat consumption for healthcare reasons. Our study provides guidance on the methods and procedures of how to conduct an exploratory sequential mixed-methods observational study that aims to identify people's health-related values and preferences. Future research is needed to replicate this study in other populations with higher meat intake and in other settings and cultures. The design we used could be applicable to other foods and/or nutrients, settings and/or nutritional contexts.

5. Conclusions

When informed about the cancer incidence and mortality risks of meat consumption, most respondents would not reduce their intake. Organizations developing public health and clinical nutrition guidelines should ensure their recommendations are consistent with population values and preferences.

Supplementary Materials: The following are available online at https://www.mdpi.com/article/10.3390/ijerph182111585/s1, Figure S1: Types of unprocessed read meat consumed (N = 304); Figure S2: Types of processed read meats consumed (N = 304); Figure S3: Meat consumptionfrequency behaviour in the semi-structured interviews; Table S1: Reasons for meat consumption for unprocessed red meat and processed meat; Table S2: Characteristics of semi-structured interview participants. Spanish version of the online survey available here (https://es.surveymonkey.com/r/CZF2DF9 accessed on 26 November 2020).

Author Contributions: Conceptualization: C.V., A.P.-D., B.C.J., V.H., J.Z., M.-A.H., A.P., F.K.N., G.H.G., M.M.B., P.A.-C., M.R. Data curation: C.V., M.S., P.A.-C., M.R. Formal analysis: C.V., M.S. Investigation: C.V., M.S., A.P.-D., B.C.J., A.P., F.K.N., G.H.G., M.M.B., P.A.-C., M.R. Methodology: C.V., A.P.-D., B.C.J., V.H., J.Z., F.K.N., G.H.G., M.M.B., P.A.-C., M.R. Project administration: C.V., A.P.-D., B.C.J., V.H., J.Z., M.-A.H., A.P., F.K.N., G.H.G., M.M.B., P.A.-C., M.R. Supervision: C.V., A.P.-D., B.C.J., J.Z., G.H.G., M.M.B., P.A.-C., M.R. Validation: C.V., A.P.-D., B.C.J., V.H., J.Z., A.P., F.K.N., G.H.G., M.M.B., P.A.-C., M.R. Writing—original draft: C.V., M.S., P.A.-C., M.R. Writing—review and editing: C.V., M.S., A.P.-D., B.C.J., V.H., J.Z., M.-A.H., A.P., F.K.N., G.H.G., M.M.B., P.A.-C., M.R. All authors have read and agreed to the published version of the manuscript.

Funding: This research received no external funding.

Institutional Review Board Statement: The Comitè Ètic d'Investigació Clínica de l'IDIAP Jordi Gol (19/121-P) approved the research protocol. Participation in the study was voluntary and participants could withdraw from the study at any time without penalty. Participants' answers were confidential; the treatment, communication and transfer of personal data of all the participating subjects was in accordance with the provisions of the Organic Law 3/2018, of December 5, on Data Protection and Guarantee of Digital Rights and the Regulation (EU) 2016/679, General Data Protection (RGPD).

Informed Consent Statement: Informed consent was obtained from all subjects involved in the study.

Data Availability Statement: All data generated or analysed during this study are included in this published article and its Supplementary Materials.

Acknowledgments: The authors thank Natalie Soto and Ignasi J. Gich for helping with the statistical analysis. Claudia Valli is a doctoral candidate for the PhD in Methodology of Biomedical Research and Public Health (Department of Paediatrics, Obstetrics, Gynaecology and Preventive Medicine), Universitat Autònoma de Barcelona, Barcelona, Spain. This direct-choice exercise was conducted using MagicApp software (http://magicproject.org/research-projects/share-it/ (accessed on 3 November 2021)). MAGIC (Making GRADE the Irresistible Choice) is a non-profit Foundation, aiming to increase value and reduce waste in healthcare through a digital and trustworthy evidence ecosystem. MAGICapp is the core platform in the evidence ecosystem bringing digitally structured guidelines, evidence summaries and decision aids to clinicians and patients.

Conflicts of Interest: M.R. is funded by a Sara Borrell post-doctoral contract (CD16/00157) from the Carlos III Institute of Health and the European Social Fund (ESF). B.C.J. has received a grant from Texas A&M AgriLife Research to fund investigator-initiated research related to saturated and polyunsaturated fats. The grant was from Texas A&M AgriLife institutional funds from interest and investment earnings, not a sponsoring organization, industry, or company. The rest of the authors conducted this study independently without involvement of a funder. No further competing interests were disclosed. The authors declared that no funding grants were involved in supporting this work.

Abbreviations

IARC	International Agency for Research in Cancer
IQR	inter-quartile-range
SR	systematic review
URM	unprocessed red meat
PM	processed meat

References

1. Stok, F.M.; Hoffmann, S.; Volkert, D.; Boeing, H.; Ensenauer, R.; Stelmach-Mardas, M.; Kiesswetter, E.; Weber, A.; Rohm, H.; Lien, N.; et al. The DONE framework: Creation, evaluation, and updating of an interdisciplinary, dynamic framework 2.0 of determinants of nutrition and eating. *PLoS ONE* **2017**, *12*, e0171077. [CrossRef]
2. Rabassa, M.; Ruiz, S.G.-R.; Solà, I.; Pardo-Hernandez, H.; Alonso-Coello, P.; García, L.M. Nutrition guidelines vary widely in methodological quality: An overview of reviews. *J. Clin. Epidemiol.* **2018**, *104*, 62–72. [CrossRef]
3. Blake, P.; Durão, S.; E Naude, C.; Bero, L. An analysis of methods used to synthesize evidence and grade recommendations in food-based dietary guidelines. *Nutr. Rev.* **2018**, *76*, 290–300. [CrossRef] [PubMed]
4. Bouvard, V.; Loomis, D.; Guyton, K.Z.; Grosse, Y.; El Ghissassi, F.; Benbrahim-Tallaa, L.; Guha, N.; Mattock, H.; Straif, K. Carcinogenicity of consumption of red and processed meat. *Lancet Oncol.* **2015**, *16*, 1599–1600. [CrossRef]
5. Canada's Food Guide. 2019. Available online: https://food-guide.canada.ca/en/ (accessed on 26 November 2020).
6. US Department of Health and Human Services and US Department of Agriculture. *2015–2020 Dietary Guidelines for Americans*, 8th ed.; US Department of Health and Human Services and US Department of Agriculture: Washington, DC, USA, 2015.
7. Public Health England: The Eat Well Guide. 2016. Available online: https://www.nhs.uk/live-well/eat-well/the-eatwell-guide/ (accessed on 26 November 2020).
8. Valli, C.; Rabassa, M.; Johnston, B.C.; Kuijpers, R.; Prokop-Dorner, A.; Zajac, J.; Storman, D.; Storman, M.; Bala, M.M.; Solà, I.; et al. Health-Related Values and Preferences Regarding Meat Consumption: A Mixed-Methods Systematic Review. *Ann. Intern. Med.* **2019**, *171*, 742–755. [CrossRef] [PubMed]
9. Han, M.A.; Zeraatkar, D.; Guyatt, G.H.; Vernooij, R.W.M.; Dib, R.E.; Zhang, Y.; Algarni, A.; Leung, G.; Storman, D.; Valli, C.; et al. Reduction of Red and Processed Meat Intake and Cancer Mortality and Incidence: A Systematic Review and Meta-analysis of Cohort Studies. *Ann. Intern. Med.* **2019**, *171*, 711–720. [CrossRef] [PubMed]
10. Wiseman, M. The second World Cancer Research Fund/American Institute for Cancer Research expert report. Food, nutrition, physical activity, and the prevention of cancer: A global perspective. *Proc. Nutr. Soc.* **2008**, *67*, 253–256. [CrossRef] [PubMed]
11. Valli, C.; Howatt, V.; Prokop-Dorner, A.; Rabassa, M.; Johnston, B.C.; Zajac, J.; Han, M.A.; Nampo, F.K.; Guyatt, G.H.; Bala, M.M.; et al. Evaluating adults' health-related values and preferences about unprocessed red meat and processed meat consumption: Protocol for a cross-sectional mixed-methods study [version 2; peer review: 2 approved]. *F1000Research* **2021**, *9*, 346. [CrossRef] [PubMed]
12. Von Elm, E.; Altman, D.G.; Egger, M.; Pocock, S.J.; Gøtzsche, P.C.; Vandenbroucke, J.P. The Strengthening the Reporting of Observational Studies in Epidemiology (STROBE)statement: Guidelines for reporting observational studies. *J. Clin. Epidemiol.* **2008**, *61*, 344–349. [CrossRef] [PubMed]

13. Johnston, B.C.; Alonso-Coello, P.; Bala, M.M.; Zeraatkar, D.; Rabassa, M.; Valli, C.; Marshall, C.; Dib, R.E.; Vernooij, R.W.M.; Vandvik, P.O.; et al. Methods for trustworthy nutritional recommendations NutriRECS (Nutritional Recommendations and accessible Evidence summaries Composed of Systematic reviews): A protocol. *BMC Med. Res. Methodol.* **2018**, *18*, 162. [CrossRef] [PubMed]
14. Howatt, V.; Prokop-Dorner, A.; Valli, C.; Zajac, J.; Bala, M.M.; Alonso-Coello, P.; Guyatt, G.H.; Johnston, B.C. Values and Preferences Related to Cancer Risk among Red and Processed Meat Eaters: A Pilot Cross-Sectional Study with Semi-Structured Interviews. *Foods* **2021**, *10*, 2182. [CrossRef] [PubMed]
15. *R: A Language and Environment for Statistical Computing*; R Foundation for Statistical Computing: Vienna, Austria, 2013; Available online: https://www.R-project.org/ (accessed on 8 March 2021).
16. Braun, V.; Clarke, V. Using thematic analysis in psychology. *Qual. Res. Psychol.* **2006**, *3*, 77–101. [CrossRef]
17. Cathain, A.; Murphy, E.; Nicholl, J. Three techniques for integrating data in mixed methods studies. *Br. Med. J.* **2010**, *341*, c4587. [CrossRef] [PubMed]
18. Guetterman, T.C.; Fetters, M.D.; Creswell, J.W. Integrating quantitative and qualitative results in health science mixed methods research through joint displays. *Ann. Fam. Med.* **2015**, *13*, 6554–6561. [CrossRef] [PubMed]
19. Suarez, M.V.; Mañas, R.J.; Fernández, S.R.; de Robledo, D. *Spanish National Dietary Survey in Adults, Elderly and Pregnant Women*; EFSA Supporting Publications: Parma, Italy, 2016.
20. Prokop-Dorner, A.; Piłat, A.; Zając, J.; Luśtyk, M.; Valli, C.; Łapczuk, A.; Brzyska, M.; Johnston, B.C.; Alonso-Coello, P.; Zera, D.; et al. Health-Related Values and Preferences Linked to Red and Processed Meat Consumption: An Advanced Online Survey and Semi-Structured Interviews. *J. Public Health Nutr.* **2021**, *171*, 742–755. [CrossRef]
21. Cheah, I.; Shimul, A.S.; Liang, J.; Phau, I. Drivers and barriers toward reducing meat consumption. *Appetite* **2020**, *149*, 104636. [CrossRef] [PubMed]
22. Sanchez-Sabate, R.; Sabaté, J. Consumer Attitudes Towards Environmental Concerns of Meat Consumption: A Systematic Review. *Int. J. Environ. Res. Public Health* **2019**, *16*, 1220. [CrossRef] [PubMed]

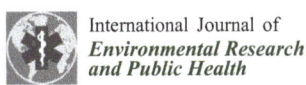

Article

In the Labyrinth of Dietary Patterns and Well-Being—When Eating Healthy Is Not Enough to Be Well

Renata Nestorowicz, Ewa Jerzyk and Anna Rogala *

Institute of Marketing, Department of Marketing Strategies, Poznań University of Economics and Business (PUEB), Niepodległości Av. 10, 61-875 Poznań, Poland; renata.nestorowicz@ue.poznan.pl (R.N.); ewa.jerzyk@ue.poznan.pl (E.J.)
* Correspondence: anna.rogala@ue.poznan.pl; Tel.: +48-61-854-37-74

Abstract: This paper aims to identify the relation between food consumption and well-being, and the level of well-being depending on a diet followed. Moreover, we analyze whether people driven by single motives, such as the health, pleasure or social dimension of food declare the lower or higher level of well-being than those motivated by a larger number of factors. The survey was conducted online (CAWI, $n = 1067$). The following scales were used: Satisfaction With Life Scale (SWLS), Satisfaction with Food-related Life Scale (SWFL), Health Taste Attitude Scales (HTAS) and Social Dimension of Food Meaning. The data analysis was carried out with the application of one-way analysis of variance (ANOVA), partial eta squared, a t-Student's test, the Hochberg test, the Games-Howell test, and Pearson's correlation. Levels of Subjective Well-Being (SWB) and Food Well-Being (FWB) are strongly correlated with consumers' dietary pattern. The frequency of consumption of organic food and following vegan, low salt, and low sugar diets leads to higher levels of SWB, while FWB is additionally affected by the regular consumption of low-fat products and foods that improve one's mood. The level of well-being is linked with the motivation to follow specific diets and attentiveness related to dietary patterns. People paying attention to the health aspects, pleasure and social dimension of food meaning show higher level of FWB than people focusing exclusively on health aspects.

Keywords: food consumption; well-being; dietary patterns; sustainable consumption; consumer behaviour; food well-being; subjective well-being

1. Introduction

In well-being studies, there are two different approaches to analysing the contribution of food consumption to the individual's life satisfaction. In subjective well-being (SWB) studies, food consumption is considered to be one of the factors contributing to the overall quality of life satisfaction e.g., [1–3], whereas food well-being (FWB) studies provide an insight into the perception of the quality of life resulting from food consumption in general, e.g., [4–11]. Subjective well-being is understood as the subjective evaluation of one's life from both an affective and a cognitive perspective [12]. On the other hand, food well-being is defined as the "positive psychological, physical, emotional, and social relationship with food at both the individual and societal levels" [4]. The findings of numerous studies prove that there is a link between food consumption and the well-being of an individual e.g., [7,13–16]. Moreover, a diet influences FWB and it is also a source of pleasure-related emotions [17].

This paper aimed to examine the relations between food consumption and subjective and food well-being. We undertook identifying consumers' well-being from the perspective of consumption of specific food categories, such as organic, ethical, convenient, sugar-free, gluten-free, and fat-reduced food, and discover which dietary patterns lead to increasing FWB and SWB. We also examined relations between FWB and SWB among Polish consumers, referring the obtained results to the findings of international studies. So far, only a few studies have been carried out to discover the impact of diets that reduce or exclude the consumption of specific product categories on one's well-being. Thus, our study fills this gap as it concerns dietary patterns and well-being.

At present, consumers show a wide variety of attitudes to diets—from the overconsumption of processed food, through a moderate and balanced diet, to reducing the consumption of specific groups of products or ingredients. At the same time, dietary guidelines worldwide include similar recommendations concerning healthy eating: one should eat diverse grocery products in proper proportions, more fruit, vegetables and whole-grain foods, less sugar, fat and salt [18]. In recent years, some new guidelines have been added to this list. They are related to the influence of a diet on the environment and to the adjustment of dietary patterns to more sustainable consumption [19]. The production of the food of animal origin, such as meat and dairy products, is identified as the key factor in soil degradation, loss of diversity and climate change. According to Vieux et al. [20], the adoption of a healthy diet, which reduces greenhouse gas emissions by thirty per cent, would require replacing of fifty per cent of the current food consumption with other food products. We are observing the fast growth of the segment of ethical consumers, who make their dietary decisions motivated by environmental considerations (cruelty and exploitation of animals, greenhouse gases) and by problems of social inequality when it comes to access to environmental resources by the present and future generations [21]. A vegetarian diet is becoming increasingly popular in Western societies, where it is preferred by the estimated number of one to nine per cent of consumers [22,23].

There is also a phenomenon of food fashions in the market, including diets based on so-called superfoods, such as chia seeds, goji berry, spirulina, linseed, walnut or kale. This phenomenon is observed among consumers following a gluten-free diet, who, having no diagnosed coeliac disease or gluten sensitivity, choose this diet despite it being more expensive and less nutritious. It is estimated that only about one per cent of the population suffer from coeliac disease and from three to six per cent are gluten sensitive. Still, as many as 20 per cent of the population choose a gluten-free diet without any medical indications [24]. Moreover, the market offers a wide range of organic, "free from" products, weight management articles, and fortified and functional products, which constitute the basis for composing diets and lifestyle, thus shaping its quality and the consumer's well-being [25].

The growing concern about the impact of dietary choices on the condition of the environment [21,26–28], food safety [29], and an increase in incidence rates of civilization diseases resulting from the poor-quality diets, [30,31], indicate the need for recognizing the importance of diets in the context of broadly defined life quality identified with well-being. An increasing number of researchers dealing with the issue of well-being recognize the important role of dietary behaviours [2,13,32–35]. In 2009, the concept of FWB appeared in scientific discourse [4]. It led to the reorientation in the approach to food consumption processes, with emphasis put on the need for developing proper attitudes and behaviours, focused not only on health, but also on overall well-being. As a result, food consumption ceased to be perceived only as the provision of nutrients, but the psychological [6,14,36–39]; and social [29,40,41] implications of this process for an individual were also recognized. The holistic approach to the role of food and dietary practices in human life takes into account the social and psychological dimension of consumption, abandoning the orientation which stems from the biomedical model of health [42]. Research carried out in this field shows that food consumption and its impact on well-being are related to the perception of health condition, a sense of pleasure and emotional aspects [8,13,17].

According to some authors, well-being may both be the effect of consumption and determine purchasing patterns [43]. Research into the influence of a diet on a person's well-being brings ambiguous results. Oke et al. [44] point out that ethical food consumption is motivated by personal health and well-being. Forestell and Nezlek [45] have found that vegetarians and semi-vegetarians are more neurotic and depressed than omnivores. As the findings of the study by Pfeiler and Egloff [46] show, a vegetarian diet does not affect

SWB whatsoever. In turn, Seconda et al. [47] found that the consumption of organic food impacts life satisfaction, while Apaolaza et al. [48] argue that it may be related to the label effect rather than the actual improvement of well-being.

The findings of the previously mentioned analyses indicate that people's well-being is related to the categories and quality of the food they consume. Those studies were conducted mainly with reference to the influence of the frequency of organic food consumption on well-being, i.e., [48–50]. They have proven that the more frequently organic food is consumed, the higher the perceived well-being level is (in the physical, psychological, and social sphere). This concerns, among others, vegetarians, vegans and people on a gluten-free diet. What is more, consumers choosing organic food are also more sensitive to the health benefits of a diet. Springfield et al. [51] point to the quality of a diet and its impact on consumers' health, while Pandya [52] argues that food allergies and elimination diets have a negative influence on the quality of life. On the other hand, Norwood et al. [53] indicate that the necessity of maintaining dietary discipline (even restrictive) does not have to entail lowered psychological well-being. In our research we also deal with diets with special regime, and we name them "exclusionary diets". By this term we mean diets excluding or reducing specific food products ingredients, such as animal source components (dairy, meat), gluten, salt, fat, or sugar. We decided to take this approach as there is no universal expression for this type of diet, and elimination or reducing diets are medical expressions with specific definitions. Thus, our contribution to the research is the inclusion of other diets and categories of food consumed as a correlate of the level of FWB and SWB perceived by consumers. In this paper, we pose a question whether the type of food consumed, i.e., a specific diet, is related to the level of SWB and FWB.

We also analysed issues of health motivation to the consumption of specific food categories and the relationship between food consumed and the level of well-being. The results of studies carried out by Ares, de Saldamando, Giménez, and Deliza's [13] and Ares et al. [8] concerning the evaluation of well-being with regard to specific products or food categories show that the influence of a diet on well-being refers to issues connected with perceived physical health, pleasure and emotional aspects. Moreover, motivation to the consumption of organic food rises under the influence of attitudes toward health-related and psychological consequences of consuming organic foods [50]. In turn, Apaolaza et al. [48] have proven that health-concerned consumers may enhance their well-being level by including organic foods in their diet. Thus, we decided to check whether such relationships occur in the case of other diets, too. Since the choice of a specific diet is dependent on consumers' various motivations, we wanted to check if this issue is also related to the level of FWB and SWB. We were particularly interested whether people driven by single motives, such as the health, pleasure or social dimension of food declared the lower/higher level of SWB and FWB than those motivated by a larger number of factors.

Only a few researchers have adopted a holistic approach to the analyses of consumers' food patterns, preferring the identification of the influence of specific diets or changes in them on well-being [54]. What is more, the existing body of literature provides a large number of examples of diets which are difficult to classify [55]. In our research we aim to identify consumers' well-being from the perspective of following a specific diet (organic, ethical, convenient, sugar-free, gluten-free, and fat-reduced food), and to discover whether the particular dietary patterns are related with increased FWB and SWB. Additionally, we examine relations between FWB and SWB among Polish consumers, referring the results to the findings of international studies.

Based on the presented literature review we formulated the following hypotheses in our study:

Hypothesis 1 (H1). *Regular consumers of organic food, or food that improves mood, or specific exclusionary diets declare higher levels of SWB and FWB than people who do not follow such diets or follow them occasionally.*

Hypothesis 2 (H2). *Consumers who regularly eat convenient food declare the lower level of SWB and FWB than people who do not eat it at all or eat it occasionally.*

Hypothesis 3 (H3). *People who pay attention to the health, pleasure and social dimension of food while choosing a specific diet declare the higher level of SWB and FWB than those selecting a dietary pattern based on only one motive.*

2. Materials and Methods

2.1. Procedure and Participants

The study was conducted using an Internet research panel of the research company Biostat. The panel covers a nationwide database of consumers and allows for the sample to be selected according to specific characteristics, while ensuring the representativeness of the Polish population. The panelists were invited to the survey by e-mail generated by the system with a button directing to the questionnaire or the push notification in mobile application. The respondents completed the questionnaire using a web application or a mobile application. The needed sample size was calculated. The first 1067 respondents who completed the questionnaire in 100% and fit into the sample distribution assumed in the study were eligible for the study. The survey was conducted in agreement with the Declaration of Helsinki. The data was encrypted and is stored according to the General Data Protection Regulation.

1067 respondents took part in the study. The sample was representative for Polish citizens in the age of 18–54 divided according to gender, age, and place of residence (confidence interval 95 per cent, maximum random error 3%). Table 1 shows the sample characteristics.

Table 1. The profile of respondents.

Variables	Frequency (%)
Total	1067 (100.0)
Gender	
Female	504 (47.2)
Male	563 (52.8)
Age	
18–24 years old	186 (17.4)
25–34 years old	351 (32.9)
35–44 years old	327 (30.6)
45–54 years old	203 (19.0)
Level of education	
Primary	30 (2.8)
basic vocational	115 (10.8)
Secondary	474 (44.4)
Higher	448 (42.0)
Place of residence	
Village	425 (39.8)
city up to 20,000 inhabitants	139 (13.0)
city from 20,000 to 100,000 inhabitants	205 (19.2)
city from 100,000 to 200,000 inhabitants	85 (8.0)
city from 200,000 to 500,000 inhabitants	90 (8.4)
city over 500,000 inhabitants	123 (11.5)
The assessment of the financial situation	
very bad or bad	66 (6.2)
Average	489 (45.8)
Good	458 (42.9)
very good	54 (5.1)

Table 1. Cont.

Variables	Frequency (%)
The assessment of the overall health condition	
definitely bad or rather bad	88 (8.2)
neither poor nor good	197 (18.5)
quite good	627 (58.8)
definitely good	155 (14.5)
BMI	
Underweight	37 (3.5)
normal weight	555 (52.0)
overweight	344 (32.2)
Obesity	131 (12.3)
Number of dietary patterns followed	
None	191 (17.9)
One	177 (16.6)
Two	241 (22.6)
Three	136 (12.7)
Four	127 (11.9)
five or more	195 (18.3)

2.2. Instruments

In order to verify our hypotheses, we applied scales which measure both SWB and FWB, as well as scales that allow for identifying consumers' attitudes to food:

- The Satisfaction With Life Scale (SWLS) developed by Diener et al. [12] is a five-item scale that measures global cognitive judgement of SWB on a seven-point scale. After summing up, individual scores produce the overall score reflecting the level of life satisfaction. The possible range of scores is 5–35—the higher the score is, the higher the level of satisfaction with life is. This scale showed good internal consistency with Cronbach's α between 0.79 and 0.89 [11,12,56–58]. Studies conducted in Poland reported high internal consistency of the scale (0.81) in its Polish version [59]. In our study, the Cronbach's alpha of the SWL scale was 0.89.
- The scale measuring the level of satisfaction with life related to food [2]—Satisfaction with Food-related Life Scale (SWFL). SWFL scale consists of five items concerning different aspects of food consumption. The respondents must indicate their degree of agreement with the statements using a six-level Likert scale. Scores obtained on this scale range from 5 to 35 and the higher the score is the higher FWB is. The Polish version of the scale was used in the original study conducted by [2]. This scale showed good internal consistency with Cronbach's α between 0.79 and 0.90 in studies conducted in European countries [2], South American country Chile [60] and in China [11]. In our study, SWFL's Cronbach's α was 0.86 presenting an adequate level of internal consistency.
- HTAS (Health Taste Attitude Scales) developed by Roininen, Lähteenmäki and Tuorila [61] measures the importance of health and taste aspects of a diet in the food choice process. We applied the general health interest subscale (hHTAS) with eight items and the pleasure sub-scale (pHTAS) with six items. All responses were measured on the seven-level Likert scale. The Polish version of HTAS scale was prepared by [62]. In our study, hHTAS's Cronbach's α was 0.74 presenting an adequate level of internal consistency. pHTAS's Cronbach's α was 0.55, therefore, in order to increase the scale's consistency, we removed the three items of low contribution to the Cronbach α. The three-item pHTAS scale was related to taking pleasure from the taste of food and showed a good internal consistency with Cronbach's α 0.73.
- Social dimension of food meaning (SMFL) taken from the scale developed by Arbit, Ruby and Rozin [63], measuring the meaning of food in life (MFL). In this scale, we used four statements evaluated on the seven-level Likert scale. The items of SMFL scale

were translated into Polish and back translated to ensure a valid translation. Afterwards the Polish version of the scale was consulted with three independent scientists, experts in the field of food consumption research. The Cronbach's alpha of the SMFL scale in this study was 0.84, what proves about high internal consistency of the scale.

All scales can be found in Appendix A.

The questionnaire included other questions related to the frequency of consumption of various food categories as well. Finally, questions for socio-demographic classification were included (gender, age, financial status, level of education, weight, growth, the assessment of overall health condition).

2.3. Data Analysis

In the data analysis process we applied descriptive techniques: measures of location, diversification, asymmetry and concentration, which were used for the preliminary analyses and description of the examined sample. At this stage, we also used the χ^2 test. For the comparison of the mean scores of SWB and FWB in the specific groups of respondents we used one-way analysis of variance (ANOVA) and partial eta squared as a measure of effect. For the data which meet the assumption of the homogeneity of variance (based on Levene's test), we applied post-hoc Hochberg's GT2 test, while with reference to data which do not meet this assumption, we applied the Games–Howell test, because both of them can be used for non-equipotent groups. By using one-way ANOVA we were able to show the influence of independent variables on the dependent ones, but no relationships between independent variables were taken into account. To verify whether people who pay attention to the health, pleasure and social dimension of food declare higher levels of SWB and FWB than people who only care about one motive, we used independent-samples t-Test and Cohen's d. Pearson's correlation analysis was used to investigate the relationship between SWB and FWB. The results were analysed using the SPSS Statistics vs. 26.0. programme for Windows.

3. Results

The first objective of this study was to analyse the existence of a positive relation between Satisfaction with Life (SWB) and Satisfaction with Food-related Life (FWB) among Polish consumers. To this end, we calculated satisfaction levels for all respondents, with the application of SWFL and SWLS scales (Table 2).

Table 2. Basic data concerning the level of SWB and FWB.

Measure		SWB	FWB
N		1067	1067
Average		21.14	20.59
Median		22.00	21.00
Mode		25.00	22.00
Standard deviation		6.45	4.94
Minimum		5.00	5.00
Maximum		35.00	30.00
Percentile	25	17.00	17.00
	50	21.00	22.00
	75	24.00	26.00

SWB: Satisfaction with Life; FWB: Satisfaction with Food-related Life.

In this research stage, we verified the first two hypotheses. As the first step, we analysed the frequency of consumption of the specific food categories, and then calculated the levels of SWB and FWB in the particular groups of respondents, who differ in frequency of the use of individual diets and compared mean scores with the application of one-way ANOVA along with respective post-hoc tests (Table 3).

Table 3. Frequency of consumption different food category and the level of FWB and SWB.

Dietary Pattern	Regularity	Frequency (%)	Mean SWB	Mean FWB
Organic $n = 979$	Regularly	301 (30.7)	22.82 [a]	22.09 [a]
	sometimes	612 (62.5)	20.99 [b]	20.45 [b]
	Never	66 (6.74)	19.17 [b]	18.45 [c]
ANOVA; post hoc; η^2		\multicolumn{3}{l}{$F_{SWB}(2, 976) = 13.471, p < 0.001$, GT2H; $\eta^2 = 0.027$; $F_{FWB}(2, 976) = 21.054, p < 0.001$, GT2H; $\eta^2 = 0.041$}		
Vegetarian $n = 967$	Regularly	190 (19.6)	21.52	21.42
	sometimes	503 (52.0)	21.57	20.65
	Never	274 (28.3)	20.84	20.60
ANOVA; post hoc		\multicolumn{3}{l}{$F_{SWB}(2, 964) = 1.267; p > 0.05$; $F_{FWB}(2, 964) = 2.010; p > 0.05$}		
Vegan $n = 929$	Regularly	85 (9.1)	21.23 [a,b]	21.80 [a]
	sometimes	422 (45.4)	22.16 [a]	20.95 [a,b]
	Never	422 (45.4)	20.81 [b]	20.43 [b]
ANOVA; post hoc; η^2		\multicolumn{3}{l}{$F_{SWB}(2, 926) = 4.872; p < 0.01$; GT2H; $\eta^2 = 0.01$; $F_{FWB}(2, 926) = 3.297; p < 0.05$; GH}		
Low fat diet $n = 924$	Regularly	324 (35.1)	21.95	21.87 [a]
	sometimes	521 (56.4)	21.24	20.23 [b]
	Never	79 (8.5)	20.66	19.42 [b]
ANOVA; post hoc; η^2		\multicolumn{3}{l}{$F_{SWB}(2, 921) = 1.958; p > 0.05$; $F_{FWB}(2, 921) = 15.054; p < 0.001$; GT2H; $\eta^2 = 0.031$}		
Gluten-free $n = 866$	Regularly	87 (10.0)	22.54 [a]	21.46
	sometimes	396 (45.7)	21.75 [a,b]	20.74
	Never	383 (44.2)	20.75 [b]	20.64
ANOVA; post hoc		\multicolumn{3}{l}{$F_{SWB}(2, 863) = 4.034; p < 0.05$; GT2H; $F_{FWB}(2, 863) = 1.025; p > 0.05$}		
Lactose-free $n = 856$	Regularly	88 (10.3)	21.83	21.22
	sometimes	347 (40.5)	21.52	20.58
	Never	421 (49.2)	21.22	20.76
ANOVA; post hoc		\multicolumn{3}{l}{$F_{SWB}(2, 853) = 0.450; p > 0.05$; $F_{FWB}(2, 853) = 0.626; p > 0.05$}		
Low-salt diet $n = 882$	Regularly	276 (31.3)	22.12 [a]	21.75 [a]
	sometimes	464 (52.6)	21.35 [a,b]	20.45 [b]
	Never	142 (16.1)	20.16 [b]	19.82 [b]
ANOVA; post hoc; η^2		\multicolumn{3}{l}{$F_{SWB}(2, 879) = 4.587; p < 0.05$; GT2H; $\eta^2 = 0.01$; $F_{FWB}(2, 879) = 9.436; p < 0.001$; GH; $\eta^2 = 0.021$}		
Low-sugar diet $n = 930$	Regularly	378 (40.6)	22.17 [a]	21.51 [a]
	sometimes	436 (46.9)	21.01 [b]	20.23 [b]
	Never	116 (12.5)	19.49 [b]	19.96 [b]
ANOVA; post hoc; η^2		\multicolumn{3}{l}{$F_{SWB}(2, 927) = 8.930; p < 0.001$; GT2H; $\eta^2 = 0.019$; $F_{FWB}(2, 927) = 8.913; p < 0.001$; GT2H; $\eta^2 = 0.019$}		
Improving mood $n = 965$	Regularly	505 (52.3)	21.37	21.34 [a]
	sometimes	414 (42.9)	20.94	19.91 [b]
	Never	46 (4.8)	20.83	19.54 [b]
ANOVA; post hoc; η^2		\multicolumn{3}{l}{$F_{SWB}(2, 962) = 0.593; p > 0.05$; $F_{FWB}(2, 962) = 11.132; p < 0.001$; GT2H; $\eta^2 = 0.023$}		
Convenient $n = 1018$	Regularly	506 (49.7)	20.37 [a]	20.35
	sometimes	481 (47.2)	21.89 [b]	20.82
	Never	31 (3.0)	21.58 [ab]	20.87
ANOVA; post hoc; η^2		\multicolumn{3}{l}{$F_{SWB}(2, 1015) = 6.978; p < 0.01$; GH; $\eta^2 = 0.02$; $F_{FWB}(2, 1015) = 1.144; p > 0.05$}		

Note: The analyses and the table took into consideration η^2, which explains at least one per cent of the variability of the SWB and FWB. Mean values with different superscripts differ significantly (GH: Games-Howell test; $p < 0.05$, GT2H: GT2 Hochberg test; $p < 0.05$). The means for a given dietary pattern differ statistically significantly only when marked with different letters (e.g., FWB mean for the regular followers of a vegan diet (M = 21.80 [a]) is statistically different from the mean for people who never pursue this diet (M = 20.43 [b]). The mean for people who sometimes observe this diet does not differ statistically significantly from the other groups (M = 20.95 [a,b]).

Results of the verification of detailed hypotheses concerning the influence of diets on the level of SWB and FWB are as follows:

- Differences in the level of SWB and FWB among people declaring different frequencies of the consumption of organic food are statistically significant on the level $p < 0.001$. The regular consumers of organic food declare the higher level of SWB and FWB than the respondents who do not follow such a diet or follow it occasionally.
- The regular consumers of the food which improves mood showed the higher level of FWB than people who eat it irregularly or do not eat it at all. Differences between the mean scores of FWB observed in these groups were statistically significant on the level $p < 0.001$. Differences in mean scores (SWB) were not statistically significant.
- With regard to the relationship between the frequency of exclusionary diets and the level of SWB it can be concluded that the regular followers of some exclusionary diets (low-salt, low-sugar, gluten-free) have the higher level of SWB than those who do not follow them at all. Differences between the levels of SWB in the groups of regular and occasional consumers were statistically significant only in the case of the consumption of low sugar products consumption.
- The regular users of the following diets: low-fat, low-salt and low-sugar showed the higher level of FWB than those who do not follow them at all or use them occasionally. In the case of vegans, significant differences were observed only between the groups of regular consumers and non-consumers. Differences in the levels of FWB concerning the frequency of consumption of vegetarian, lactose-free and gluten-free food were not statistically significant. It can therefore be concluded that the FWB level was higher for people regularly using some exclusionary diets.
- For the SWB, H1 was supported by the data only for organic and low-sugar diets. Concerning FWB, H1 was verified for the low-salt diet, low-fat diet, and the food improving mood food as well. It can thus be confirmed that more dietary patterns are related to the level of FWB than to the level of SWB. In both aspects, the consumption of organic food has a positive impact, while the influence of exclusionary diets is ambiguous. That is why, in further analysis we analysed how the combination of a few exclusionary diets correlates with SWB and FWB.
- The regular consumers of convenient food exhibited the lower level of SWB than the respondents who eat such food only occasionally. With reference to FWB, the examined relationship was not statistically significant at all. The H2 was not supported by the data.

Seeking further relationships between dietary patterns and the level of well-being, we undertook discovering the relationship between the number of diets excluding or reducing specific ingredients of food products followed and the levels of FWB and SWB. The highest levels of FWB and SWB were observed in the groups of people who regularly follow at least four exclusionary diets, while the lowest were among the consumers who do not regularly use any diet and those who follow only one diet. The ANOVA analysis and Hochberg GT2 post hoc test revealed that people following a variety of diets differed statistically significantly in terms of the declared level of SWB and FWB: $F_{SWB}(3.1063) = 4.491; p < 0.01$; $\eta^2 = 0.013$ and $F_{FWB}(3.1063) = 12.754, p < 0.001, \eta^2 = 0.035$. Table 4 presents the comparison of homogeneous groups of SWB and FWB means. The means in each distinguished group (column) do not significantly differ from each other. Thus, with regard to SWB, people who do not follow any exclusionary diet and those who pursue at least four such diets are statistically significantly different. In the case of FWB, three homogeneous groups were established: people who do not follow such a diet, people who pursue one to three exclusionary diets and those who use at least four diets.

Table 4. SWB and FWB levels in the groups of respondents distinguished according to the number of diets followed.

Number of Exclusionary Diets	n	Mean SWB Subset for α = 0.05		Mean FWB Subset for α = 0.05		
		1	2	1	2	3
Four and more diets	112	22.36		22.49		
Two or three diets	287	21.70	21.70		21.12	
One diet	186	21.52	21.52		20.97	
No diets	482		20.39			19.69
Sig.		0.219	0.714	1.00	1.00	1.00

Note: Subset for α = 0.05 means that subgroups between which means differ with statistical significance α = 0.05 were marked. Sig. refers to the significance of differences between means inside the column.

So far it has been shown that the regular consumption of organic food is associated with increased SWB and FWB. Other diets had similar effects, although it was difficult to find any regularities (e.g., diet restrictiveness), which would allow us to make some general statements concerning exclusionary diets. That is why we decided to analyse consumers' attitudes affecting the choice of a diet.

In order to verify hypothesis H3, we conducted Student's t-test for independent samples. The groups were distinguished on the basis of quartiles. In the analysis, we took into consideration people belonging to the highest quartiles according to hHTAS, reduced pHTAS and SMFL. As regards SWB, the analysis showed that the average level of SWB of those who pay attention to the health, pleasure and social dimension of food is statistically significantly higher (M = 25.00; SD = 6.17) than the SWB level of people who only care about the health issues (M = 20.96; SD = 6.22; t(203) = 4.40; $p < 0.001$, d = 0.650) or pleasure (M = 21.56; SD = 6.77; t(150) = 3.625, $p < 0.001$, d = 0.591) or social dimension of food (M = 22.34; SD = 6.68; t(163) = 2.601, $p = 0.01$, d = 0.411). The same relationships were observed in the case of FWB. The average level of FWB of those who pay attention to the health, pleasure and social dimension of food is statistically significantly higher (M = 24.93; SD = 3.73) than the FWB level of people who only care about the health issues (M = 21.21; SD = 3.97; t(203) = 6.46; $p < 0.001$, d = 0.954) or pleasure (M = 21.66; SD = 4.51; t(150) = 4.796, $p < 0.001$, d = 0.781) or social dimension of food (M = 21.31; SD = 4.75; t(163) = 5.256, $p < 0.001$, d = 0.830 (Table 5). This means that hypothesis H3 was positively verified.

Table 5. The comparison of the average SWB and FWB levels of people driven by three motives and those motivated exclusively by the health issues or pleasure or social dimension of food.

Type of Well-Being	Motives	M	SD
SWB	Health + Pleasure + Social dimension of food	25.00	6.17
	Health	20.96	6.22
	Pleasure	21.56	6.77
	Social dimension of food	22.34	6.68
FWB	Health + Pleasure + Social dimension of food	24.93	3.73
	Health	21.21	3.97
	Pleasure	21.66	4.51
	Social dimension of food	21.31	4.75

Effect size (Cohen's d) in the case of health was higher than for the other single motives, which means that adding the remaining motives to health increased SWB and FWB more than adding two motives to pleasure or social dimension. This influence was more significant with regard to FWB than SWB.

4. Discussion

In our study, we examined whether there is a link between consumption and motivations to follow specific diets (organic, vegetarian, vegan, convenient, lactose-free, gluten-free, salt-reduced, sugar-reduced and fat-reduced food) and the levels of FWB and SWB.

Our research results show that there is a strong relation between life satisfaction measured on the SWLS scale and satisfaction connected with the area of food consumption, measured on the SWFL scale (r-Pearson correlation between SWB and FWB was $r = 0.59$ and was statistically significant on the level $p < 0.01$ (both ways). The correlation between SWB and FWB in the present study is similar to those obtained in China [11], which was 0.58, in Chile: 0.53 [60], and higher than in Ecuador: 0.39 [64] and in European countries [2], which was 0.36. It should be pointed out that not only the overall scores of SWLS and SWFL, but also all statements from both scales are correlated. This means that nutrition and satisfaction or dissatisfaction with food consumption are associated with the broadly defined well-being. These findings are in line with the current state of knowledge and are consistent with the results of studies of, among others [11,60,64,65].

A novelty in our study is that we referred the levels of SWB and FWB to the use of different diets defined as dietary patterns. A positive relationship occurs mainly with regard to the consumption of organic food, which confirms the findings of previous studies in this area e.g., [48,50]. The regular consumption of organic food does not mean eliminating some product categories, but it involves the selection of food with additional quality benefits. That is why this positive relationship between the frequency of consumption of high-quality food and the higher perceived satisfaction with life is easy to understand. What is striking is the observed dependency between adopting exclusionary diets and well-being. The abandonment of specific food product categories may increase a sense of discomfort after all. It turns out, however, that the use of diets involving different kinds of eliminations or reductions does not have to make a consumer feel limited in their food choice, thus be less satisfied with life. In many cases, the opposite is the case. The regular use of vegan, low-salt and low-sugar diets is related to high SWB, while, in addition to these diets, the frequent consumption of low-fat products correlates with the high level of FWB. The influence of the regular use of specific exclusionary diets on the levels of FWB and SWB is not homogeneous. One of the reasons could be the trigger to adopting such a diet—whether it was because a consumer wanted it or whether he or she was forced to it because of his or her physical condition.

When analysing consumers' dietary choices, the motivation to make them is an important area that should be taken into account. An individual's physical condition and health, but also the pleasure and social dimension of food consumption are a few among many other motives. Therefore, these motivations for choosing different diets are key. A specific diet can be chosen because of the same or of the various motives. However, in our research, it turned out that single motives are less important for the levels of FWB and SWB than their combination. We proved in our research that people who pay attention to the health, pleasure and social dimension of food while choosing a specific diet, declared the higher level of SWB and FWB than those selecting a dietary pattern based on only one motive. These results should be used to encourage consumers to adopt specific diets. It is only the combination of all these areas in the promotion of dietary patterns that may lead to a permanent change in people's eating habits. Therefore, we have to educate consumers to raise awareness that a diet can be tasty and that its observance can become a positive element of social relations, because, apart from pro-health aspects, it is equally important to take pleasure from having meals together and have the support of a family. Like other studies, ours also has some limitations, which, at the same time, offer some clues regarding the directions of further research. We did not perform the evaluation of the quality of diets used by the respondents, but we used their declarations concerning the diet they observed. In future research, more precise tools may be applied, such as the Stanford Wellness Living Laboratory (WELL) or Food Frequency Questionnaire (FFQ). They will make it possible to assess different diets more accurately [51]. Moreover, we compared the levels of SWB and FWB between the respondents following or not following a particular diet. Because of the design of our research, we could not compare the levels of SWB and FWB between the groups following different dietary patterns, as these groups were not distinct. Another limitation is that because we removed the three items of low contribution to the Cronbach α from the original pHTAS scale to increase the scale's consistency, our results are less comparable with other studies using the original version.

In our study, we examined the orientation on health, pleasure and socialization as a motivation to follow a diet, so the number of the analysed motives was limited by including a larger number of motives, we would be able to distinguish, among others, people who are on a diet by choice (beliefs, fashion) from those who follow them because of allergies or food intolerance. This would contribute to the broadening of knowledge connected with FWB and SWB. That is why further research is needed in the area of consumers' motivation to adopt a particular dietary pattern, with special attention given to the complexity and interdependence of motives. Knowing the reasons behind the nutritional choices which contribute to increasing the level of life satisfaction, we can be more effective in adjusting argumentation encouraging consumers to make dietary decisions that would benefit them. If we only appeal to pro-health aspects, we will not achieve the expected results. We also need to pay attention to the social dimension and pleasure.

In order to identify changes of motivation and behaviour in time, it will also be worth introducing longitudinal studies [66]. For the sake of deepening knowledge concerning dietary patterns and the resulting well-being, future research should take into consideration the situational and cultural context in which food and diets are chosen. The effective change of a diet is determined by the support of a family, friends, schoolmates and of the whole society. This positive change can be also encouraged with the help of new technology-based solutions as well, such as mobile applications. Given the above, future studies should also explain the role of the different sources of support in fostering dietary habits characteristic of specific diets.

5. Conclusions

What is the main contribution of this paper is that it provides empirical evidence that the relationship between dietary patterns and food consumption motivations and consumers' food and subjective well-being exists? The dietary choices we make, and the reasons behind them are therefore important correlates of our well-being. Previous studies of the influence of food consumption on SWB and FWB to a limited extent took into account the motivation to adopt a diet as a factor differentiating an individual's SWB and FWB levels. Our paper fills this gap and provides conclusions concerning the shaping of dietary patterns desired from the point of view of both the individual and the society.

Dieticians usually recommend various food choices that contribute to the better health of the individual. On the other hand, consumers are guided in their decisions by various motivations related to, inter alia the pleasure of eating, the social dimension of consumption, but also the desire to decrease the environmental impact of food consumption practices. Our research shows that coexisting differentiated motivations show a positive relationship with food and subjective well-being. A consumer engaged in various nutritional goals, using a wider range of diets, experiences the higher level of satisfaction with the quality of his or her life.

Knowledge concerning people's motivation to follow specific diets, as well as the occurrence of the relationships between food consumption and an individual's overall well-being may be used for creating communication to support proper dietary decisions. According to our research, food products' communication based on health values and benefits may not bring optimal results in terms of the growth of well-being. It is necessary to take into consideration the psychological and social aspects of SBW [50]. The findings of our study shed light on the important aspects that should be taken into account when communicating these issues to society. This communication should include not only health benefits and effects, but also references to the social aspects of consumption and happiness because consumers are motivated not only by their concern about health, but also by pleasure and the social dimension of consumption.

Author Contributions: Conceptualization R.N., E.J. and A.R.; methodology R.N., E.J. and A.R.; software R.N. and A.R.; validation R.N.; formal analysis A.R.; investigation R.N., E.J. and A.R.; resources R.N., E.J. and A.R.; data curation R.N.; writing—original draft preparation E.J., A.R. and R.N.; writing—review and editing A.R. and R.N.; visualization R.N.; supervision A.R.; project administration A.R.; funding acquisition, A.R., R.N. and E.J. All authors have read and agreed to the published version of the manuscript.

Funding: The project financed within the Regional Initiative for Excellence programme of the Minister of Science and Higher Education of Poland, years 2019–2022, grant no. 004/RID/2018/19, financing 3,000,000 PLN.

Institutional Review Board Statement: The study was conducted according to the guidelines of the Declaration of Helsinki and the General Data Protection Regulation. The data was collected by BIOSTAT, a certificated research and scientific agency.

Informed Consent Statement: Informed consent was obtained from all subjects involved in the study.

Data Availability Statement: The datasets analysed during the current study are available from the corresponding author on a request.

Acknowledgments: Authors would like to thank two anonymous reviewers and Iwona Olejnik for their remarks and comments that helped to improve the paper.

Conflicts of Interest: The authors declare no conflict of interest.

Appendix A

A. Satisfaction with Life Scale (SWLS), 7-point Likert Scale (1: disagree completely, 7: agree completely) [12], Polish version [59]

1. In most ways my life is close to my ideal.
2. The conditions of my life are excellent.
3. I am satisfied with my life.
4. So far I have gotten the important things I want in life.
5. If I could live my life over, I would change almost nothing.

B. Satisfaction with Food-related Life Scale (SWFL), 6-point Likert scale (1: disagree completely, 6: agree completely) Polish version used in original research of [2]

1. Food and meals are positive elements
2. I am generally pleased with my food
3. My life in relation to food and meals is close to ideal
4. With regard to food, the conditions of my life are excellent
5. Food and meals give me satisfaction in daily life

C. Health Taste Attitude Scales—health (hHTAS) 7-point Likert (1: disagree completely, 7: agree completely) [61]; Polish version [62]

1. The healthiness of food has little impact on my food choices.
2. I am very particular about the healthiness of food I eat.
3. I eat what I like and I do not worry much about the healthiness of food.
4. It is important for me that my diet is low in fat.
5. I always follow a healthy and balanced diet.
6. It is important for me that my daily diet contains a lot of vitamins and minerals.
7. The healthiness of snacks makes no difference to me.
8. I do not avoid foods, even if they may raise my cholesterol.

D. Pleasure Health Taste Attitude Scales (pHTAS), 7-point Likert Scale (1: strongly disagree, 7: strongly agree) scale [61]; Polish version [62]

1. I do not believe that food should always be source of pleasure.
2. The appearance of food makes no difference to me

3. When I eat, I concentrate on enjoying the taste of food.
4. It is important for me to eat delicious food on weekdays as well as weekends.
5. An essential part of my weekend is eating delicious food.
6. I finish my meal even when I do not like.

E. Social Dimension of Food Meaning (SMFL), 7-point Likert Scale (1: disagree completely, 7: agree completely) [63]; Polish version: own translation)

1. Sharing food with others makes me feel closer to them
2. When I eat food I feel connected with the people I am eating with
3. Food is closely tied to my relationships with others
4. Making food for others is a main way I show care for them

References

1. Rozin, P. The meaning of food in our lives: A cross-cultural perspective on eating and well-being. *J. Nutr. Educ. Behav.* **2005**, *37*, 107–112. [CrossRef]
2. Grunert, K.; Dean, D.; Raats, M.; Nielsen, N.; Lumbers, M. A measure of satisfaction with food-related life. *Appetite* **2007**, *49*, 486–493. [CrossRef] [PubMed]
3. Reeves, S.; Halsey, L.G.; McMeel, Y.; Huber, J.W. Breakfast habits, beliefs and measures of health and wellbeing in a nationally representative UK sample. *Appetite* **2013**, *60*, 51–57. [CrossRef] [PubMed]
4. Block, L.G.; Grier, S.A.; Childers, T.L.; Davis, B.; Ebert, J.E.J.; Kumanyika, S.; Laczniak, R.N.; Machin, J.E.; Motley, C.M.; Peracchio, L.; et al. From nutrients to nurturance: A conceptual introduction to food well-being. *J. Public Policy Mark.* **2011**, *30*, 5–13. [CrossRef]
5. Bublitz, M.G.; Peracchio, L.A.; Andreasen, A.R.; Kees, J.; Kidwell, B.; Miller, E.G.; Motley, C.M.; Peter, P.C.; Rajagopal, P.; Scott, M.L.; et al. The Quest for Eating Right: Advancing Food Well-being. *J. Res. Consum.* **2011**, *19*, 1–12.
6. Bublitz, M.G.; Peracchio, L.A.; Andreasen, A.R.; Kees, J.; Kidwell, B.; Miller, E.G.; Motley, C.M.; Peter, P.C.; Rajagopal, P.; Scott, M.L.; et al. Promoting positive change: Advancing the food well-being paradigm. *J. Bus. Res.* **2013**, *66*, 1211–1218. [CrossRef]
7. Schnettler, B.; Miranda, H.; Lobos, G.; Orellana, L.; Sepúlveda, J.; Denegri, M.; Etchebarne, S.; Mora, M.; Grunert, K.G. Eating habits and subjective well-being. A typology of students in Chilean state universities. *Appetite* **2015**, *89*, 203–214. [CrossRef]
8. Ares, G.; de Saldamando, L.; Giménez, A.; Claret, A.; Cunha, L.M.; Guerrero, L.; Pinto de Moura, A.; Oliveira, D.C.R.; Symoneaux, R.; Deliza, R.; et al. Consumers' associations with wellbeing in a food-related context: A cross-cultural study. *Food Qual. Pref.* **2015**, *40*, 304–315. [CrossRef]
9. Ares, G.; Giménez, A.; Vidal, L.; Zhou, Y.; Krystallis, A.; Tsalis, G.; Symoneaux, R.; Cunha, L.M.; de Moura, A.P.; Claret, A.; et al. Do we all perceive food-related wellbeing in the same way? Results from an exploratory cross-cultural study. *Food Qual. Pref.* **2016**, *52*, 62–73. [CrossRef]
10. Batat, W.; Peter, P.C.; Moscato, E.M.; Castro, I.A.; Chan, S.; Chugani, S.K.; Muldrow, A.F. The experiential pleasure of food: A savoring journey to food well-being. *J. Bus. Res.* **2019**, *100*, 392–399. [CrossRef]
11. Liu, R.; Grunert, K.G. Satisfaction with food-related life and beliefs about food health, safety, freshness and taste among the elderly in China: A segmentation analysis. *Food Qual. Pref.* **2020**, *79*, 103775. [CrossRef]
12. Diener, E.; Emmons, R.A.; Larsen, R.J.; Griffin, S. The Satisfaction with Life Scale. *J. Personal. Assess.* **1985**, *49*, 71–75. [CrossRef] [PubMed]
13. Ares, G.; de Saldamando, L.; Giménez, A.; Deliza, R. Food and wellbeing. Towards a consumer-based approach. *Appetite* **2014**, *74*, 61–69. [CrossRef] [PubMed]
14. Bradford, T.W.; Grier, S. Restricted pleasure for healthy eating and food well-being. *Qual. Mark. Res.* **2019**, *22*, 557–569. [CrossRef]
15. Grao-Cruces, A.N.; Nuviala, A.; Fernández-Martínez, A.; Porcel-Gálvez, A.; Moral-García, J.; Martínez-López, E.J. Adherencia a La Dieta Mediterránea En Adolescentes Rurales Y Urbanos. *Nutr. Hosp.* **2013**, *1*, 1129–1135. [CrossRef]
16. Blanchflower, D.G.; Oswald, A.J.; Stewart-Brown, S. Is psychological well-being linked to the consumption of fruit and vegetables? *Soc. Indic. Res.* **2013**, *114*, 785–801. [CrossRef]
17. Guillemin, I.; Marrel, A.; Arnould, B.; Capuron, L.; Dupuy, A.; Ginon, E.; Layé, S.; Lecerf, J.M.; Prost, M.; Rogeaux, M.; et al. How French subjects describe well-being from food and eating habits? Development, item reduction and scoring definition of the Well-Being related to Food Questionnaire (Well-BFQ©). *Appetite* **2016**, *96*, 333–346. [CrossRef]
18. Herforth, A.; Arimond, M.; Álvarez-Sánchez, C.; Coates, J.; Christianson, K.; Muehlhoff, E. A global review of food-based dietary guidelines. *Adv. Nutr.* **2019**, *10*, 590–605. [CrossRef]
19. Steenson, S.; Buttriss, J.L. The challenges of defining a healthy and 'sustainable' diet. *Nutr. Bull.* **2020**, *45*, 206–222. [CrossRef]
20. Vieux, F.; Perignon, M.; Gazan, R.; Darmon, N. Dietary changes needed to improve diet sustainability: Are they similar across Europe? *Eur. J. Clin. Nutr.* **2018**, *72*, 951–960. [CrossRef]
21. Vermeir, I.; Weijters, B.; De Houwer, J.; Geuens, M.; Slabbinck, H.; Spruyt, A.; Van Kerckhove, A.; Van Lippevelde, W.; De Steur, H.; Verbeke, W. Environmentally Sustainable Food Consumption: A Review and Research Agenda From a Goal-Directed Perspective. *Front. Psychol.* **2020**, *11*, 1603. [CrossRef] [PubMed]

22. Dorard, G.; Mathieu, S. Vegetarian and omnivorous diets: A cross-sectional study of motivation, eating disorders, and body shape perception. *Appetite* **2021**, *156*, 104972. [CrossRef] [PubMed]
23. Ruby, M.B. Vegetarianism. A blossoming field of study. *Appetite* **2012**, *58*, 141–150. [CrossRef] [PubMed]
24. Arslain, K.; Gustafson, C.R.; Baishya, P.; Rose, D.J. Determinants of gluten-free diet adoption among individuals without celiac disease or non-celiac gluten sensitivity. *Appetite* **2021**, *156*, 104958. [CrossRef]
25. Duarte, P.; Costa e Silva, S.; Sintra Pisco, A.M.; Moreira de Campos, J. Orthorexia Nervosa: Can Healthy Eating Food Trends Impact Food Companies Marketing Strategies? *J. Food Prod. Mark.* **2019**, *25*, 754–770. [CrossRef]
26. Baudry, J.; Péneau, S.; Allès, B.; Touvier, M.; Hercberg, S.; Galan, P.; Amiot, M.J.; Lairon, D.; Méjean, C.; Kesse-Guyot, E. Food Choice Motives When Purchasing in Organic and Conventional Consumer Clusters: Focus on Sustainable Concerns (The NutriNet-Santé Cohort Study). *Nutrients* **2017**, *9*, 88. [CrossRef]
27. Strassner, C.; Cavoski, I.; Di Cagno, R.; Kahl, J.; Kesse-Guyot, E.; Lairon, D.; Lampkin, N.; Løes, A.K.; Matt, D.; Niggli, U.; et al. How the Organic Food System Supports Sustainable Diets and Translates These into Practice. *Front. Nutr.* **2015**, *2*, 19. [CrossRef]
28. Carrus, G.; Pirchio, S.; Mastandrea, S. Social-Cultural Processes and Urban Affordances for Healthy and Sustainable Food Consumption. *Front. Psychol.* **2018**, *9*, 2407. [CrossRef]
29. Voola, A.P.; Voola, R.; Wyllie, J.; Carlson, J.; Sridharan, S. Families and food: Exploring food well-being in poverty. *Eur. J. Mark.* **2018**, *52*, 2423–2448. [CrossRef]
30. Koss-Mikołajczyk, I.; Baranowska, M.; Todorovic, V.; Albini, A.; Sansone, C.; Andreoletti, P.; Cherkaoui-Malki, M.; Lizard, G.; Noonan, D.; Sobajic, S.; et al. Prophylaxis of Non-communicable Diseases: Why Fruits and Vegetables may be Better Chemopreventive Agents than Dietary Supplements Based on Isolated Phytochemicals? *Curr. Pharm. Des.* **2019**, *25*, 1847–1860. [CrossRef]
31. Kupka, R.; Siekmans, K.; Beal, T. The diets of children: Overview of available data for children and adolescents. *Glob. Food Secur.* **2020**, *27*, 100442. [CrossRef]
32. Schnettler, B.; Miranda, H.; Sepúlveda, J.; Denegri, M.; Mora, M.; Lobos, G.; Grunert, K.G. Psychometric properties of the satisfaction with food-related life scale: Application in Southern Chile. *J. Nutr. Educ. Behav.* **2013**, *45*, 443–449. [CrossRef] [PubMed]
33. Mugel, O.; Gurviez, P.; Decrop, A. Eudaimonia Around the Kitchen: A Hermeneutic Approach to Understanding Food Well-Being in Consumers' Lived Experiences. *J. Public Policy Mark.* **2019**, *38*, 280–295. [CrossRef]
34. Hémar-Nicolas, V.; Ezan, P. How do children make sense of food well-being? Food for thought for responsible retailers. *Int. J. Retail. Distrib. Manag.* **2019**, *47*, 605–622. [CrossRef]
35. Bodunrin, T.S.; Stone, T. Consuming well-being and happiness through epicurean ingestion. *Qual. Mark. Res.* **2019**, *22*, 595–607. [CrossRef]
36. Cornil, Y.; Chandon, P. Pleasure as an ally of healthy eating? Contrasting visceral and Epicurean eating pleasure and their association with portion size preference and wellbeing. *Appetite* **2016**, *104*, 52–59. [CrossRef]
37. Mujcic, R.; Oswald, A.J. Evolution of Well-Being and Happiness After Increases in Consumption of Fruit and Vegetables. *AJPH Res.* **2016**, *106*, 1504–1510. [CrossRef]
38. Wahl, D.R.; Villinger, K.; König, L.M.; Ziesemer, K.; Schupp, H.T.; Renner, B. Healthy food choices are happy food choices: Evidence from a real life sample using smartphone based assessments. *Science* **2017**, *7*, 17069. [CrossRef]
39. Landry, M.; Lemieux, S.; Lapointe, A.; Bédard, A.; Bélanger-Gravel, A.; Bégin, C.; Provencher, V.; Desroches, S. Is eating pleasure compatible with healthy eating? A qualitative study on Quebecers' perceptions. *Appetite* **2018**, *125*, 537–547. [CrossRef]
40. Batat, W.; Paula, P.C.; Handen, V.; Valerie, M.; Ebru, U.; Emre, U.; Soonkwan, H. Alternative food consumption (AFC): Idiocentric and allocentric factors of influence among low socio-economic status (SES) consumers. *J. Mark. Manag.* **2017**, *33*, 580–601. [CrossRef]
41. De Rosis, S.; Pennucci, F.; Seghieri, C. Segmenting Adolescents Around Social Influences on Their Eating Behavior: Findings from Italy. *Soc. Mark. Q.* **2019**, *25*, 256–274. [CrossRef]
42. Biltekoff, C. Consumer response: The paradoxes of food and health. *Ann. N. Y. Acad. Sci.* **2010**, *1190*, 174–178. [CrossRef] [PubMed]
43. Gangdmair-Wooliscroft, A.; Wooliscroft, B. Well-being and everyday ethical consumption. *J. Happiness Stud.* **2017**, *20*, 141–163. [CrossRef]
44. Oke, A.; Ladas, J.; Bailey, M. Ethical consumers: An exploratory investigation of the ethical food consumption behaviour of young adults in the North East of Scotland. *Br. Food J.* **2020**, *122*, 3623–3638. [CrossRef]
45. Forestell, C.A.; Nezlek, J.B. Vegetarianism, depression, and the five factor model of personality. *Ecol. Food Nutr.* **2018**, *57*, 246–259. [CrossRef]
46. Pfeiler, T.M.; Egloff, B. Do vegetarians feel bad? Examining the association between eating vegetarian and subjective well-being in two representative samples. *Food Qual. Pref.* **2020**, *86*, 104018. [CrossRef]
47. Seconda, L.; Péneau, S.; Bénard, M.; Allès, B.; Hercberg, S.; Galan, P.; Lairon, D.; Baudry, J.; Kesse-Guyot, E. Is organic food consumption associated with life satisfaction? A cross-sectional analysis from the NutriNet-Santé study. *Prev. Med. Rep.* **2017**, *8*, 190–196. [CrossRef]
48. Apaolaza, V.; Hartmann, P.; D'Souza, C.; López, C. Eat organic—Feel good? The relationship between organic food consumption, health concern and subjective wellbeing. *Food Qual. Pref.* **2018**, *63*, 51–62. [CrossRef]

49. Bauer, H.H.; Heinrich, D.; Schäfer, D.B. The effects of organic labels on global, local, and private brands: More hype than substance? *J. Bus. Res.* **2013**, *66*, 1035–1043. [CrossRef]
50. Lee, H.J. Does Consumption of Organic Foods Contribute to Korean Consumers' Subjective Well-Being? *Sustainability* **2019**, *11*, 5496. [CrossRef]
51. Springfield, S.; Cunanan, K.; Heaney, C.; Peng, K.; Gardner, C. The WELL diet score correlates with the alternative healthy eating index-2010. *Food Sci. Nutr.* **2020**, *8*, 2710–2718. [CrossRef] [PubMed]
52. Pandya, S.P. Adolescents Living with Food Allergies in Select Global Cities: Does a WhatsApp-Based Mindful Eating Intervention Promote Wellbeing and Enhance their Self-Concept? *J. Pediatr. Nurs.* **2020**, *55*, 83–94. [CrossRef] [PubMed]
53. Norwood, R.; Cruwys, T.; Chachay, V.S.; Sheffield, J. The psychological characteristics of people consuming vegetarian, vegan, paleo, gluten free and weight loss dietary patterns. *Obes. Sci. Pract.* **2019**, *5*, 148–158. [CrossRef] [PubMed]
54. Vermeulen, S.J.; Park, T.; Khoury, C.K.; Béné, C. Changing diets and the transformation of the global food system. *Ann. N. Y. Acad. Sci.* **2020**, *22*, 3–17. [CrossRef] [PubMed]
55. Modi, N.; Priefer, R. Effectiveness of mainstream diets. *Obes. Med.* **2020**, *18*, 100239. [CrossRef]
56. Pavot, W.; Diener, E. Review of the Satisfaction with Life Scale. *Psychol. Assess.* **1993**, *5*, 164–172. [CrossRef]
57. Pavot, W.; Diener, E. The Satisfaction with Life Scale and the emerging construct of life satisfaction. *J. Posit. Psychol.* **2008**, *3*, 137–152. [CrossRef]
58. Esnaola, I.; Benito, M.; Antonio-Agirre, I.; Freeman, J.; Sarasa, M. Measurement invariance of the Satisfaction with Life Scale (SWLS) by country, gender and age. *Psicothema* **2017**, *29*, 596–601. [CrossRef]
59. Juczyński, Z. *Narzędzia Pomiaru w Promocji i Psychologii Zdrowia*; Pracownia Testów Psychologicznych Polskiego Towarzystwa Psychologicznego: Warsaw, Poland, 2001.
60. Schnettler Morales, B.; Coria, M.D.; Vargas, H.M.; Maldonado, J.S.; González, M.M.; Andrade, G.L. Satisfaction with life and with food-related life in central Chile. *Psicothema* **2014**, *26*, 200–206. [CrossRef]
61. Roininen, K.; Lähteenmäki, L.; Tuorila, H. Quantification of consumer attitudes to health and hedonic characteristics of foods. *Appetite* **1999**, *33*, 71–88. [CrossRef]
62. Czarnocińska, J.; Jeżewska-Zychowicz, M.; Babicz-Zielińska, E.; Joanna, K.; Lidia, W. *Postawy Względem Żywności, Żywienia i Zdrowia a Zachowania Żywieniowe Dziewcząt i Młodych Kobiet w Polsce*, 1st ed.; UWM: Olsztyn, Poland, 2013.
63. Arbit, N.; Ruby, M.; Rozin, P. Development and validation of the meaning of food in life questionnaire (MFLQ): Evidence for a new construct to explain eating behaviour. *Food Qual. Pref.* **2017**, *59*, 35–45. [CrossRef]
64. Schnettler, B.; Miranda-Zapata, E.; Lobos, G.; Lapo, M.; Grunert, K.G.; Adasme-Berríos, C.; Hueche, C. Cross-cultural measurement invariance in the satisfaction with food-related life scale in older adults from two developing countries. *Health Qual. Life Outcomes* **2017**, *15*. [CrossRef] [PubMed]
65. Schnettler, B.; Miranda-Zapata, E.; Grunert, K.G.; Lobos, G.; Denegri, M.; Hueche, C.; Poblete, H. Life Satisfaction of University Students in Relation to Family and Food in a Developing Country. *Front. Psychol.* **2017**, *8*, 1522. [CrossRef] [PubMed]
66. Martín-María, N.; Caballero, F.F.; Moreno-Agostino, D.; Olaya, B.; Haro, J.M.; Ayuso-Mateos, J.L.; Miret, M. Relationship between subjective well-being and healthy lifestyle behaviours in older adults: A longitudinal study. *Aging Ment. Health* **2020**, *24*, 611–619. [CrossRef] [PubMed]

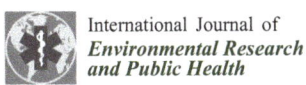

Article

Central Persons in Sustainable (Food) Consumption

Carolin V. Zorell

School of Humanities, Education and Social Sciences, Örebro University, 701 82 Örebro, Sweden; carolin.zorell@oru.se

Abstract: What people eat has become a highly political issue, closely intertwined with public health, environmental concerns, and climate change. Individuals' consumption decisions tend to be greatly influenced by the people that surround them, and this seems to be especially true when it comes to food. In recent years, alongside close contacts, such as family and friends, a myriad of social influencers have appeared on the screens, sharing opinions on what (not) to eat. Presenting results from a youth survey conducted in Sweden in 2019 (N = 443), this paper shows that social media have become the primary source of *information* about food and eating for youths, followed by schools and families. However, primary sources of *influence* continue to be parents and the family at large. Furthermore, the study shows that it is possible to identify *'central persons'*, i.e., relatively clear-cut groups of people whose food choices—measured as tendency to eat climate friendly—is mirrored by the youths, both in their everyday food preferences and in their broader political awareness as expressed through political consumerism. A conclusion from this is that certain people can be particularly successful at inspiring larger numbers of other people to engage with healthier and environmentally friendlier (food) consumption in a society.

Keywords: social influence; food choice; climate-friendly eating; social media; political consumerism; children's health

Citation: Zorell, C.V. Central Persons in Sustainable (Food) Consumption. *Int. J. Environ. Res. Public Health* **2022**, *19*, 3139. https://doi.org/10.3390/ijerph19053139

Academic Editors: F. Xavier Medina, Francesc Fusté-Forné and Nela Filimon

Received: 3 January 2022
Accepted: 28 February 2022
Published: 7 March 2022

Publisher's Note: MDPI stays neutral with regard to jurisdictional claims in published maps and institutional affiliations.

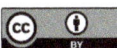

Copyright: © 2022 by the author. Licensee MDPI, Basel, Switzerland. This article is an open access article distributed under the terms and conditions of the Creative Commons Attribution (CC BY) license (https://creativecommons.org/licenses/by/4.0/).

1. Introduction

What food is consumed, in what way, and with whom, has fundamentally changed over the last decades. On average, today individuals eat more [1], more out of home [2], and more sugary, processed, and in general unhealthy food [1]. This is a major and continuously increasing problem, causing a rise in preventable diseases and premature deaths in countries worldwide [3,4]. Likewise, it is causing great harm to the environment and climate [3,5,6]. The food sector has thus been identified as one of the most important sectors to be urgently changed in order to reach sustainability goals and climate targets [3,5,6].

A key ambition stated across countries is therefore to encourage citizens to choose more ecological, climate-friendly, and healthy food. Especially children and adolescents seem to have been identified as key target group for such endeavour [7–9]. They are the adults of tomorrow, and thus whether they develop environmentally- and climate-friendly food habits today will determine the food sector's long-term success at performing within the Earths' "planetary boundaries" [10,11].

A common finding is that food choices are related to individual-level factors (e.g., attitudes, tastes, biological and demographic factors) and purchasing contexts (e.g., food availability). It is also increasingly recognised that food choices and behaviours are very much related to what peers and parents eat and drink [12,13], and, in a broader sense, to those sharing a social identity [14,15]. However, in a massively growing media landscape, the sources of information and the ways of communicating about food have changed fundamentally. B/vlogs, YouTube channels, (pseudo-)documentaries, social media posts, and food influencers have mushroomed, spreading recommendations about what to eat or not to eat. Digital spheres seem to have become an ever more important source of information about food, diets, and their implications for both health and the environment, especially—though by no means exclusively—for adolescents and young adults [16,17].

Hence, the number of potential sources of influence on when, where, and what a person eats seems to have exploded. However, just because people get information from certain sources, this must not necessarily mean that it translates into behaviour [18]. Initial studies suggest that digital media influence food choice and intake of children and youths [16,19]. How their influence compares to non-digital sources, such as parents or friends, remains unclear though. A strand of literature in social psychology and economics highlights that certain people have more influence on their peers than others in making them adopt certain attitudes or behaviours. Crucially, these studies suggest that on the basis of certain relationship characteristics or attributes, one can identify such "central persons" [20] or "social referents" [21]. Additionally, having such central persons changing behaviour and disseminating information about it seems to effectively achieve behaviour change of individuals and in larger populations [20,21].

This paper aims to study if such 'central persons' can also be identified in the context of sustainable consumption and eating (meaning, ethical, environmentally- and climate-friendly). This is done through addressing three sets of questions which stem from the above-mentioned:

RQ1: To what degree do digital sources of information about food influence the food choices of youths, and how does their influence compare to that of close ones such as parents or friends?

RQ2: Can the idea of 'central persons' be applied to the sphere of food, that is, can we identify certain kinds of people that are particularly central to (youths') everyday food choices and influence what they eat, and if so, how can they be identified?

From this, a third question follows. As described above, food is tied to great socio-political challenges. Analogous, eating ethical, ecological, and 'climate-friendly' food has become political, expressed among other things through so-called political consumerism [22,23]. Additionally, the individual responsibility to be considerate about the wider societal and environmental implications of consumption choices is hotly debated, highlighted, and gradually acknowledged across spheres and people [24]. This raises the question:

RQ3: Can the behaviours and recommendations of central persons be 'catalysts' of a broader political engagement, such as boycotting and buycotting products for ethical, environmental, or other political reasons?

In keeping with this last question, the paper focuses on environmental and climate aspects of food. To investigate into the various questions, it uses data from a high school survey conducted in Sweden in 2019 ($N = 443$). Next to questions about everyday food habits and sources of information about food, health, and ecology/climate, it contains an original measure to identify 'central' persons and their perceived eating habits. However, before presenting the data, methods, and results in detail, the paper starts with a review of current knowledge on the roots of eating patterns and food influence(r)s. Afterwards, it proceeds with presenting the empirical results. The paper concludes by discussing its contribution to the understanding of the role of social influence(r)s in defining eating patterns in the context of acute needs for more ecological and, generally, sustainable food choices.

2. Theoretical Background

2.1. Food Information and Influence

Individual preferences, attitudes, tastes, biological traits, and demographic backgrounds play a major role in determining when, what, and how much a person eats. Considerations such as convenience, price, taste, certain dietary requirements, health objectives or environmental values can guide what an individual is interested in knowing about food, where they search for information about food, and what they eventually buy and eat [13,25].

However, there are multiple other sources from the social and physical environments which inform and direct individual food choices [26–32] (see for a review [12]).

Parents play a particularly crucial role. By way of how and what parents provide for eating, what they encourage (not) to eat, and what they eat themselves, parents influence what their children eat, from early childhood throughout adolescence into adulthood [2,33–36]. Peer groups are another place where individuals discuss, get informed about, and mimic food preferences and habits. What and how much peers eat and weigh, especially close friends, has been shown to be tightly correlated with individual eating habits and weight [32,37,38] (but see also [33]). This points to much time being spent together consuming food, possibly talking about food, and influencing each other's food habits.

A third important factor shaping where and how food is purchased and consumed is physical and socio-cultural contexts. Such contexts cultivate socio-cultural norms, values, and traditions, and they typically build on certain policy and regulatory frameworks. These shape what is produced and imported in a country [12] and how individuals and media communicate about food (e.g., through advertising laws [39,40]). Thus, they determine what kind of food is made available, in which quantities, and what is socially accepted and encouraged to buy and eat (e.g., [40]). Furthermore, cultural belongings and social identities can influence, e.g., customs and tastes, and thus choices [14].

In modern everyday lives, these individual predispositions and immediate social and physical influences compete with multiple other aspects. In print and digital media, schools, and other outlets, individuals encounter a wide array of news and information about impacts of food on health and the environment. Some advocate certain diets for reasons of, e.g., attaining a certain body shape or look, or on how to 'comfort' the self through food. Others connect the advertised foods or diets to certain social images and groups [41], conveying the impression that for becoming or remaining a certain person or part of a social group, one should eat this or that [42]. Simultaneously, food advertisements surround individuals everywhere, most commonly for snacks and food that can be considered unhealthy [19,43–45]. Given their usually processed and plastic-packaged nature, they typically cannot be considered environmentally friendly either. Taking the multitude of messages about diets and lifestyles together, they are often contradictory and give rise to conflicting recommendations, desires, and needs.

As it becomes difficult to ascertain what food choice is the 'right' one, individuals find themselves in recurrent situations of uncertainty. Here, they likely look for orientation. Numerous studies show that exposure to advertisements, recommendations, and to less obvious marketing of products, especially in social media, has a discernible impact on attitudes towards the products and the likelihood to consume them [42,46,47], see also [12] (p. S66). This is found even when individuals disapprove or are unwilling to acknowledge such influence [47]. The interaction between different users in their roles as individuals seems to be an important driver of such influences [48,49]. In a recent randomised experimental study, Coates and colleagues [16] show how seeing social media influencers that eat unhealthy food successfully purports consumption of unhealthy food (measured in terms of calories) among children. Other research comes to the same conclusion. Media and advertisements, including user-generated content, predominantly focus on food that can be considered unhealthy; and, as a whole, it is mainly the intake of unhealthy food which is purported *successfully* in (social) media [43,50]. The information and messages surrounding an individual in these spheres thus seem to serve as anchors that give orientation in the decision what to eat.

Research yet also suggests that for being granted attention and successfully influencing an audience, individuals, brands, and their relationship towards a person need to satisfy certain criteria. For instance, they need to be able to raise feelings of accessibility and a "warm personal relationship" [49] (p. 5). Additionally, the ability to establish and maintain a trusting relationship seems to be of crucial importance [51], which can enable and be enabled through interpersonal contacts [52]. Correspondingly, personal closeness (family, close friends) and trust in the counterparts' competence in food matters (schools, teachers, doctors) play a key role in developing food preferences and choice [35,53].

However, social media very much build on such principles, too. Certain styles of language and images are used to raise feelings of closeness and shared social identities, with the ambition to influence peers and followers. Groups are created (e.g., in Facebook) or imagined (e.g., the following community of an Instagram influencer) and some seem to influence thousands (or millions) of followers to adopt certain diets, try recipes, or purchase certain (food) products.

A general contention thus is that social media is increasingly outdoing parents and other close ones as sources of information and influence about what to eat, especially for young people. Yet, how the various 'channels' of information and potential influence fare compared to each other remains largely uncharted. The knowledge gap is even greater when one includes other sources that spread information about food, health, or climate-friendly eating, such as TV, magazines, and civil society actors. One may agree with the contention and expect that (hypothesis h1) *social media have become the most important source of information about food*. Yet, parents, schools, and friends are the daily interaction partners of youths. An alternative hypothesis thus is that (ha1) *parents, friends, and schools are the most important sources of information about food*.

2.2. Central Persons and Food Habits

Transmitting information to people does not necessarily entail getting them to do something [54]. Some researchers studying social influence and imitation differentiate between different kinds of persons and strengths of influence. As they highlight, some persons are more influential—or 'central'—in opinion and behaviour formation than others are [21,54–57].

Crucially, Banjeree and colleagues [20] show that it is possible to identify concrete persons in a community who are better at spreading messages (e.g., gossips) and calls for action (i.e., getting people to get inoculated). Similarly, Paluck and her colleagues [21,56,58] could identify certain individuals that were more apt than others at instigating changes in attitudes and behaviours (in their case, harassment behaviour at schools) by changing perceptions of collective norms. Food consumption and the development and change of food preferences and habits tend to occur in social settings. Hence, the food individuals choose in their everyday lives may be similarly influenced.

Importantly, observing 'central persons' engaging with aspects such as ecology and climate change in relation to their food choices could motivate an individual—be it an adolescent or an adult—to do the same. Central persons can work as a source of information about food, food habits, and food norms in general, as well as about sustainable and climate-friendly eating in particular. In conversations and as living examples, they may inspire others to reflect upon their food habits, and to try and adopt new ones. In other words, observing central persons engaging with sustainable consumption and eating, e.g., eating climate friendly, could be an effective way through which more people get drawn into sustainable consumption.

Hence, the insights by Banjeree, Paluck, and their colleagues suggest that some people may be more powerful at influencing others' food preferences than others, and with this, at drawing people into sustainable eating. Hence, hypothesis 2 is that (h2) *it is possible to identify certain kinds of persons that are more 'central' than others at influencing people's food preferences*.

Moreover, this could work as an entry point into broader engagements with politics. By raising interest in the political implications of food, it may stir a broader sociopolitical awareness. In this vein, political scientists have consistently shown that political participation—mainly studied in terms of voting—is connected to what surrounding people say and do (e.g., [59–63]). Correspondingly, what central persons eat may not only affect individual food preferences. If individuals perceive their central person focus on political issues such as climate friendliness of food, they may become interested in politics in a broader sense. That is, they may engage with the politics of consumption, e.g., through deliberately choosing to buy or boycotting certain foods, diets, and other products for ecological, ethical, or other political reasons [64,65]. Put simply, a last hypothesis is that (h3) *an individual's boycotting and buycotting engagement correlates with the perceived tendency of their central persons to ground food choices on political considerations.*

3. Materials and Methods

The subsequent empirical study uses data collected as part of a survey of Swedish pupils in their last semester at senior high in 2019. The selection of schools was guided by a combined sample strategy of strategic sampling, where the aim was to cover classes with different subject specialisations (natural sciences, social sciences), orientations (aiming for further education or practical work after school), and from towns of different sizes in mid-Sweden (five in total, ranging from Stockholm as a big city, to Hallsberg municipality as a small town area). Yet, regardless of this strategic approach, the sample needs to be seen as a convenience sample.

Before the survey, the teachers made available the information about the study aim and ethical issues in their school's internal information system, so the pupils had time to go through the material. Data collection took place in the classrooms, for anonymity and quality reasons without the teachers. Trained study assistants distributed again information about the study and ethics and collected informed consent before students would receive a link to the electronic questionnaire (a few answered in paper format). The assistants remained in the classroom while the students filled in the questionnaire, which took about 90 min (with a break in between). The students did not get any reward for answering the questionnaire. Those who did not want to participate did schoolwork instead. The final sample consisted of 443 pupils aged 16–22; this excludes ca. 40 respondents who provided answers that gave reason to suspect systematic misreporting. In total, 59% of the respondents were girls, 39% boys, and 1% youth identifying with another gender.

To measure the most important *source of information* (hypothesis 1), the youths were asked from where they usually get information about food, eating, and ecology/climate. To this end, they were presented a list of six kinds of social ties and media (family, friends, school, social media, TV, newspaper) plus an open answer field and asked to assign to each of them a rank describing to what extent they usually get information about food from that source. Given the setup of the questionnaire, the participants assigned to each of the seven potential sources of information a number between 1 (least usual) and 7 (most usual). This resulted in seven variables with seven categories, i.e., scale values. For each value, the frequency of responses indicates the number of people who ranked the source of information on the respective rank. Comparing these frequencies permits drawing conclusions about the comparative importance of the distinct kinds of social ties and media as sources of information for the youth. However, in many cases, the ranking was not entirely 'neatly' done, but respondents assigned same ranks to more than one source and no source to single ranks. Since the focus of measurement is on identifying the *most important* source of information, the analysis focuses on the frequency to which each source was ranked first (i.e., as main/most important); if single individuals ranked more than one with "1", all of them are counted as "most important". This renders a comparative assessment of the various sources' importance.

The dependent variable for hypothesis 2 grounds on a validated questionnaire capturing *everyday food preferences*. It asks respondents what is important to them that the food they eat on a typical day fulfils. Through 24 response items, individuals can indicate on a 7-point scale whether a trait is not at all (1) to very (7) important to them [66–68]. The items include price, various health-related, sensory, and popularity aspects, as well as ecological and ethical criteria. A factor analysis provides five distinct factors, of which one discernibly relates to 'sustainable' eating (Cronbach's $\alpha = 0.934$; see Appendix A). It covers that the food should be organic, fair traded, produced and packaged environmentally friendly, be in harmony with one's ethical values, and climate friendly. On its basis, an additive index is created that captures the degree to which an individual puts weight on the fact that their everyday food choices are 'sustainable'.

To capture *central persons*, a measure was adapted from Åmna and colleagues [69] (see Appendix B). Respondents were asked whether certain kinds of persons have a greater influence on their food choices than others, and if so, to freely mention one or two such persons. To make the question simpler to understand, the wording further specified "who this person is, for example a person [they] follow on social media, [their] best friend, [their] mom or dad, a celebrity, the leader of an organization".

As a second independent variable (*climate-friendly eating of central persons*), the youths were asked if and to what extent one or the two of these persons themselves "buy/eat climate-friendly food". Here, the answer options included (1) "No, they do not", "Yes, one does so (2) sporadically/(3) most of the time", "Yes, the two do so (4) sporadically/ (5) most of the time", as well as a (6) "I do not know" (see also Appendix B). Despite the question referring to the prior question, examining the data revealed that the youths did not necessarily refrain from answering this question despite previously having answered that there is no central person. In total, 19 individuals answered that one or two central persons are eating climate friendly, despite not having named any central person beforehand. This might be due to the additional effort that writing down a central person implies (first question), whereas ticking a box (second question) requires less cognitive effort. A check showed that these responses do not change the general conclusions. Nonetheless, in the following analysis the two variables are treated as separated from each other.

For hypothesis 3, two questions gauged the regularity of political consumerism. Adapted from commonly employed measures [63] (p. 9), they ask how often it occurred in the last 12 months that the person (1) boycotted and (2) bought food or other products for ecological or ethical reasons. Respondents then indicated on a 6-point scale whether they did so never (1) to every day (6). The *boycotting* and *buycotting* variables are correlated (r_p = 0.546; p = 0.000; N = 432), yet there are differences across individuals and thus the two are considered as separate dependent variables.

Finally, *age* (measured in years of age) and *gender* (girl (0), boy (1), other (0)) were included in all models as control variables. Table 1 summarises the descriptive statistics for all variables.

Table 1. Descriptive statistics for dependent and independent variables.

Variable	Obs.	Mean	Std. Dev.	Min	Max
Additive index everyday food choices must be sustainable	442	3.89	1.41	1	6.78
Boycotting	432	2.78	1.76	1	6
Buycotting	439	3.39	1.29	1	6
Source of information:					
Family	430	4.15	1.80	1	7
Friends	429	3.52	1.68	1	7
School	429	4.03	1.72	1	7
TV	428	3.66	1.73	1	7
Newspaper	428	2.83	1.71	1	7
Social media	431	5.16	1.77	1	7
Other	162	2.78	2.29	1	7
Central person(s)	432	1.38	0.49	1	2
Climate-friendly eating of central persons	194	3.33	1.40	1	5
Gender	436	0.40	0.49	0	1
Age	440	17.92	0.66	16	22

The methodological approach starts with descriptive and correlation analysis. This is combined with non-parametric group tests (Kruskal–Wallis H test) to compare groups of people with and without central persons that eat in a certain way (i.e., climate friendly).

4. Results

4.1. Identifying Central Persons Influencing Food Preferences

To map the terrain, the enquiry starts with a look at the principle factors that the youths mention as guiding their food choices. Figure 1 reports the mean values for the five overarching categories (which, according to a non-parametric Friedman test, are statistically different from each other; $\chi^2(4) = 492.77$, $p < 0.001$). The principal factor are sensory and emotional aspects, i.e., taste, texture, and mood. This is closely followed by price and, with some distance, health criteria. All three are not different for girls and boys. For the third gender, given the small number of respondents, a discussion would be speculative in character and is therefore excluded from this comparison.

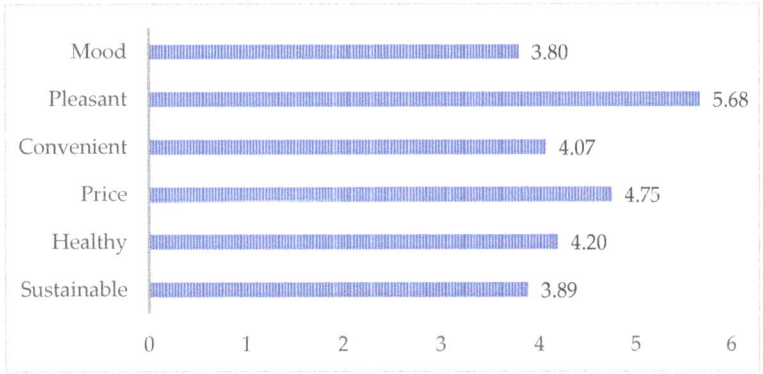

Figure 1. Food properties guiding food choice of youths, mean values.

Ecological criteria range lowest in influence on food choice. However, they are notably different between girls and boys. Girls show a greater tendency to consider sustainability important than boys. This difference fits in with multiple other studies on environmental behaviours, showing that across all age groups, women tend to be more considerate of ecological and ethical consumption aspects than men (even though the gap has narrowed over the past years; cf. [70] p. 132). Overall, however, it seems clear that the issue of food choices remains complex, and the youths are far from all being "Greta", that is, young environmental activists who have changed their lifestyles entirely.

Such differences in the priorities can be rooted in various kinds of personal circumstances. A main one as suggested in this paper is where individuals get information about food and the people with whom they interact discussing food-related matters. Looking into this question, Figure 2 summarises the ranking provided by the respondents of the sources through which they usually receive information about "food, eating, and climate matters". Their comparative ranking is interpreted as an indication of their comparative importance; that is, the sources were the youths state to get information most (usually) are here understood as being the most important sources of information.

Visibly, social media headed the ranking with a mean value of 5.16 on a 7-point scale. With notable distance, this is followed by the family and school. After this, TV and friends follow. Newspapers and other sources rank as least usual sources of information. Some respondents also specified what they mean with "other" sources; those named by several respondents include statistics, (online) documentaries, and podcasts. A single respondent named politicians. According to a non-parametric Friedman test, these mean values are different from each other to a statistically significant extent ($\chi^2(6) = 189.87$, $p < 0.001$).

Digital media outlets, especially social media, are thus the principal 'channel' through which youths receive information about matters relating to food. This confirms hypothesis 1. Of the non-remote sources, schools, teachers, and the family can be considered important, while friends less so. Overall, however, they do not seem to be the most important sources of information about food, which disproves the alternative hypothesis (ha1).

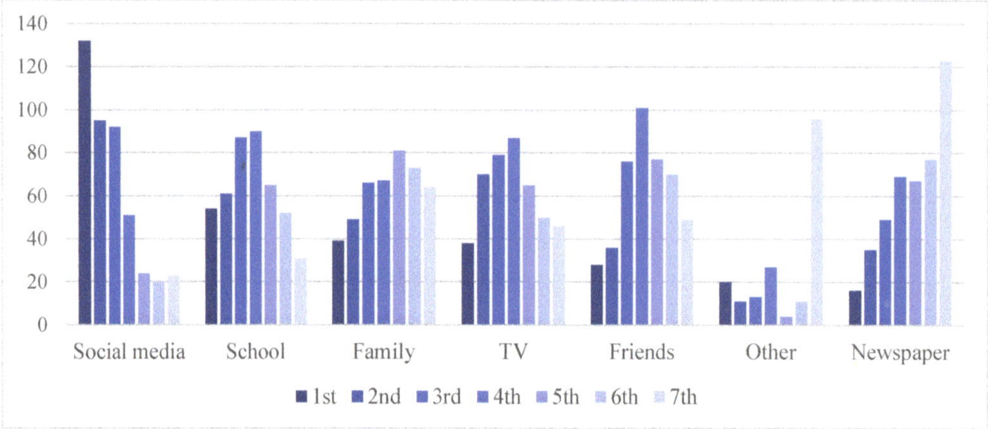

Figure 2. Most usual sources of information about food (numbers of respondents ranking source 1st to 7th). Note: Ordered from left to right according to source that was most to least often ranked as most important.

Influencers on social media and teachers at school may advocate certain healthy diets. However, this does not automatically and necessarily mean that the receivers of the messages adopt their dietary recommendations. This leads to the question whether there are certain kinds of people who are particularly central at *influencing* a person's everyday food choices. This can be gauged in two ways. By directly asking about the existence of central persons; and indirectly, by observing if a potentially central person has an influence on what a person eats.

The survey includes a direct question. Furthermore, while it provides only cross-sectional data, which does not allow for studying a causal connection between eating patterns, the questionnaire includes questions that allow for comparing the eating patterns of a group of youth whose central persons eat climate friendly with that of a group whose central persons do not eat climate friendly. This way, we can study if the patterns of climate-friendly eating of central persons correspond with the eating patterns of the respondents.

About 38% of the youth state that there is a specific person that has especially affected what they buy and choose when it comes to food. Correspondingly, a majority states that they *cannot* name anyone that has a central role in influencing their food choices. While this does not necessarily mean that there is no one affecting their choices, it yet means that they have no one who consciously and distinctively affects them, and who can be named off the top of their head.

Figure 3 reports the sorted answers to the open question about who the central persons are (i.e., responses given by 38% of respondents). Instagram, influencers, etc., are not directly grouped under the label of social media to illustrate the variation in answers. Besides, it gives an impression of the various sub-types and variety that the label 'social media' actually covers.

The graph renders a relatively clear picture, which slightly diverges from the results regarding sources of information. When it comes to actual influence on food choice, it seems that family members, and especially parents, range similarly high in importance as social media, even after subsuming the different sub-types of social media into one category. Hence, parents may not be considered primary sources of information about food, but they are primary sources of influence. Admittedly, this is not entirely surprising as most youths live at home (91% of the respondents), and hence may find their parents choosing what food is bought and served to begin with. This also likely influences the food tastes and habits in situations where the youths make choices on their own. However, parents are also central for those who do not live at home, thus pointing to an additional kind of influence besides that of owning the decision-making authority.

Best friends are important too, ranging on the same level as influencers. Schools and teachers, in turn, seem to be important sources of information, but according to this descriptive result, they appear to lack influence on what is eaten.

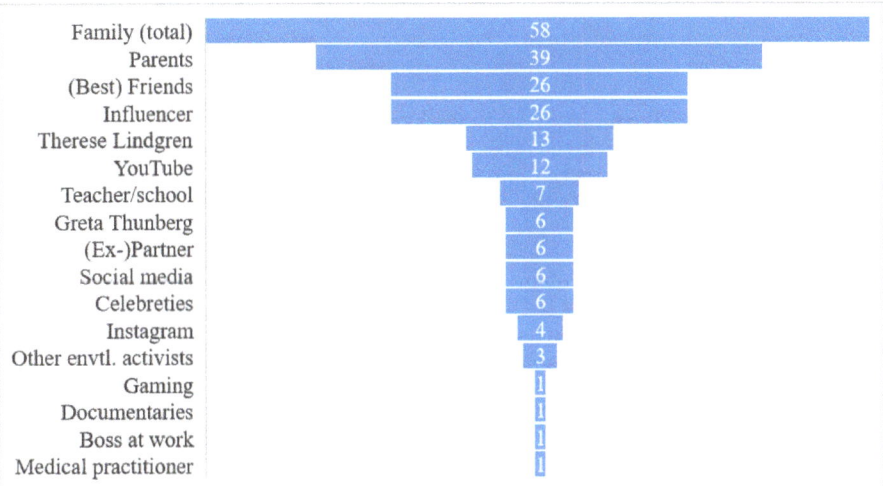

Figure 3. Central persons affecting food purchase and choice, frequencies of mentions. Note: Family (total) includes parents plus any other kind of family tie. Therese Lindgren is a Swedish influencer on lifestyle issues in general. The figure reflects the responses provided by 38% of participants, i.e., 166 individuals. In total, 12 persons provided answers that could not be classified. A total of 89 individuals named one central person, the rest named two and a few named a combination of several categories in relation to a single central person, e.g., Therese Lindgren *and* YouTube *and* influencer; in the graph, these cases are counted, respectively, with a value for each of the different categories.

Table 2 reports the responses to whether one or two central persons eat climate friendly. A clear majority reports perceiving at least one doing so. What is more, they are perceived to be doing it more regularly than sometimes. This is surprising, since it suggests a disproportionately large fraction of people eating climate friendly. An alternative reason may be that the respondents observe it consciously precisely *because* it stands out. In any of the two cases, the figures should not compromise the later conclusions, but they will be kept in mind when drawing general conclusions from the results.

Table 2. Central persons eating climate friendly.

Central Persons Eating Climate Friendly	Frequencies	Percentage
None of them	27	13.92
One of them sometimes	23	11.86
One of them regularly	66	34.02
Both of them sometimes	15	7.73
Both of them regularly	63	32.47
Total	194	100

Note: Next to these 194 individuals and the ones who said they have no central person, another 46 individuals answered with "I do not know".

According to the theory of central persons, if an individual perceives that their central person(s) focuses on something such as the climate friendliness of what they eat, the individual would be expected to reproduce it in their everyday food choices. To test this theory, one can look at the overlap between the frequency with which an individual perceives their central person(s) is (are) grounding food choices on certain aspects (i.e., climate-friendly eating) and the individual's own frequency of doing so. The variable assessing perceived central persons' climate-friendly eating is treated as an ordinal variable in the analysis, i.e., the influence of two persons eating sometimes climate friendly is considered to be stronger than one person doing so regularly. This assumption is based on research into social influence and behaviour spread, suggesting that several influences tend to reinforce each other and therewith strengthen the influencing effect [54]).

The test statistics of a Kruskal–Wallis H test indicate that there is a statistically significant difference in the median focus that respondents put on sustainability aspects of their food depending on the degree to which they perceive their central persons to be doing so (i.e., the independent variable as reported in Table 2) ($\chi^2(4) = 24.934, p < 0.001$). Hence, the youths' focus on sustainable eating seems to indeed vary along with what they perceive their central persons are doing. Non-parametric correlation analysis further specifies that what central persons are perceived to be doing is *positively* related to what the youths themselves do ($r\tau = 0.235, p < 0.001, N = 194$). However, when differentiating according to gender, the effect is again different among girls and boys. For girls, the correlation coefficient does not reach statistical significance ($r\tau = 0.099, p = 0.163, N = 120$), while for boys it is moderately strong ($r\tau = 0.312, p < 0.001, N = 69$).

A bar chart visualises this difference (Figure 4). Girls' inclination to consider it important that their everyday food choices are sustainable is high throughout. The mean values are slightly higher among those reporting that one or two of the central persons are eating climate friendly on a regular basis. Yet, the confidence intervals overlap with the other categories. Thus, their inclination seems to be relatively independent of what their central persons are perceived to be doing. In contrast, boys who do not perceive any central person to be eating climate friendly do not either. Yet, if one or two central persons sometime or regularly eat climate friendly, they tend to do so as well. Moreover, the inclination increases quasi-linear along with the increased number and frequency of central persons eating climate friendly (although the confidence intervals overlap, suggesting that this last interpretation must be taken with caution).

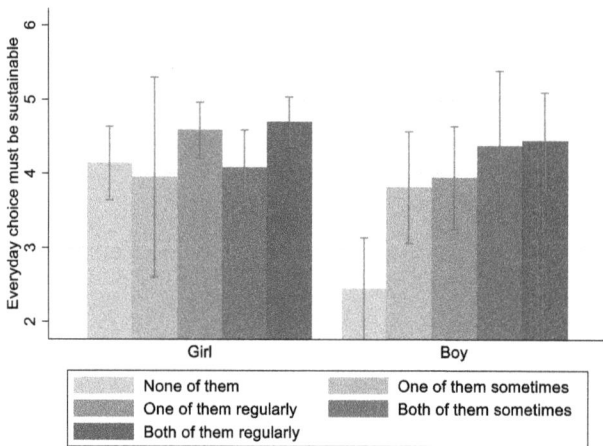

Figure 4. Central persons and youths eating climate friendly. Lines show 95% confidence intervals.

In sum, the results suggest that there are central persons. These central persons seem to belong to relatively clear-cut groups of people, who can be characterised by a distinct type of affiliation to the individual (e.g., family, friends, social media influencer). Yet, perceived centrality does not necessarily mean behavioural centrality. For girls, influence seems to happen mainly if central persons eat climate friendly on a notable, i.e., regular basis. Boys, in turn, the more frequently they perceive their central persons to be grounding food choices on climate considerations, the more frequent they ground their everyday food choices on such criteria as well. This association can be interpreted as a potential influence coming from the central person, which allows for confirming hypothesis 2.

4.2. Central Persons and Political Consumerism

The last hypothesis (h3) states that what central persons are perceived to be doing can affect more than eating habits. If they are perceived to be grounding food choices on climate considerations, this may get the ones to whom they are central to engage with the politics of food and consumption more widely. In other words, central persons' behaviour may instigate broader political awareness and motivate political engagements, especially political consumerism. Two dependent variables are used to measure such engagement: boycotting and buycotting. The independent variable is the degrees of climate-friendly eating of central persons.

The results of a Kruskal–Wallis H test indicate that there is a statistically significant difference in buycotting between the youth within the five different degrees of perceived climate-friendly eating of their central persons ($\chi^2(4) = 43.370, p < 0.000$). Non-parametric correlation analysis further points to a positive relationship, for both girls ($r\tau = 0.212$, $p = 0.006, N = 120$) and boys ($r\tau = 0.431, p < 0.000, N = 67$). For boycotting, the group test also reveals a statistically significant difference between the five degrees of what central persons are perceived to be doing ($\chi^2(4) = 19.122, p < 0.000$). Yet, according to correlation analysis, this holds only for boys ($r\tau = 0.273, p = 0.006, N = 66$), while not for girls ($r\tau = 0.100$, $p = 0.187, N = 120$).

Figure 5 specifies the patterns. Girls' tendency to buycott is connected to central persons' engagement with climate-friendly eating if the central persons do so regularly, but not if they are perceived to be doing so only sometimes or not at all. An explanation may be that the baseline for girls is higher as they have generally a higher tendency towards being already engaged with the politics of food and consumption. Hence, they may note and be influenced only by those cases that stand out through great regularity of climate-friendly consumption. Girls' boycotting engagement does not appear to be related to what their central persons do.

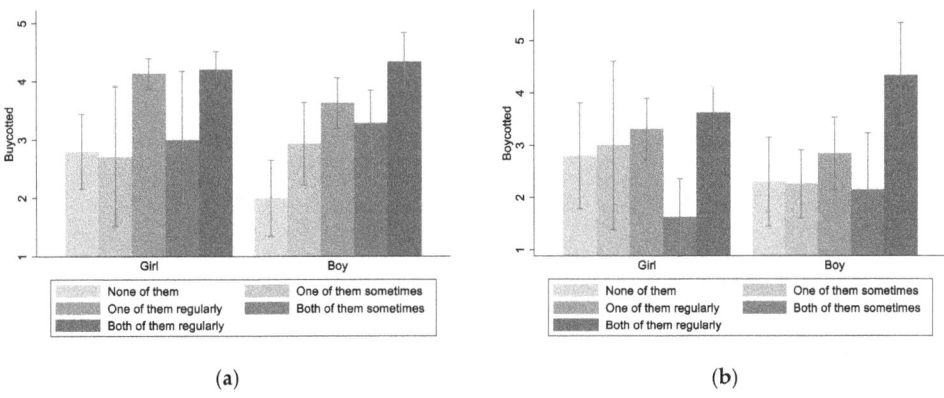

Figure 5. Central persons and youths' political consumer engagements, (a) buycotting and (b) boycotting. Lines show 95% confidence intervals.

Conversely, boys' engagement with buycotting is more closely related to what their central persons are perceived to be doing. If they are perceived to never eat climate friendly, the boys do the same. If they are perceived to focus on climate-friendly eating sporadically or frequently, the boys respectively buycott sporadically or frequently. Boycotting, however, seems to need a stronger engagement on the central persons' side to uncover an effect. That is, a potential influence seems to be observable only if central persons, be it one or two, are perceived to *regularly* engage with climate-friendly eating. Overall, it seems reasonable to confirm the part of hypothesis 3 relating to buycotting. The youths' buycotting engagement is closely related to what they observe of their central persons, and this is especially strong for boys. Boycotting, in turn, seems to be related only for boys and only provided central persons send strong signals through regular engagements with the politics of eating.

5. Conclusions

The consumption of unhealthy and unecological food is a major and continuously increasing problem, causing a rise in preventable diseases, premature deaths, and ecological disasters in countries worldwide [3–6]. With the ambition to contribute knowledge to advance ambitions to get citizens choose more ecological food, this paper provides insights which suggest that gaining certain kinds of people adopting climate-friendly diets can act as multiplier inspiring other people to do the same.

In a study of Swedish high school students, the paper could identify relatively clear-cut groups of people who show to be particularly central for what youths prefer to eat. These groups are characterised by a distinct type of affiliation to the individual: the family, friends, or influencer on social media. Depending on whether these central persons are seen to eat climate friendly or not, the youth respectively consider environmental and ethical aspects important in their food choices as well, or they do not. This influence of central persons seems to be particularly great on boys, and although to a lesser extent, also on girls. Moreover, their influence seems to extend beyond everyday food habits and come along with broadened political awareness that is expressed through political consumerism.

From a more general perspective, adults tend to like to see themselves as less vulnerable to others' influences, yet research suggests otherwise (e.g., [48,71]). Hence, while these findings rest on a youth sample, we can expect that similar tendencies would be observable in other age groups. Nonetheless, a limitation is that the youth may not always buy food for themselves and need to eat what is served. This can imply that we are observing a larger influence of especially parents in this study as what would be observed in a study of the general population. In addition, it carries the possibility that there are various kinds of influence observed in the present study, again especially of parents on their kids, as they may not only 'inspire' their kids towards certain food choices, but also choose the food they get to begin with. Future studies, therefore, need to explore more in detail what happens within families, and to what extent the influence of the family is temporary.

The findings illustrate two other things. First, there seems to be an important distinction between sources of information and sources of influence. Schools and teachers, for example, are important sources of information for the youth, while they seem to have little actual influence on food choice. The reverse holds for parents and friends. Social media, in turn, fare high on both aspects, but more so on the provision of information.

A common contention is that social media are more relevant in youths' lives than in that of adults. However, the findings suggest that even among the youth, social media influence seems to be on average lower than that of family and friends. This allows for concluding that findings regarding influence may be quite similar in a study of the general population. That is, close ties such as family and friends are principal influencers. This includes the possibility of a recursive link where youths influence their parents.

The findings further suggest that to successfully promote changes in diets, it is important to focus on addressing and convincing those who can actually influence others to change what they eat, i.e., *central persons*, rather than only disseminate information through, e.g., leaflets and educational programmes. The paper also provides a methodological tool for it: one can identify certain kinds of 'central' people based on easily observable characteristics (e.g., being a parent or a v/blogger). Hence, knowing about such ties can work as a methodological shortcut to identify persons who can influence eating patterns particularly well. Campaigns and broader strategies aimed at promoting ecological and healthy eating may then not need to start each time by categorising and assessing each individual's very personal conception of their social influencers. Instead, they can build on those easily identifiable relationship characteristics and explicitly target those groups, who can act as multipliers.

Second, the observations underscore how supposedly small everyday actions such as food activism can multiply and trigger broader engagements with the politics of consumption, climate change, and political issues more in general. Thinking one step further, this process may not only unfold at the level of the individual who engages in gradually more ways with such issues, but also at the level of a society, where engagements of some can 'tip over' to others, inspiring them to engage with the politics of, e.g., food and climate change. Future studies may apply social network approaches to dive deeper into this idea and study whether the influence of certain people can especially effectively advance sustainable consumption in a larger population.

These future studies may then also cover aspects which represent limitations of this study: the cross-sectional nature of the data, the small sample size, and the focus on youths and only one country. Additionally, there is the possibility of reporting bias due to the potential desire of respondents to put themselves in a better light when reporting what they care for and tend to consume. Future studies may include more systematic measures to control for such biases. Likewise, they may focus on further age groups (also to study who are the central persons of those central persons) and include more socio-demographic and economic background variables, as well as longitudinal measures.

This paper made a first effort to compare roles of different kinds of people in the process of changing consumption patterns. It reconfirms that eating is deeply connected to social environments. Yet, it adds the insight that not all social ties are equally relevant. Additionally, while the findings are based on a youth sample, there are reasons to expect that it also applies to adults. This is an invaluable insight for those aiming to transform current food consumption patterns. Specifically, gaining central persons for the purpose may be a key to reach social tipping points at which 'sustainable' consumption choices become the 'new normal'.

Funding: The collection of data for this research was funded by the Swedish Research Council for Sustainable Development Formas through project 2017-00880, led by Maria Ojala (Örebro University).

Institutional Review Board Statement: The study was conducted in accordance with the Declaration of Helsinki, and approved by the Swedish National Ethics Committee national ethics committee under protocol number 2019-03857.

Informed Consent Statement: Informed consent was obtained from all subjects involved in the study.

Data Availability Statement: The data presented in this study are available on request from the corresponding author.

Acknowledgments: I would like to thank the participants of the 2021 paper workshop from the Centre for Environmental and Sustainability Social Science (CESSS) at Örebro University for their valuable comments. Furthermore, my special thanks go to Maria Ojala, for offering me to add questions to her survey study.

Conflicts of Interest: The author declares no conflict of interest. The funders had no role in the design of the study; in the collection, analyses, or interpretation of data; in the writing of the manuscript, or in the decision to publish the results.

Appendix A

Table A1. Factor analysis for important aspects in everyday food consumption. Principal Component Analysis. Varimax with Kaiser Normalization. Only loadings > 0.400 are shown. KMO: 0.906, Chi-sq.: 5,484,406. Explained Variance: 69.40%, Cronbach's Alpha: 0.934, 0.895, 0.731, 0.492, and 0.431, for components 1–5, respectively. Components 1 and 2 are moderately-strong correlated (0.504), while all other correlations range between 0.043 (components 1 and 4) and 0.293 (components 2 and 5).

	Component					
	Sustainable	Healthy	Price	Convenience	Sensations	Mood
Produced in an environmentally friendly way	0.894					
Climate friendly	0.885					
Packaged in an environmentally friendly way	0.868					
Environmentally friendly	0.849					
Organic	0.848					
Fairtrade	0.810					
Animal friendly	0.712					
In line with my ethical values	0.661					
Natural	0.469					
Nutritious		0.827				
Much protein		0.816				
Keeps me healthy		0.809				
Much fibre		0.806				
Vitamins and minerals		0.780				
Good for the teeth/hair/nails etc.		0.690				
Healthy		0.639				
Helps me control my weight		0.506				
Not too expensive			0.851			
Affordable			0.833			
Well-known				0.805		
Convenient/simple				0.649		
Pleasant sensations					0.805	
Tasty					0.739	
Mood						0.869

Appendix B

Questions gauging central persons:

Q1: Is there someone who has particularly influenced what you buy and choose when it comes to food and drink? If so, please state who this person is, e.g., a person you follow on social media, your best friend, your mom or dad, a celebrity, the leader of an organisation.

Please specify one or two of the most important persons.

0 = No one
1 = Yes, my (1) _____
(2) _____

Q2: If you have specified at least one person, does any of them buy/eat climate friendly food?

1 = No, they do not
2 = Yes, one does so sporadically
3 = Yes, one does so most of the time
4 = Yes, the two do so sporadically
5 = Yes, the two do so most of the time
6 = I do not know

References

1. Popkin, B.M.; Adair, L.S.; Ng, S.W. Global Nutrition Transition and the Pandemic of Obesity in Developing Countries. *Nutr. Rev.* **2012**, *70*, 3–21. [CrossRef] [PubMed]
2. Savage, J.S.; Fisher, J.O.; Birch, L.L. Parental Influence on Eating Behavior. *J. Law Med. Ethics* **2007**, *35*, 22–34. [CrossRef] [PubMed]
3. Clark, M.A.; Springmann, M.; Hill, J.; Tilman, D. Multiple Health and Environmental Impacts of Foods. *Proc. Natl. Acad. Sci. USA* **2019**, *116*, 23357–23362. [CrossRef]
4. Forouzanfar, M.H.; Alexander, L.; Anderson, H.R.; Bachman, V.F.; Biryukov, S.; Brauer, M.; Burnett, R.; Casey, D.; Coates, M.M.; Cohen, A.; et al. Global, Regional, and National Comparative Risk Assessment of 79 Behavioural, Environmental and Occupational, and Metabolic Risks or Clusters of Risks in 188 Countries, 1990–2013: A Systematic Analysis for the Global Burden of Disease Study 2013. *Lancet* **2015**, *386*, 2287–2323. [CrossRef]
5. Clark, M.A.; Domingo, N.G.G.; Colgan, K.; Thakrar, S.K.; Tilman, D.; Lynch, J.; Azevedo, I.L.; Hill, J.D. Global Food System Emissions Could Preclude Achieving the 1.5° and 2 °C Climate Change Targets. *Science* **2020**, *370*, 705–708. [CrossRef]
6. Willett, W.; Rockström, J.; Loken, B.; Springmann, M.; Lang, T.; Vermeulen, S.; Garnett, T.; Tilman, D.; DeClerck, F.; Wood, A.; et al. Food in the Anthropocene: The EAT–Lancet Commission on Healthy Diets from Sustainable Food Systems. *Lancet* **2019**, *393*, 447–492. [CrossRef]
7. Galli, F.; Brunori, G.; Di Iacovo, F.; Innocenti, S. Co-producing sustainability: Involving parents and civil society in the governance of school meal services. A case study from Pisa, Italy. *Sustainability* **2014**, *6*, 1643–1666. [CrossRef]
8. Morgan, K.; Sonnino, R. Empowering consumers: The creative procurement of school meals in Italy and the UK. *Int. J. Consum. Stud.* **2007**, *31*, 19–25. [CrossRef]
9. UNICEF. *The State of the World's Children 2019. Children, Food and Nutrition: Growing Well in a Changing World*; UNICEF: New York, NY, USA, 2019.
10. Steffen, W.; Richardson, K.; Rockström, J.; Cornell, S.E.; Fetzer, I.; Bennett, E.M.; Biggs, R.; Carpenter, S.R.; De Vries, W.; De Wit, C.A.; et al. Planetary Boundaries: Guiding Human Development on a Changing Planet. *Science* **2015**, *347*, 1259855. [CrossRef]
11. Rockström, J.; Steffen, W.; Noone, K.; Persson, Å.; Stuart Chapin, F.; Lambin, E.F.; Lenton, T.M.; Scheffer, M.; Folke, C.; Schellnhuber, H.J.; et al. A Safe Operation Space for Humanity. *Nature* **2009**, *461*, 472–475. [CrossRef]
12. Larson, N.; Story, M. A Review of Environmental Influences on Food Choices. *Ann. Behav. Med.* **2009**, *38*, 56–73. [CrossRef] [PubMed]
13. Neumark-Sztainer, D.; Story, M.; Perry, C.; Casey, M.A. Factors Influencing Food Choices of Adolescents: Findings from Focus-group Discussions with Adolescents. *J. Am. Diet. Assoc.* **1999**, *99*, 929–937. [CrossRef]
14. Hackel, L.M.; Coppin, G.; Wohl, M.J.A.; Van Bavel, J.J. From Groups to Grits: Social Identity Shapes Evaluations of Food Pleasantness. *J. Exp. Soc. Psychol.* **2018**, *74*, 270–280. [CrossRef]
15. Oyserman, D.; Fryberg, S.A.; Yoder, N. Identity-Based Motivation and Health. *J. Pers. Soc. Psychol.* **2007**, *93*, 1011–1027. [CrossRef] [PubMed]
16. Coates, A.E.; Hardman, C.A.; Halford, J.C.G.; Christiansen, P.; Boyland, E.J. Social Media Influencer Marketing and Children's Food Intake: A Randomized Trial. *Pediatrics* **2019**. [CrossRef]
17. Potvin Kent, M.; Pauzé, E.; Roy, E.A.; de Billy, N.; Czoli, C. Children and Adolescents' Exposure to Food and Beverage Marketing in Social Media Apps. *Pediatr. Obes.* **2019**, *14*, e12508. [CrossRef]
18. Brown, K.; Mcilveen, H.; Strugnell, C. Nutritional Awareness and Food Preferences of Young Consumers. *Nutr. Food Sci.* **2000**, *30*, 230–235. [CrossRef]
19. Coates, A.E.; Hardman, C.A.; Halford, J.C.G.; Christiansen, P.; Boyland, E.J. Food and Beverage Cues Featured in YouTube Videos of Social Media Influencers Popular With Children: An Exploratory Study. *Front. Psychol.* **2019**, *10*, 1–14. [CrossRef]
20. Banjeree, A.V.; Chandrasekhar, A.G.; Duflo, E.; Jackson, M.O. *Using Gossips to Spread Information: Theory and Evidence from two Randomized Controlled Trials*. MIT Department of Economics Working Paper. 2018. Available online: https://papers.ssrn.com/sol3/papers.cfm?abstract_id=2425379 (accessed on 2 January 2022).
21. Paluck, E.L.; Shepherd, H.S. The Salience of Social Referents: A Field Experiment on Collective Norms and Harassment Behavior in a School Social Network. *J. Pers. Soc. Psychol.* **2012**, *103*, 899–915. [CrossRef]
22. Stolle, D.; Hooghe, M.; Micheletti, M. Politics in the Supermarket: Political Consumerism as a Form of Political Participation. *Int. Polit. Sci. Rev.* **2005**, *26*, 245–269. [CrossRef]
23. Theocharis, Y.; van Deth, J.W. The Continuous Expansion of Citizen Participation: A New Taxonomy. *Eur. Polit. Sci. Rev.* **2018**, *10*, 139–163. [CrossRef]
24. Schnaudt, C.; van Deth, J.W.; Zorell, C.V.; Theocharis, Y. Revisiting norms of citizenship in times of democratic change. *Politics* **2021**. [CrossRef]
25. Aertsens, J.; Verbeke, W.; Mondelaers, K.; van Huylenbroeck, G. Personal Determinants of Organic Food Consumption: A Review. *Br. Food J.* **2009**, *111*, 1140–1167. [CrossRef]
26. Cioffi, C.E.; Levitsky, D.A.; Pacanowski, C.R.; Bertz, F. A nudge in a healthy direction. The effect of nutrition labels on food purchasing behaviors in university dining facilities. *Appetite* **2015**, *92*, 7–14. [CrossRef]
27. Higgs, S.; Thomas, J. Social Influences on Eating. *Curr. Opin. Behav. Sci.* **2016**, *9*, 1–6. [CrossRef]
28. Miller, G.F.; Gupta, S.; Kropp, J.D.; Grogan, K.A.; Mathews, A. The Effects of Pre-ordering and Behavioral Nudges on National School Lunch Program Participants' Food Item Selection. *J. Econ. Psychol.* **2016**, *55*, 4–16. [CrossRef]

29. Robinson, E.; Tobias, T.; Shaw, L.; Freeman, E.; Higgs, S. Social Matching of Food Intake and the Need for Social Acceptance. *Appetite* **2011**, *56*, 747–752. [CrossRef]
30. Rozin, P.; Scott, S.; Dingley, M.; Urbanek, J.K.; Jiang, H.; Kaltenbach, M. Nudge to Nobesity I: Minor Changes in Accessibility Decrease Food Intake. *Judgm. Decis. Mak.* **2011**, *6*, 323–332.
31. Salvy, S.J.; de la Haye, K.; Bowker, J.C.; Hermans, R.C.J. Influence of Peers and Friends on Children's and Adolescents' Eating and Activity Behaviors. *Physiol. Behav.* **2012**, *106*, 369–378. [CrossRef]
32. Wansink, B.; Sobal, J. Mindless Eating: The 200 Daily Food Decisions we Overlook. *Environ. Behav.* **2007**, *39*, 106–123. [CrossRef]
33. Feunekes, G.I.J.; De Graaf, C.; Meyboom, S.; Van Staveren, W.A. Food Choice and Fat Intake of Adolescents and Adults: Associations of Intakes Within Social Networks. *Prev. Med.* **1998**, *27*, 645–656. [CrossRef] [PubMed]
34. Sharps, M.; Higgs, S.; Blissett, J.; Nouwen, A.; Chechlacz, M.; Allen, H.A.; Robinson, E. Examining Evidence for Behavioural Mimicry of Parental Eating by Adolescent Females. An Observational Study. *Appetite* **2015**, *89*, 56–61. [CrossRef] [PubMed]
35. van der Horst, K.; Oenema, A.; Ferreira, I.; Wendel-Vos, W.; Giskes, K.; Van Lenthe, F.; Brug, J. A Systematic Review of Environmental Correlates of Obesity-related Dietary Behaviors in Youth. *Health Educ. Res.* **2007**, *22*, 203–226. [CrossRef] [PubMed]
36. Bruening, M.; Eisenberg, M.; MacLehose, R.; Nanney, M.S.; Story, M.; Neumark-Sztainer, D. Relationship between Adolescents' and Their Friends' Eating Behaviors: Breakfast, Fruit, Vegetable, Whole-Grain, and Dairy Intake. *J. Acad. Nutr. Diet.* **2012**, *112*, 1608–1613. [CrossRef]
37. De la Haye, K.; Robins, G.; Mohr, P.; Wilson, C. Adolescents' Intake of Junk Food: Processes and Mechanisms Driving Consumption Similarities Among Friends. *J. Res. Adolesc.* **2013**, *23*, 524–536. [CrossRef]
38. Caraher, M.; Landon, J.; Dalmeny, K. Television Advertising and Children: Lessons from Policy Development. *Public Health Nutr.* **2006**, *9*, 596–605. [CrossRef]
39. Radesky, J.; Chassiakos, Y.R.; Ameenuddin, N.; Navsaria, D.; Ameenuddin, N.; Boyd, R.; Selkie, E.; Radesky, J.; Patrick, M.; Friedman, J.; et al. Digital Advertising to Children. *Pediatrics* **2020**, *146*, e20201681. [CrossRef]
40. Kubik, M.Y.; Lytle, L.A.; Hannan, P.J.; Perry, C.L.; Story, M. The Association of the School Food Environment with Dietary Behaviors of Young Adolescents. *Am. J. Public Health* **2003**, *93*, 1168–1173. [CrossRef]
41. Qutteina, Y.; Hallez, L.; Mennes, N.; De Backer, C.; Smits, T. What Do Adolescents See on Social Media? A Diary Study of Food Marketing Images on Social Media. *Front. Psychol.* **2019**, *10*, 2637. [CrossRef]
42. Dittmar, H. *Consumer Culture, Identity and Well-Being: The Search for the "Good Life" and the "Body Perfect"*; Psychology Press: Hove, UK, 2008; ISBN 9781135420161.
43. Fleming-Milici, F.; Harris, J.L. Adolescents' Engagement With Unhealthy Food and Beverage Brands on Social Media. *Appetite* **2020**, *146*, 104501. [CrossRef]
44. Reagan, R.; Filice, S.; Santarossa, S.; Woodruff, S.J. #ad on Instagram: Investigating the Promotion of Food and Beverage Products. *J. Soc. Media Soc.* **2020**, *9*, 1–28.
45. Coates, A.E.; Hardman, C.A.; Halford Grovenor Jason, C.; Christiansen, P.; Boyland, E.J. "It's Just Addictive People That Make Addictive Videos": Children's Understanding of and Attitudes Towards Influencer Marketing of Food and Beverages by YouTube Video Bloggers. *Int. J. Environ. Res. Public Health* **2020**, *17*, 449. [CrossRef] [PubMed]
46. Kostygina, G.; Tran, H.; Binns, S.; Szczypka, G.; Emery, S.; Vallone, D.; Hair, E. Boosting Health Campaign Reach and Engagement Through Use of Social Media Influencers and Memes. *Soc. Media Soc.* **2020**, *6*, 2056305120912475. [CrossRef]
47. Spanos, S.; Vartanian, L.R.; Herman, C.P.; Polivy, J. Personality, Perceived Appropriateness, and Acknowledgement of Social Influences on Food Intake. *Pers. Individ. Dif.* **2015**, *87*, 110–115. [CrossRef]
48. Cheung, M.L.; Pires, G.D.; Rosenberger, P.J.; Leung, W.K.S.; Salehhuddin Sharipudin, M.N. The Role of Consumer-consumer Interaction and Consumer-brand Interaction in Driving Consumer-brand Engagement and Behavioral Intentions. *J. Retail. Consum. Serv.* **2021**, *61*, 102574. [CrossRef]
49. Tajvidi, M.; Wang, Y.; Hajli, N.; Love, P.E.D. Brand value Co-creation in social commerce: The role of interactivity, social support, and relationship quality. *Comput. Hum. Behav.* **2021**, *115*, 105238. [CrossRef]
50. Folkvord, F.; de Bruijne, M. The Effect of the Promotion of Vegetables by a Social Influencer on Adolescents' Subsequent Vegetable Intake: A Pilot Study. *Int. J. Environ. Res. Public Health* **2020**, *17*, 2243. [CrossRef]
51. Folkvord, F.; Roes, E.; Bevelander, K. Promoting Healthy Foods in the New Digital Era on Instagram: An Experimental Study on the Effect of a Popular Real Versus Fictitious Fit Influencer on Brand Attitude and Purchase Intentions. *BMC Public Health* **2020**, *20*, 1677. [CrossRef]
52. Harrigan, M.; Feddema, K.; Wang, S.; Harrigan, P.; Diot, E. How Trust Leads to Online Purchase Intention Founded in Perceived Usefulness and Peer Communication. *J. Consum. Behav.* **2021**, *20*, 1297–1312. [CrossRef]
53. Schilke, O.; Huang, L. Worthy of Swift Trust? How Brief Interpersonal Contact Affects Trust Accuracy. *J. Appl. Psychol.* **2018**, *103*, 1181–1197. [CrossRef]
54. Oostindjer, M.; Aschemann-Witzel, J.; Wang, Q.; Skuland, S.E.; Egelandsdal, B.; Amdam, G.V.; Schjøll, A.; Pachucki, M.C.; Rozin, P.; Stein, J.; et al. Are School Meals a Viable and Sustainable Tool to Improve the Healthiness and Sustainability of Children's Diet and Food Consumption? A Cross-national Comparative Perspective. *Crit. Rev. Food Sci. Nutr.* **2017**, *57*, 3942–3958. [CrossRef] [PubMed]
55. Centola, D. *How Behaviour Spreads: The Science of Complex Contagions*; Princeton University Press: Princeton, NJ, USA; Oxford, UK, 2018.

56. Prentice, D.; Paluck, E.L. Engineering Social Change Using Social Norms: Lessons from the Study of Collective Action. *Curr. Opin. Psychol.* **2020**, *35*, 138–142. [CrossRef] [PubMed]
57. Earls, M. *Herd. How to Change Mass Behaviour By Harnessing Our True Nature*, 2nd ed.; Wiley & Sons: Chichester, UK, 2009.
58. Tankard, M.E.; Paluck, E.L. Norm Perception as a Vehicle for Social Change. *Soc. Issues Policy Rev.* **2016**, *10*, 181–211. [CrossRef]
59. Kuran, T. *Private Truths, Public Lies: The Social Consequences of Preference Falsification*; Harvard University Press: Cambridge, MA, USA, 1997.
60. Nickerson, D.W. Is voting contagious? Evidence from two field experiments. *Am. Polit. Sci. Rev.* **2008**, *102*, 49–57. [CrossRef]
61. Partheymüller, J.; Schmitt-Beck, R. A "Social Logic" of Demobilization: The Influence of Political Discussants on Electoral Participation at the 2009 German Federal Election. *J. Elect. Public Opin. Parties* **2012**, *22*, 457–478. [CrossRef]
62. Schlozman, K.L.; Verba, S.; Brady, H.E. *The Unheavenly Chorus: Unequal Political Voice and the Broken Promise of American Democracy*; Princeton University Press: Princeton, NJ, USA, 2012.
63. Zorell, C.V.; Denk, T. Political Consumerism and Interpersonal Discussion Patterns. *Scan. Polit. Stud.* **2021**, *44*, 392–415. [CrossRef]
64. Micheletti, M.; Stolle, D. Vegetarianism—A Lifestyle Politics? In *Creative Participation: Responsibility-Taking in the Political World*; Micheletti, M., Mcfarland, A.S., Eds.; Paradigm: Boulder, CO, USA, 2010; pp. 125–145.
65. Micheletti, M.; Stolle, D. Sustainable Citizenship and the New Politics of Consumption. *Ann. Am. Acad. Pol. Soc. Sci.* **2012**, *644*, 88–120. [CrossRef]
66. Onwezen, M.C.; Reinders, M.J.; Verain, M.C.D.; Snoek, H.M. The development of a single-item Food Choice Questionnaire. *Food Qual. Prefer.* **2019**, *71*, 34–45. [CrossRef]
67. Lindeman, M.; Väänänen, M. Measurement of Ethical Food Choice Motives. *Appetite* **2000**, *34*, 55–59. [CrossRef]
68. Verain, M.C.D.; Onwezen, M.C.; Sijtsema, S.J.; Dagevos, H. The Added Value of Sustainability Motivations in Understanding Sustainable Food Choices. *Appl. Stud. Agribus. Commer.* **2017**, *10*, 67–76. [CrossRef]
69. Åmnå, E.; Ekström, M.; Kerr, M.; Stattin, H. *Codebook: The Political Socialization Program*; Örebro universitet: Örebro, Sweden, 2010.
70. Zorell, C.V. *Varieties of Political Consumerism. From Boycotting to Buycotting*; Palgrave Macmillan: Basingstoke, UK, 2019.
71. Spanos, S.; Vartanian, L.R.; Herman, C.P.; Polivy, J. Failure to Report Social Influences on Food Intake: Lack of Awareness or Motivated Denial? *Health Psychol.* **2014**, *33*, 1487–1494. [CrossRef] [PubMed]

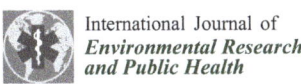

Article

The Impact of Interpretive Packaged Food Labels on Consumer Purchase Intention: The Comparative Analysis of Efficacy and Inefficiency of Food Labels

Muhammad Zeeshan Zafar [1], Xiangjiao Shi [2,3], Hailan Yang [2], Jaffar Abbas [4] and Jiakui Chen [5,*]

1. Department of Business Administration, University of Chakwal, Chakwal 48800, Pakistan
2. Business School, Shandong Jianzhu University, Jinan 250101, China
3. Institute of Business Administration, Shandong University of Finance and Economics, Jinan 250014, China
4. School of Media and Communication & Antai College of Economics and Management, Shanghai Jiao Tong University, Shanghai 200240, China
5. School of Economics and Management (Cooperative College), Qingdao Agricultural University, Qingdao 266109, China
* Correspondence: chenjiakui@126.com

Abstract: The objectives of this study are twofold. Firstly, the current study elucidates the impact and efficacy of food labels in developing consumers' attitudes and intentions towards the selection of nutritional food. Secondly, the inefficacy of labels in developing consumers' attitudes and intentions towards healthy packaged food selection is demonstrated. The supportive theories of the current model are those of reasoned action and protection motivation. The data of 797 respondents have been collected from four major grocery stores in Pakistan. The structural equation model has been employed for the analysis of data. The results indicate that the efficacy of food labels has a positive significant effect on attitudes towards familiar and unfamiliar foods. In contrast to this, inefficacy in labelling has shown a positive significant effect on familiar foods but is insignificant for unfamiliar foods. The user-friendly food labels significantly affect unfamiliar foods in terms promoting consumer attitudes. Reciprocally, the inefficacy of labels creates a hindrance to the reading of unfamiliar labels while purchasing food items. The study findings reveal the fact that food label information and its format influences consumer attitudes and intentions at the point of purchase.

Keywords: food label; consumer purchase intention; attitude

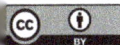

1. Introduction

Numerous studies have explored public health issues and the reported results have revealed that they often relate to consumers' irrational behaviors toward the selection of unhealthy food items [1]. The cause of unhealthy food intake is the profound change in individual eating behaviors over the last five decades [2]. Globally, it has been observed that individuals' food intake habits have been transformed from home-cooked foods to ready-to-eat, packaged food items [3]. The increasing tendency towards packaged food has affected the medical expenses of individuals on a national scale. A worldwide survey has identified the fact that a poor diet is the major cause of increasing medical expenses, not only for individuals but for the national economy [4]. Therefore, researchers have emphasized the need to investigate the effects of food on the lives and well-being of consumers [5,6]. Additionally, scholars have suggested introducing effective and scalable interventions for consumer awareness to encourage the selection of healthy food items [3].

To achieve food system sustainability regarding healthy food consumption, both food and nutrient literacy play pivotal roles [7]. Education regarding nutrients motivates individuals to make healthy food choices [8]. There is no formal education system to create awareness among individuals regarding healthy packaged food besides food label information. Intuitively, food label information is the most effective tool to guide consumers in the food selection process [9]. The objective of food label information is to provide information about product ingredients and in turn allow the consumer to select healthier food items at the point of purchase [10]. Additionally, the nutritional label is a tool that informs the public about healthy foods, protects the consumer from unsafe foods, and discourages food manufacturers from producing unhealthy and defective food items [11]. There is a need to motivate consumers to consult label information at the point of purchase [5,12]. If they are not motivated to consult label information, as previously mentioned studies have found, the impact of food label information is void because the decisions are made without the customer engaging with the available information [13]. Although food label information is the most widely proposed tool for educating consumers at the point of purchase [14], the reported results regarding the usefulness of food labels at the point of purchase are contradictory.

The reading and understanding of food label information requires special proficiency. Therefore, studies have suggested the design of food labels which reduce label complexity, provide simple and meaningful numeric information and simple text, reduce the use of percentages, and use easy-to-understand label presentation [15,16]. The friendly label allows the consumer to read it before putting a food item into their shopping cart. Similarly, the research also highlights factors that cause consumers to avoid the food label information at the point of purchase, e.g., a lack of understanding, lack of usefulness, lack of trustworthiness, and technical label information [17]. These factors lead to the inefficacy of food labels at the point of selection. However, several authors have reported the effectiveness of food labels for raising the awareness of consumers [18]. Owing to convenience, packaged food products attract consumer attention and have gained a substantial market share. It is very difficult to motivate consumers to stop consuming processed foods, and creating awareness in order to reduce the quantity is one of the only options available [19]. A substantial amount of scientific literature has indicated that the consumer selects food items on the basis of taste [20,21]. Reciprocally, a common notion prevails among consumers that healthier food is less palatable [22,23]. Hence, informative and unique food labels are required to attract consumers' attention when choosing the appropriate food items. Moreover, familiar and unfamiliar food labels influence the behavior of consumers differently [23,24], because familiar food labels can easily attract consumers' attention, whereas unfamiliar food labels require further effort to have an impact on consumers' minds, as well as building their trust [25].

The prior studies' inconsistent results have motivated the current researchers to investigate the impact of food label efficacy and inefficacy in developing individuals' attitudes towards familiar and unfamiliar food labels. Reciprocally, the objectives of the present study are twofold. The first is to study the efficacy of the food label information on the attitudes of consumers when consulting familiar and unfamiliar food labels to make nutritional food choices. The second is examining the impact of the inefficacy of the food label information on the consumers' intentions when consulting familiar and unfamiliar food labels for healthy food selection.

2. Literature Review and Hypothesis Development

There are multiple causes of early death, and a poor diet is one of them [26]. Although food-processing companies print detailed information regarding food ingredients and nutrients, food companies are, nevertheless, the drivers of obesity and non-communicable diseases [27]. In contrast to this, food labels allow consumers to make appropriate decisions by providing the necessary information regarding healthy and hygienic food products, and they are an essential tool to provide consumers with knowledge about food ingredients [28,29]. The primary source of communication between consumers and organizations is food labeling, which often influences consumers' purchase decisions [30,31]. Moreover, food label guides consumers in making right choices [32]. The aforementioned studies have revealed that well-written and detailed information at label is necessary for consumer products [33]. The information written at labels makes an individual able to evaluate the characteristics of food products, interpret correct information and later choose products according to their lifestyle, preference, and health condition [34]. It noticed in the past few years that consumers become more conscious regarding their health and selection of food items. Therefore, consumer's demand for more transparent food label information increased about nutrients, health benefits, and ingredients [35,36].

Furthermore, to promote their products food processing companies utilize the food labels as promotional tool. [15,37]. In this modern era of consumerism, consumers are becoming more alert and conscious about the nutritional value of the food items [28,38]. Consumers' decision regarding food selection has mainly influenced by some factors like; the quality, packaging, and labeling of the food products [39,40]. Nevertheless, past studies have observed contradictory results regarding the decisiveness of label. There are numerous scholars in the past, who have examined the influence of label fonts, colors, information and formats on consumer perception [41]. Reciprocally, the marketing activities of food processing companies shape consumer's opinion. Moreover, studies have accounted that individuals are least interested towards label information. The cause of consumer's least interest towards food label information is lack of understanding, lack of confidence, proficiency about written nutrients, and lifestyle [42,43]. Therefore, it is necessary to examine the factors that motivate and demotivate consumers to consult food label information at the point of purchase [30].

2.1. Efficacy of Food Label Effect on Familiar and Unfamiliar Label and Selection Intention

Efficacy of food label schemes is an important tool. It evaluates the nutritional content at the point of purchase [44–46]. Besides, the frequent purchase of packaged food items make consumer familiar with label information. Additionally, the food label information needs numeric proficiency. In continuation with, familiarity and efficacy of food label is helpful for healthy food choice [47]. Reciprocally, to understand the information at food label with familiar food label assistant individual in making healthy packaged food intention [48]. The aforementioned studies have unfolded that, when individual intend to purchase unusual packaged food item, the efficacy of food label information play vital role [49]. The easy to read food label information makes individual confident while purchasing new packaged food item. The food label is a promotional tool. The presentation of food label information regarding nutrients, manufacturing and expiry dates and companies basic information develop trust among consumers [50].

Furthermore, food label information is the fundamental means to communicate information to customers about characteristics of food. Hence, the useful attributes of food label information has investigated multiple times [51]. Studies have suggested to examine the effects of familiarity and unfamiliarity of food labeling on various food products [52]. The aforementioned studies have unfolded the fact that the primary concern of researchers regarding food labeling is nutrition composition and the way nutritional information has displayed at food labels [53]. The European Food Information Council has indicated that consumers in the United Kingdom (UK) are habitual to seek for labels' information before purchasing the food items for both the familiar or unfamiliar food labels. However, in comparison to the UK, the results are inconsistent in the rest of the world regarding the consultation of food labels for healthy food selection [51]. Besides, some formats of food label could not convince individuals in changing their packaged food choices. The cause of avoiding food label is lack of numeracy about food label contents [54]. Nevertheless, food processing companies and retailers have put collective efforts in devising attractive and easy to read labels for the convenience of consumers. Therefore, the current study has examined the efficacy of food labels in influencing consumers' purchase decisions. Hence, the current study proposed the hypothesis.

H1. *Efficacy of food label positively affects consumer's intention and attitude for familiar label mediates in making this relationship significant.*

H2. *Efficacy of food label positively affects consumer's intention and attitude for unfamiliar label mediates in making this relationship significant.*

2.2. Label Inefficacy Effects on Familiar and Unfamiliar Label Reading Attitude and Selection Intention

It is an unequivocal fact that food label is useful for educating consumer for the healthier product selection. On the other hand the display of nutritional information with scientific terminologies create hindrance for individual to consult the label at point of purchase for healthy food selection [55]. The effect of inefficacy of food label on unfamiliar food label is significant. Hence, consumers tend to believe in the label while purchasing products [56]. More specifically, the decisiveness of food label information becomes more prominent for unfamiliar food label products. Most often individual is intend to add some newly introduced packaged food items in their shopping list, therefore, individual keenly observe the food label which is unfamiliar to them. Therefore, sometimes unfamiliarity is not the cause of individual demotivation [57]. Hence, the nutritional table is quite confusing that cause the avoidance to read unfamiliar food label [58]. The most common reasons to avoid food label information are reading difficulties, complicated comprehension, lack of time, and lack of information search behavior [59]. Reciprocally, studies have witnessed the effect of inefficacy of food label at familiar food label reading is weak as compare to unfamiliar food label [60]. The packaged food items, which are in regular use of consumer, are familiar with the information given at food label. On the other hand, some of the studies have reported that familiar and unfamiliar food labels have some common information and individual read that text and can select the required packaged food item [61]. In contrary to that past literature have revealed that the impact of food label efficacy and inefficacy are vital in using familiar and unfamiliar label reading while choosing right amount of packaged items. Furthermore, studies have also reported that consumer's exposure towards food labels also depends upon their household size, purchase pattern of household members, and household composition. The verity of products have consumed by different household members and how many multiple food choices exist in one family member can also be the cause of food label familiarity and unfamiliarity [62]. Hence, the current study has hypothesized that:

H3. *Inefficacy of food label positively affects consumer's intention and attitude for familiar label mediates in making this relationship significant.*

H4. *Inefficacy of food label positively affects consumer's intention and attitude for unfamiliar label mediates in making this relationship significant.*

The intention of an individual towards any objective is the consequences of an attitude [63]. Reciprocally, the attitude is use to explain the change behavior of an individual [64]. Past literature has revealed that in making a strong intention of an individual attitude play vital role [65]. Therefore, consumer moods most often varies while selecting food related products. Hence, there is a dire need to examine that which factors affect individual's attitude to consult label information while making a decision regarding food items. Moreover, studies have revealed that label information is basic source of guidance for consumers at purchase point [66]. Besides, the reading attitude of food labels has associated with the highest quality of diets [67,68]. Numerous scholars have reported that most of the time individual's reported figures regarding reading of label information contradicts from actual behavior [69,70]. There is substantial percentage of packaged food items exists in shopping list of consumers. Therefore, due to routine purchase of the packaged food products consumer become familiar with the label information. Hence, to encourage consumer to read familiar food label is an easy task. In contrary to that, to motivate consumer attitude to consult unfamiliar food label is necessary to make healthy and right amount of food selection intention [71]. The nutritional information, which has mentioned at food label, has most often found confusing. Nevertheless, food label has considered a standard for promoting healthy food items among individuals [59]. To empirically test the above assertions, the current study has put forward the following hypotheses.

H5. *Attitude towards familiar food label significantly effect on nutritional food selection intention.*

H6. *Attitude towards unfamiliar food label significantly effect on nutritional food selection intention.*

2.3. Theoretical Framework

The proposed model has underpinned with reasoned action theory (TRA) and theory of Protection motivation (PMT). Moreover, to investigate the volitional behavior, the reasoned action theory has most often employed. More specifically past scholars have rendered the services of reasoned action to examine the volitional behavior of food consumption, sustainable and ethical consumption, and organic food selection [72]. Reciprocally, the theory of reasoned action predicts consumer probability, purchase intention and a sensible effort for buying any product [73]. Theory of reasoned action assists scholars in examining whether external factors directly effect on individual's behavioral intention or not [74]. Furthermore, according to theory of reasoned action, intention is the strong predictor of actual behavior and intention of an individual depends on strong attitude. Additionally, TRA investigates that how individual behave with pre-existing attitude [75]. Although TRA investigates individual intention towards any object but the purpose of present study was to examine the motivational features, which build strong intention about selection of nutritional food items.

Therefore, the current study has rendered the services of Protection Motivation Theory [76]. Protection motivation theory seeks the clarity in cognitive process of an individual while taking any decision. According to the definition of PMT "*Protection Motivation Theory (PMT) emphasis on the cognitive processes mediating attitudinal and behavioral change*" [76]. Besides, PMT posits two processes; one is the arousal of threat and second is the coping of threat. These two characteristics of PMT support current authors to achieve the objective of study. The available information at food label states a threatening situation for an individual if it is not useful for making healthy food selection. Similarly, it also states a coping situation for individual if it is easily understandable and makes consumer intention for healthy package food product. Therefore, the effect of efficacy and inefficacy of food label in making individual attitude to consult familiar and unfamiliar food label at point of purchase is very decisive for healthy packaged food selection intention. Moreover, according to the definition of the protection motivation theory the behavior discusses to motivate or demotivate individual with the belief that the use of preventive measure for any behavior reduces the risk factors. Likewise, the efficacy and inefficacy of food label motivate and de-motivate individuals to read familiar and unfamiliar food label. The researchers of the present study have examined that food label develop individual's attitude to read food label and strong attitude effect on individual's intention. Additionally, the food label reading attitude move forward in making intention of an individual to consult label information at the time of food item selection. Figure 1 is the graphical representation of proposed model.

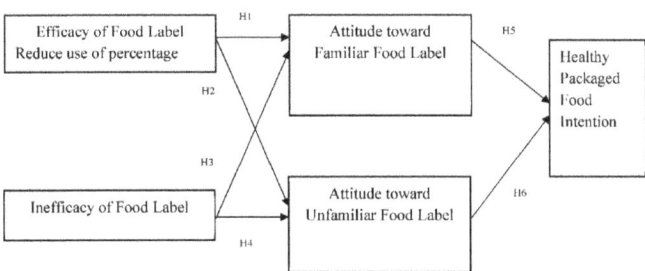

Figure 1. Food labeling and consumer intention for healthy package food.

3. Methods

The objective of the study is to find the effect of efficacy and inefficacy of food label information in making consumer attitude with familiar and unfamiliar food label. To achieve the objective of the study respondents' point of purchase opinion is decisive. Besides, authors of the study have intended to explore impact of food labels efficacy on unfamiliar food label information. Reciprocally, studies have reported that consumer's responses at the time of shopping most often validate their actual behavior [77]. Therefore, for data collection authors of the study selected four retail outlets. The authors of the study have devised selection criteria for the selection of four retail stores such as the daily footfall of customers, verity of packaged food displayed at their shelves, the population of city where theses outlets have situated, the diversity of customers with respect to gender and age and the income level of customers.

The convenience sampling technique has used to collect data from grocery stores. The convenience sampling technique has supported authors for finding relevant respondents who can willingly participate in research survey. Because the results reported in past literature has evidence that most often customers get offended if someone interferes during shopping [78]. Therefore, the convenience sampling technique has used which demonstrate that respondents have shown their consent to participate. Furthermore, authors of the study have tested their objective with empirical data therefore the data collected using a structured questionnaire. It was adapted questionnaire. The detail of instruments has reported in Table 1.

The distribution of questionnaire among respondents is very technical. Therefore, authors of the study have contacted store managers. The detail of study and objective has discussed with managers. As per the guidance of managers, a written request forwarded for final approval. Besides, due to the customer safety policy, store managers have placed the questionnaire at payment counter and instructed to the employee that take customer consent for the participation in survey and then handover the questionnaire to customer with request to return in next possible visit. The period for data collection was from September 2021 to December 2021. Furthermore, the questionnaire has comprised of questions about each variable and a brief description about objective of survey. Name of the participants was optional.

Sample of the study is very significant for generalizing the outcome of study. The current study has set the sample size using Uma Sekaran Table method and the sample size was 385. Besides, various scholars have suggested different sample sizes like; according to [79] recommended that in marketing studies sample size of 200–500 are valid. In continuation with some of the scholars have suggested that 50 is poor, 300 is good, 500 is very good and 1000 is an excellent sample size [80]. To achieve the minimum sample standard distributed questionnaires were 1000.

Table 1. Measurement Items.

Variables	Authors	Items
Inefficacy	[81]	Most food products' labels are not clear, so I cannot purchase them
		Most food products need specific proficiency therefore, I avoid these food products
		It is difficult to identify food products that have complex labels.
		I do not trust on the crowded food product labels.
		To read label information I need technical proficiency.
Efficacy	[81]	Easy to read label information is necessary for the right choice of nutritional food.
		It is compulsory to provide information which explain ethical dimension of packaged food
		Packaged food label must be environmental friendly.

Table 1. Cont.

Variables	Authors	Items
Intention	[81]	Food processing companies should adhere national rules and regulations for food packaging and ingredients.
		I have intend to purchase a processed food product
		I have plan to purchase processed food products
		I am willing to purchase processed food products
Attitude towards Familiar food label	[82]	The detail given at familiar food label guides individual at the time of shopping and for me it is significant.
		The available information on familiar labels is appropriate for the selection of healthy processed food and for me it is important.
		A familiar label is an appropriate source for healthy processed food selection and for me it is important.
		Familiar food label is easy to understand and supportive of healthy package food selection.
Attitude towards unfamiliar food label	[82]	The unfamiliar label is not useful for nutritional food selection.
		The available information at unfamiliar labels is difficult to understand
		At unfamiliar food label individual find difficulty to search relevant information for the selection of healthy package food.
		Unfamiliar food label is difficult to understand and support for healthy package food selection.

Structural equation modeling (SEM) has become a popular analysis tool to test structural relationships instead of first-generation analysis. SEM is second generation multivariate analysis tool having several advantages in terms of convenience, efficiency, and accuracy [83,84]. The study used PLS-SEM because it has several advantages over CB-SEM for advanced research analysis [85]. PLS-SEM often preferred because it overcomes the issue of normality and outliers. PLS-SEM considered a silver bullet and holy grails due to its ability to deal with complicated relationships simultaneously [86]. Moreover, PLS-SEM heavily contributes towards exploratory studies and predicts better accuracy [87].

According to [86,88], PLS-SEM analysis the data with two stages approach, i.e., measurement model evaluation and structural model evaluation. Assessment of measurement model involves evaluation of constructs while the structure model involves evaluation of relationship analysis.

Assessment of measurement model has checked through construct reliability and validity, which involve outer loading, composite reliability, average variance extracted, and discriminant validity [89]. The superiority of the model has evaluated through the recommended value of the above mention tests. For the confirmation of convergent validity, the items loading must be greater than 0.5 [90], AVE must be higher than the recommended value of 0.5 and composite reliability greater than 0.7 [91].

There are two criteria to check discriminant validity, i.e., Heterotrait-Monotrait (HTMT) ratio and Fornell–Larcker criterion. The study used Fornell–Larcker criterion to assess discriminant validity [92]. The squared root value of AVE's (diagonal value) should be higher than the correlation between the latent construct (off-diagonal values).

The structural model evaluates the relationships of latent variables and observed variables. This evaluation has tested through series of assessments such as path coefficients (β), t-values, significance value (p-value), coefficient of determination (R^2), effect size (F^2), and predictive relevance (Q^2). The bootstrapping method (5000 resample) was used for hypotheses testing

4. Results and Discussion

Authors of the study have received 831 out of 1000 distributed questionnaires. In primary screening, usable questionnaires were 797 because some participants have filled 50% questionnaires, which excluded from the final analysis. So, 797 sample sizes considered for the studies. The detail presented in Table 2 with the title respondent profile. The data has collected at the time when individuals are shopping, because it gives better idea and opinion about the food selection intention. Additionally, researchers have obtained formal permissions to store before data collection procedure. Each store manager allocated one person as an assistant for data collection. Proper guidance provided to participants as per their demand.

Table 2. Respondent profile.

	Characteristics	Frequency	Percentage
Gender	Male	503	63.11
	Female	294	36.89
Age	18–21	241	30.24
	22–25	289	36.26
	26–29	180	22.58
	30-over	87	10.92
Education Level	Undergraduate	356	44.67
	Graduate	305	38.27
	Postgraduate	136	17.06
Shopping Method	Shopping Single	355	44.54
	Shopping with Family with kids	263	32.99
	Shopping with Family without kids	179	22.47

Moreover, the data collected at the point of purchase with the permission of shoppers therefore, the response rate was quite high. Additionally, majority of the respondents lies within the age group of 22 to 30. It indicates that young customer were more interested to participate in food related survey because the popularity of package food products is high as compare to mature population. Besides, the total population of Pakistan is 250 million. In total population the highest representation, which is 64%, belong to age group 22 to 35 [84]. Therefore, the study results can generalize.

5. Evaluation of Measurement Model

For the assessment of model authors have used various validity and reliability test. Table 3 and Figure 2 show that all values of outer loading are more significant than the recommended value of 0.5, while values for composite reliability also meet the threshold value of 0.7 ranging from 0.826 (efficacy of food label) to 0.852 (attitude toward unfamiliar food). Similarly, the AVE values are also well above the cut-off value of 0.5, ranging from 0.545 (efficacy of food label) to 0.655 (Healthy packaged food intention).

Table 3. Measurement model evaluation.

Constructs	Item	Loading	CR	AVE
Efficacy of food label	EFF1	0.647	0.826	0.545
	EFF2	0.832		
	EFF3	0.728		
	EFF4	0.733		
Inefficacy of food label	INEFF1	0.741	0.848	0.584
	INEFF2	0.828		
	INEFF3	0.715		
	INEFF4	0.768		

Table 3. *Cont.*

Constructs	Item	Loading	CR	AVE
Attitude toward Familiar food	ATFF1	0.810	0.850	0.586
	ATFF2	0.794		
	ATFF3	0.778		
	ATFF4	0.674		
Attitude toward Unfamiliar food	ATUF1	0.605	0.853	0.595
	ATUF2	0.818		
	ATUF3	0.847		
	ATUF4	0.792		
Healthy Packaged food Intention	PI1	0.850	0.850	0.655
	PI2	0.773		
	PI3	0.804		

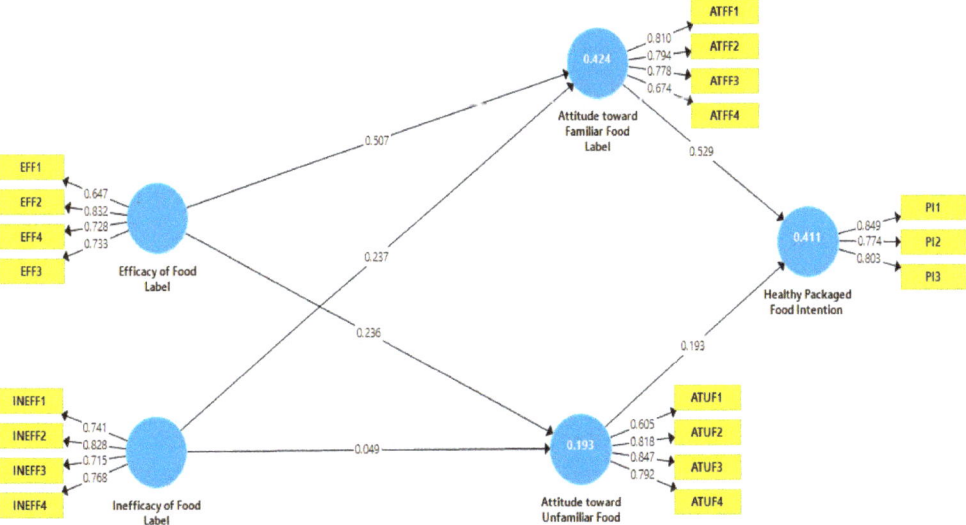

Figure 2. Outer loadings.

Table 4 shows that all diagonal values are higher than off-diagonal values, which means discriminant validly is confirmed.

Table 4. Discriminant validity (Fornell–Larcker criterion).

	ATTF	ATTUF	EFF	PI	INEFF
ATTF	0.766				
ATTUF	0.458	0.771			
EFF	0.616	0.364	0.738		
PI	0.618	0.435	0.685	0.809	
INEFF	0.470	0.387	0.459	0.406	0.764

6. Structural Model Evaluation

The results indicated that efficacy of food labels ($\beta = 0.507$, $t = 14.269 > 1.64$, $p < 0.05$) and inefficacy of food labels ($\beta = 0.237$, $t = 6.554 > 1.64$, $p < 0.05$) positively and significantly affect the attitude of the consumer towards familiar food labels. Efficacy of food labels ($\beta = 0.236$, $t = 5.040 > 1.64$, $p < 0.05$) found to have significant effect on attitude of the consumer towards unfamiliar food labels while inefficacy of food label ($\beta = 0.049$, t = 1.296 < 1.64, $p > 0.05$) found to have insignificant effect on attitude of the consumer towards unfamiliar food labels. Moreover, consumers' attitude of familiar food (β = 0.529, t = 16.015 > 1.64, $p < 0.05$) and unfamiliar food (β = 0.193, t = 5.218 > 1.64, $p < 0.05$) also positively and significantly affect consumer intentions regarding healthy food packages. The R^2 value of the model is 0.411, which means the model explains 41% variation in the intention of the consumer regarding healthy food packages. [93] suggested that any value for R^2 greater than 0.35 is substantial for any model. So our model is considered as substantial (0.414) as recommended by [93]. Moreover, [93] indicated that value of f^2 with 0.02 is poor, with 0.15 is medium, and with 0.35 is strong. The detail has presented in Table 5 and Figure 3. It is argued that if $Q^2 > 0$, the model has predictive relevance [94]. Therefore, the value of Q^2 is higher than the rule of thumb which is Q^2 = 0.266 and it indicates that the predicted value is high.

Table 5. Hypothesis testing (structure model results).

	Path Coefficients	SD	t-Value	p-Value	Supported	R^2	Q^2	F^2
EFF → ATFF	0.507	0.035	14.269	0.000	Yes	0.414	0.266	0.380
INEFF → ATFF	0.237	0.037	6.554	0.000	Yes			0.076
EFF → ATUF	0.236	0.048	5.040	0.000	Yes			0.082
INEFF → ATUF	0.049	0.047	1.296	0.183	No			0.003
ATFF → PI	0.529	0.037	16.015	0.000	Yes			0.383
ATUF → PI	0.193	0.038	5.218	0.000	Yes			0.049

EFF (Efficacy of food-label), INEFF (In-Efficacy of Food-Label), ATFF (Attitude towards Familiar Food-Label), ATUF (Attitude towards Unfamiliar Food-Label) and PI (Purchase Intention).

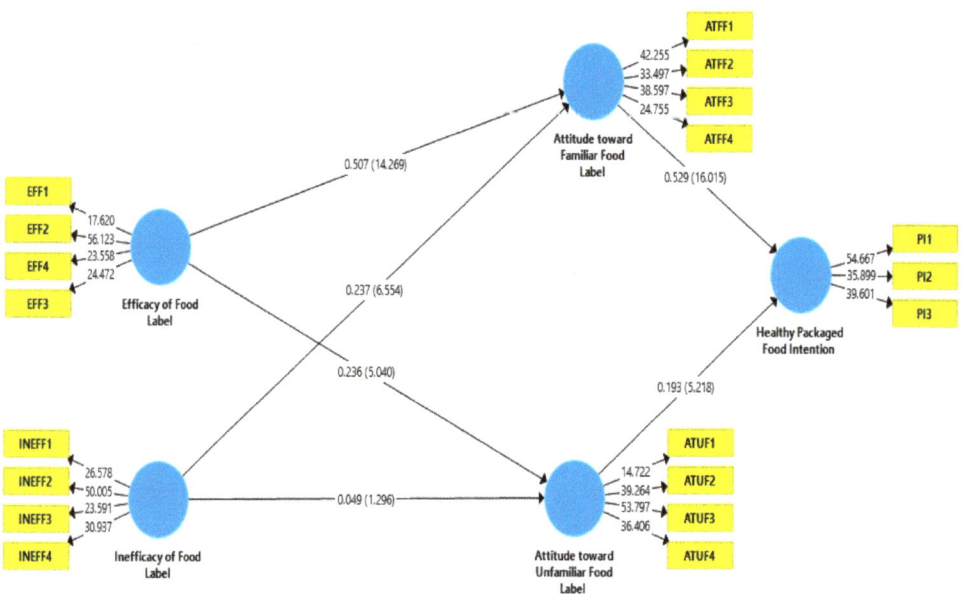

Figure 3. Hypothesis testing (Bootstrapping results).

Mediation of Attitude of Familiar and Unfamiliar Food

The study checked the mediation of attitude of the consumer regarding familiar and unfamiliar food between efficacy and inefficacy of food labels and consumer intention for health packaged goods. The results suggested that consumers attitude regarding familiar food mediates (β = 0.276, t = 9.086 > 1.64, $p < 0.05$) the relationship of efficacy of food labels and consumer intention for healthy foods. Finding also confirmed the mediation

($\beta = 0.124$, t = 6.2.2 > 1.64, $p < 0.05$) of consumer attitude of familiar food between inefficacy of food labels and consumer intention regarding healthy food packages. As hypothesize, consumer attitude regarding unfamiliar food mediates ($\beta = 0.056$, t = 3.338 > 1.64, $p < 0.05$) the relationship of efficacy of food labels and consumer intention of healthy packaged goods. Moreover, the results indicate no mediation of consumer attitude of unfamiliar food ($\beta = 0.014$, t = 1.288 < 1.64, $p > 0.05$) between inefficacy of food labels and consumer intention for healthy foods (see Table 6).

Table 6. Mediation results.

	Path Coefficients	SD	t-Value	p-Value	Supported
EFF → ATFF → PI	0.276	0.030	9.086	0.000	yes
INEFF → ATFF → PI	0.124	0.020	6.202	0.000	yes
EFF → ATUF → PI	0.056	0.017	3.338	0.000	yes
INEFF → ATUF → PI	0.014	0.011	1.288	0.198	No

7. Discussion

The purpose of the present study is to investigate the impact of food label efficacy and inefficacy to make consumer attitude towards both familiar and unfamiliar food labels. Empirical results indicate that efficacy of food label information make consumer attitude even for unfamiliar food labels. On contrary, the inefficacy of food label information has insignificant effect on unfamiliar food label. Moreover, the statistics of present study have unfolded the fact that food label efficacy has pivotal for making an attitude of consumer to consult label information at point of purchase. The efficacy also grabs consumer attention for the products, which they select first time for their shopping. The proposed model comprises of five variables. The researchers have examined how food label efficacy and inefficacy influence in making consumer attitude with familiar and unfamiliar food labels that ultimately leads to strong intention in choosing healthy packaged food. However, to guide consumers about nutrients, food label efficacy and inefficacy is significant for informed decision. The conscious consumer demands food safety. Therefore, food label information has used for informed decision at point of purchase. The most common observation of researchers is the existence of diversity in the food label. The food label is a navigator for consumers for guiding them to the right selection of food but in reality, it is becoming the cause of confusion. Multiple factors affect consumer's well-being, healthy food is one of them. The increasing trend of packaged food has transformed disease patterns from acute diseases to chronic diseases. To make healthy food selection decisions it is necessary to educate consumers. Furthermore, in the absence of formal criteria regarding the awareness of consumer food label information is an appropriate method. The information is printed at food labels enhance consumers' awareness about food nutrients like fats, saturated fats, sodium, salt, and fiber. All nutrients are necessary for consumer's well-being but their balance intake is more essential for a healthy life.

The results indicate that consumers prefer label efficacy in both familiar and unfamiliar food label. The results of present study have linked with previous studies, which suggest that consumers most often judge food products from the labeled information [95]. Reciprocally, the inefficacy and unfamiliarity of food labels create hindrance for consumers while shopping food items. Most often the unfamiliar and complicated food labels create uncertainty in consumer's minds for nutritious packaged food [96]. Consumers, most often consult food label information to get the insights about composition of these products. The products that are seldom consumed need more information to shape the favorable attitude of an individual. The inefficacy of printed information creates a hindrance to this process. Therefore, the efficacy of food label plays a vital role in developing a positive attitude of consumers to consult label information and develop favorable intentions which are often transformed into actual purchase decisions [97].

Furthermore, consumers have found comfortable with familiar label even the understanding of information is uneasy. Similar results have been examined in past studies and researcher has reported that the food label information is familiar and label format is found to be difficult to understand nevertheless consumer select healthy food items [69]. In contrast, when the food label is unfamiliar and food label information is also difficult to comprehend consumers avoid consulting such products at the point of purchase [98]. Not with standing, regular purchase and consumption make consumers get familiar with the utility of food products. Additionally, while purchasing regularly consumed items, consumers most often do not consult food labels and put them directly into the shopping carts. Though, in regularly consumed edible items, the efficacy or inefficacy of food label information with familiar and unfamiliar food labels, consumers could not make any difference at the point of purchase. As a marketing tactic, if the manufacturer changes the existing format of food labels and the format is new for the consumers still such consumers do not have any concern at the point of purchases [99].

8. Theoretical Contribution

The proposed model of the current study is supported by two theories, TRA and PMT. The PMT investigates the factors, which cause the threats and coping of the threats. The involvement of PMT to examine consumer's nutritional food selection intention has also identified which factors become the cause of threat to avoid food label inform and which factors can be used for coping of these threats. The inefficacy of food label is the threats for consumer to consult food label information, which can be cope with efficacy of food label. Reciprocally, the inefficacy and efficacy affect consumer attitude in reading or avoiding food label, which later influence consumer intention for the choice of nutritional food items.

9. Practical Contribution

The practical contribution in current study has linked with the design of the food label, which encourage consumer for healthy food selection. The familiarity of the food label has related to the easy to understandable information written on label. Besides, most of the packaged food products are in regular used items of majority of consumers. Therefore, due to experience consumer has trust on these packaged food firms. Additionally, the outcome of the study reveals that easy to read food labels are very effective. Reciprocally, the food label is the most effective tool for guiding consumers towards nutritional food intention. Therefore, food-processing companies should focus on designing better, effective, and easy to understand food labels with brief, relevant, and comprehensive information. The technical and overcrowded labels create hindrances for customers while shopping packaged food items. Moreover, the efficacy of label can also be a competitive edge for packaged food firms, because consumer will be more comfortable in purchasing package food products from the companies, which have user-friendly food labels.

10. Future Direction

The current study paves the way towards a new avenue of research by the efficacy of food labels in influencing consumers' purchasing decisions. Nevertheless, owing to time constraints, researchers could not achieve other objectives that have been left open for future researchers. Future studies may employ unstructured questionnaires and adopt in-depth interview techniques for data collection. In future, scholars must have to develop a list of processed items, which have consumed occasionally and regularly. This list can further differentiate consumer's opinions for food label efficacy and inefficacy at point of purchase. Although the current study is based on the data at the point of purchase nevertheless the structured questionnaires not provide liberty to consumers to express their opinions in detail. Therefore, a qualitative data analysis technique opted in future studies. In addition to, the past studies have claimed that strong intention transformed into actual behavior. Therefore, future researchers should involve actual behavior in the proposed model.

11. Conclusions

This research aimed to examine consumers' intention to nutritional processed food selection. Owing to the absence of proper guidance the role of label is inevitable. Food label information is mandatory but most often consumers need special proficiency and intention to understand food label information. The current study proposed a model and suggested that food label efficacy is significant for informed purchase decision.

Author Contributions: Conceptualization, M.Z.Z. and H.Y.; Software, X.S.; Formal Analysis, M.Z.Z., X.S. and H.Y.; Investigation, M.Z.Z., X.S., J.A. and J.C.; Data Curation, M.Z.Z. and J.C.; Methodology, X.S. and J.A.; Writing—Original Draft Preparation, M.Z.Z., H.Y., X.S. and J.A.; Writing—Review and Editing, M.Z.Z. and H.Y.; Visualization, X.S.; Validation, M.Z.Z.; Supervision, M.Z.Z. and H.Y.; Funding acquisition, J.C. All authors have read and agreed to the published version of the manuscript.

Funding: This research received no external funding.

Institutional Review Board Statement: Not applicable.

Informed Consent Statement: Informed consent was obtained from all subjects involved in the study.

Data Availability Statement: The primary data used for the analysis of the current study. The data collected through adapted questionnaire with the consent of respondents. All respondents have shown their consent to participate in the research.

Conflicts of Interest: The authors declared no conflict of interest.

References

1. Acton, R.B.; Kirkpatrick, S.; Hammond, D. Comparing the Effects of Four Front-of-Package Nutrition Labels on Consumer Purchases of Five Common Beverages and Snack Foods: Results from a Randomized Trial. *J. Acad. Nutr. Diet.* **2022**, *122*, 38–48. [CrossRef] [PubMed]
2. Roy, R.; Alassadi, D. Does labelling of healthy foods on menus using symbols promote better choices at the point-of-purchase? *Public Health Nutr.* **2020**, *24*, 746–754. [CrossRef] [PubMed]
3. Asbridge, S.C.M.; Pechey, E.; Marteau, T.M.; Hollands, G.J. Effects of pairing health warning labels with energy-dense snack foods on food choice and attitudes: Online experimental study. *Appetite* **2021**, *160*, 105090. [CrossRef] [PubMed]
4. Li, Z.; Zhang, L. Poverty and health-related quality of life: A cross-sectional study in rural China. *Health Qual. Life Outcomes* **2020**, *18*, 153. [CrossRef] [PubMed]
5. Ares, G.; de Saldamando, L.; Gimenez, A.; Claret, A.; Cunha, L.M.; Guerrero, L.; de Moura, A.P.; Oliveira, D.C.R.; Symoneaux, R.; Deliza, R. Consumers' associations with wellbeing in a food-related context: A cross-cultural study. *Food Qual. Prefer.* **2015**, *40*, 304–315. [CrossRef]
6. Jacobus Berlitz, S.; De Villa, D.; Maschmann Inácio, L.A.; Davies, S.; Zatta, K.C.; Guterres, S.S.; Külkamp-Guerreiro, I.C. Azelaic acid-loaded nanoemulsion with hyaluronic acid—A new strategy to treat hyperpigmentary skin disorders. *Drug Dev. Ind. Pharm.* **2019**, *45*, 642–650. [CrossRef]
7. Willett, W.; Rockstrom, J.; Loken, B.; Springmann, M.; Lang, T.; Vermeulen, S.; Garnett, T.; Tilman, D.; DeClerck, F.; Wood, A.; et al. Food in the Anthropocene: The EAT-Lancet Commission on healthy diets from sustainable food systems. *Lancet* **2019**, *393*, 447–492. [CrossRef]
8. Clarke, N.; Pechey, E.; Mantzari, E.; Blackwell, A.K.M.; De-loyde, K.; Morris, R.W.; Munafo, M.R.; Marteau, T.M.; Hollands, G.J. Impact of health warning labels on snack selection: An online experimental study. *Appetite* **2020**, *154*, 104744. [CrossRef]
9. Chandon, P. How Package Design and Packaged-based Marketing Claims Lead to Overeating. *Appl. Econ. Perspect. Policy* **2013**, *35*, 7–31. [CrossRef]
10. Pechey, E.; Clarke, N.; Mantzari, E.; Blackwell, A.K.M.; De-Loyde, K.; Morris, R.W.; Marteau, T.M.; Hollands, G.J. Image-and-text health warning labels on alcohol and food: Potential effectiveness and acceptability. *BMC Public Health* **2020**, *20*, 376. [CrossRef]
11. Ljubičić, M.; Sarić, M.M.; Rumbak, I.; Barić, I.C.; Sarić, A.; Komes, D.; Šatalić, Z.; Dželalija, B.; Guiné, R.P.F. Is Better Knowledge about Health Benefits of Dietary Fiber Related to Food Labels Reading Habits? A Croatian Overview. *Foods* **2022**, *11*, 2347. [CrossRef] [PubMed]
12. Tanner, S.A.; McCarthy, M.B.; O'Reilly, S.J. Exploring the roles of motivation and cognition in label-usage using a combined eye-tracking and retrospective think aloud approach. *Appetite* **2019**, *135*, 146–158. [CrossRef] [PubMed]
13. Liao, L.X.; Corsi, A.M.; Chrysochou, P.; Lockshin, L. Emotional responses towards food packaging: A joint application of self-report and physiological measures of emotion. *Food Qual. Prefer.* **2015**, *42*, 48–55. [CrossRef]
14. Neff, R.A.; Spiker, M.; Rice, C.; Schklair, A.; Greenberg, S.; Leib, E.B. Misunderstood food date labels and reported food discards: A survey of US consumer attitudes and behaviors. *Waste Manag.* **2019**, *86*, 123–132. [CrossRef]

15. Roberto, C.A.; Khandpur, N. Improving the design of nutrition labels to promote healthier food choices and reasonable portion sizes. *Int. J. Obes.* **2014**, *38*, S25–S33. [CrossRef]
16. Ikonen, I.; Sotgiu, F.; Aydinli, A.; Verlegh, P.W.J. Consumer effects of front-of-package nutrition labeling: An interdisciplinary meta-analysis. *J. Acad. Mark. Sci.* **2020**, *48*, 360–383. [CrossRef]
17. Festila, A.; Chrysochou, P.; Krystallis, A. Consumer response to food labels in an emerging market: The case of Romania. *Int. J. Consum. Stud.* **2014**, *38*, 166–174. [CrossRef]
18. Dominguez Diaz, L.; Fernandez-Ruiz, V.; Camara, M. An international regulatory review of food health-related claims in functional food products labeling. *J. Funct. Food* **2020**, *68*, 103896. [CrossRef]
19. Bhattacharya, S.; Saleem, S.M.; Bera, O.P. Prevention of childhood obesity through appropriate food labeling. *Clin. Nutr. ESPEN* **2022**, *47*, 418–421. [CrossRef]
20. Tanemura, N.; Hamadate, N. Association between consumers' food selection and differences in food labeling regarding efficacy health information: Food selection based on differences in labeling. *Food Control* **2022**, *131*, 108413. [CrossRef]
21. Verbeke, W. Functional foods: Consumer willingness to compromise on taste for health? *Food Qual. Prefer.* **2006**, *17*, 126–131. [CrossRef]
22. Pink, A.E.; Stylianou, K.S.; Lee, L.L.; Jolliet, O.; Cheon, B.K. The effects of presenting health and environmental impacts of food on consumption intentions. *Food Qual. Prefer.* **2022**, *98*, 104501. [CrossRef]
23. Temple, N.J. Front-of-package food labels: A narrative review. *Appetite* **2020**, *144*, 104485. [CrossRef] [PubMed]
24. Vijaykumar, S.; Lwin, M.O.; Chao, J.; Au, C. Determinants of Food Label Use among Supermarket Shoppers: A Singaporean Perspective. *J. Nutr. Educ. Behav.* **2013**, *45*, 204–212. [CrossRef] [PubMed]
25. Meijer, G.W.; Detzel, P.; Grunert, K.G.; Robert, M.-C.; Stancu, V. Towards effective labelling of foods. An international perspective on safety and nutrition. *Trends Food Sci. Technol.* **2021**, *118*, 45–56. [CrossRef]
26. Pulker, C.E.; Li, D.C.C.; Scott, J.A.; Pollard, C.M. The Impact of Voluntary Policies on Parents' Ability to Select Healthy Foods in Supermarkets: A Qualitative Study of Australian Parental Views. *Int. J. Environ. Res. Public Health* **2019**, *16*, 3377. [CrossRef]
27. Wijayaratne, S.P.; Reid, M.; Westberg, K.; Worsley, A.; Mavondo, F. Food literacy, healthy eating barriers and household diet. *Eur. J. Mark.* **2018**, *52*, 2449–2477. [CrossRef]
28. Abdul Latiff, Z.A.B.; Rezai, G.; Mohamed, Z.; Amizi Ayob, M. Food Labels' Impact Assessment on Consumer Purchasing Behavior in Malaysia. *J. Food Prod. Mark.* **2016**, *22*, 137–146. [CrossRef]
29. Bazhan, M.; Mirghotbi, M.; Amiri, Z. Food labels: An analysis of the consumers' reasons for non-use. *J. Paramed. Sci.* **2015**, *6*, 2–10.
30. Moreira, M.J.; Garcia-Diez, J.; de Almeida, J.M.M.M.; Saraiva, C. Evaluation of food labelling usefulness for consumers. *Int. J. Consum. Stud.* **2019**, *43*, 327–334. [CrossRef]
31. Pomeranz, J.L.; Wilde, P.; Mozaffarian, D.; Micha, R. Mandating front-of-package food labels in the US—What are the First Amendment obstacles? *Food Policy* **2019**, *86*, 101722. [CrossRef] [PubMed]
32. Meiselman, H.L. Quality of life, well-being and wellness: Measuring subjective health for foods and other products. *Food Qual. Prefer.* **2016**, *54*, 101–109. [CrossRef]
33. Barauskaite, D.; Gineikiene, J.; Fennis, B.M.; Auruskeviciene, V.; Yamaguchi, M.; Kondo, N. Eating healthy to impress: How conspicuous consumption, perceived self-control motivation, and descriptive normative influence determine functional food choices. *Appetite* **2018**, *131*, 59–67. [CrossRef]
34. Cecchini, M.; Warin, L. Impact of food labelling systems on food choices and eating behaviours: A systematic review and meta-analysis of randomized studies. *Obes. Rev.* **2016**, *17*, 201–210. [CrossRef]
35. Weaver, C.M.; Dwyer, J.; Fulgoni, V.L.; King, J.C.; Leveille, G.A.; MacDonald, R.S.; Ordovas, J.; Schnakenberg, D. Processed foods: Contributions to nutrition(1,2). *Am. J. Clin. Nutr.* **2014**, *99*, 1525–1542. [CrossRef] [PubMed]
36. Todd, M.; Guetterman, T.; Sigge, G.; Joubert, E. Multi-stakeholder perspectives on food labeling and health claims: Qualitative insights from South Africa. *Appetite* **2021**, *167*, 105606. [CrossRef]
37. O'Connor, E.L.; White, K.M. Willingness to trial functional foods and vitamin supplements: The role of attitudes, subjective norms, and dread of risks. *Food Qual. Prefer.* **2010**, *21*, 75–81. [CrossRef]
38. Odaman, T.A.; Bahar, R.; Şam, S.; Ilyasoğlu, H. Food label reading habits of health sciences students. *Nutr. Food Sci.* **2020**, *50*, 1021–1032. [CrossRef]
39. Bogue, J.; Yu, H. The Influence of Sociodemographic and Lifestyle Factors on Consumers' Healthy Cereal Food Choices. *J. Food Prod. Mark.* **2016**, *22*, 398–419. [CrossRef]
40. Vidal, L.; Ares, G.; Machín, L.; Jaeger, S.R. Using Twitter data for food-related consumer research: A case study on "what people say when tweeting about different eating situations". *Food Qual. Prefer.* **2015**, *45*, 58–69. [CrossRef]
41. Saha, S.; Vemula, S.R.; Mendu, V.V.R.; Gavaravarapu, S.M. Knowledge and Practices of Using Food Label Information Among Adolescents Attending Schools in Kolkata, India. *J. Nutr. Educ. Behav.* **2013**, *45*, 773–779. [CrossRef] [PubMed]
42. O'Rourke, D.; Ringer, A. The Impact of Sustainability Information on Consumer Decision Making. *J. Ind. Ecol.* **2016**, *20*, 882–892. [CrossRef]
43. Chung, J.-E.; Stoel, L.; Xu, Y.; Ren, J. Predicting Chinese consumers' purchase intentions for imported soy-based dietary supplements. *Br. Food J.* **2012**, *114*, 143–161. [CrossRef]
44. Sibbald, B. New food labels to reveal nutritional content. *Can. Med. Assoc. J.* **2000**, *163*, 1490.

45. Visschers, V.H.M.; Hess, R.; Siegrist, M. Health motivation and product design determine consumers' visual attention to nutrition information on food products. *Public Health Nutr.* **2010**, *13*, 1099–1106. [CrossRef]
46. Yee, A.Z.H.; Lwin, M.O.; Ho, S.S. The influence of parental practices on child promotive and preventive food consumption behaviors: A systematic review and meta-analysis. *Int. J. Behav. Nutr. Phys. Act.* **2017**, *14*, 47. [CrossRef]
47. Coderre, F.; Sirieix, L.; Valette-Florence, P. The facets of consumer-based food label equity: Measurement, structure and managerial relevance. *J. Retail. Consum. Serv.* **2022**, *65*, 102838. [CrossRef]
48. Pettigrew, S.; Dana, L.M.; Talati, Z.; Tian, M.; Praveen, D. The role of colour and summary indicators in influencing front-of-pack food label effectiveness across seven countries. *Public Health Nutr.* **2021**, *24*, 3566–3570. [CrossRef]
49. Van der Merwe, D.; de Beer, H.; Nel, M.; Ellis, S.M. Marketing and family-related factors affecting food label use: The mediating role of consumer knowledge. *Br. Food J.* **2022**, *124*, 3936–3952. [CrossRef]
50. Jezewska-Zychowicz, M.; Plichta, M.; Drywien, M.E.; Hamulka, J. Food Neophobia among Adults: Differences in Dietary Patterns, Food Choice Motives, and Food Labels Reading in Poles. *Nutrients* **2021**, *13*, 1590. [CrossRef]
51. Mattar, J.B.; Candido, A.C.; de Souza Vilela, D.L.; de Paula, V.L.; Vidigal Castro, L.C. Information displayed on Brazilian food bar labels points to the need to reformulate the current food labelling legislation. *Food Chem.* **2022**, *370*, 131318. [CrossRef] [PubMed]
52. Feldmann, C.; Hamm, U. Consumers' perceptions and preferences for local food: A review. *Food Qual. Prefer.* **2015**, *40*, 152–164. [CrossRef]
53. Huang, L.; Lu, J. The Impact of Package Color and the Nutrition Content Labels on the Perception of Food Healthiness and Purchase Intention. *J. Food Prod. Mark.* **2016**, *22*, 191–218. [CrossRef]
54. Mulders, M.D.G.H.; Corneille, O.; Klein, O. Label reading, numeracy and food & nutrition involvement. *Appetite* **2018**, *128*, 214–222. [CrossRef] [PubMed]
55. Zafar, M.Z.; Maqbool, A.; Cioca, L.-I.; Shah, S.G.M.; Masud, S. Accentuating the Interrelation between Consumer Intention and Healthy Packaged Food Selection during COVID-19: A Case Study of Pakistan. *Int. J. Environ. Res. Public Health* **2021**, *18*, 2846. [CrossRef] [PubMed]
56. Koenigstorfer, J.; Groeppel-Klein, A. Examining the use of nutrition labelling with photoelicitation. *Qual. Mark. Res. Int. J.* **2010**, *13*, 389–413. [CrossRef]
57. Pilla Reddy, V.; Jo, H.; Neuhoff, S. Food constituent- and herb-drug interactions in oncology: Influence of quantitative modelling on Drug labelling. *Br. J. Clin. Pharmacol.* **2021**, *87*, 3988–4000. [CrossRef]
58. Szakaly, Z.; Kovacs, S.; Peto, K.; Huszka, P.; Kiss, M. A modified model of the willingness to pay for functional foods. *Appetite* **2019**, *138*, 94–101. [CrossRef]
59. Mackey, M.A.; Metz, M. Ease of reading of mandatory information on Canadian food product labels. *Int. J. Consum. Stud.* **2009**, *33*, 369–381. [CrossRef]
60. Madilo, F.K.; Owusu-Kwarteng, J.; Kunadu, A.P.-H.; Tano-Debrah, K. Self-reported use and understanding of food label information among tertiary education students in Ghana. *Food Control* **2020**, *108*, 106841. [CrossRef]
61. Bryła, P. Who Reads Food Labels? Selected Predictors of Consumer Interest in Front-of-Package and Back-of-Package Labels during and after the Purchase. *Nutrients* **2020**, *12*, 2605. [CrossRef] [PubMed]
62. Cheah, Y.K.; Moy, F.M.; Loh, D.A. Socio-demographic and lifestyle factors associated with nutrition label use among Malaysian adults. *Br. Food J.* **2015**, *117*, 2777–2787. [CrossRef]
63. ElHaffar, G.; Durif, F.; Dube, L. Towards closing the attitude-intention-behavior gap in green consumption: A narrative review of the literature and an overview of future research directions. *J. Clean Prod.* **2020**, *275*, 122556. [CrossRef]
64. Chu, S.-C.; Chen, H.-T. Impact of consumers' corporate social responsibility-related activities in social media on brand attitude, electronic word-of-mouth intention, and purchase intention: A study of Chinese consumer behavior. *J. Consum. Behav.* **2019**, *18*, 453–462. [CrossRef]
65. Verma, V.K.; Chandra, B.; Kumar, S. Values and ascribed responsibility to predict consumers' attitude and concern towards green hotel visit intention. *J. Bus. Res.* **2019**, *96*, 206–216. [CrossRef]
66. Wang, J.; Tao, J.; Chu, M. Behind the label: Chinese consumers' trust in food certification and the effect of perceived quality on purchase intention. *Food Control* **2020**, *108*, 106825. [CrossRef]
67. Hendriks-Hartensveld, A.E.M.; Rolls, B.J.; Cunningham, P.M.; Nederkoorn, C.; Havermans, R.C. Does labelling a food as "light" vs. "filling" influence intake and sensory-specific satiation? *Appetite* **2022**, *171*, 105916. [CrossRef]
68. Kreuter, M.W.; Brennan, L.K.; Scharff, D.P.; Lukwago, S.N. Do nutrition label readers eat healthier diets? Behavioral correlates of adults' use of food labels. *Am. J. Prev. Med.* **1997**, *13*, 277–283. [CrossRef]
69. Besler, H.T.; Buyuktuncer, Z.; Uyar, M.F. Consumer Understanding and Use of Food and Nutrition Labeling in Turkey. *J. Nutr. Educ. Behav.* **2012**, *44*, 584–591. [CrossRef]
70. Lubman, N.; Doak, C.; Jasti, S. Food Label Use and Food Label Skills among Immigrants from the Former Soviet Union. *J. Nutr. Educ. Behav.* **2012**, *44*, 398–406. [CrossRef]
71. De Canio, F.; Martinelli, E. EU quality label vs organic food products: A multigroup structural equation modeling to assess consumers' intention to buy in light of sustainable motives. *Food Res. Int.* **2021**, *139*, 109846. [CrossRef] [PubMed]
72. Yadav, R.; Pathak, G.S. Intention to purchase organic food among young consumers: Evidences from a developing nation. *Appetite* **2016**, *96*, 122–128. [CrossRef] [PubMed]

73. Spears, N.; Singh, S.N. Measuring Attitude Toward the Brand and Purchase Intentions. *J. Curr. Issues Res. Advert.* **2004**, *26*, 53–66. [CrossRef]
74. Eyinade, G.A.; Mushunje, A.; Yusuf, S.F.G. The willingness to consume organic food: A review. *Food Agric. Immunol.* **2021**, *32*, 78–104. [CrossRef]
75. Ajzen, I.; Fishbein, M. Factors Influencing Intentions and the Intention-Behavior Relation. *Hum. Relat.* **1974**, *27*, 1–15. [CrossRef]
76. Rogers, R.W. A Protection Motivation Theory of Fear Appeals and Attitude Change1. *J. Psychol.* **1975**, *91*, 93–114. [CrossRef]
77. Berry, C.; Romero, M. The fair trade food labeling health halo: Effects of fair trade labeling on consumption and perceived healthfulness. *Food Qual. Prefer.* **2021**, *94*, 104321. [CrossRef]
78. Giacalone, D.; Jaeger, S.R. Consumer ratings of situational ('Item-by-use') appropriateness predict food choice responses obtained in central location tests. *Food Qual. Prefer.* **2019**, *78*, 103745. [CrossRef]
79. Churchill, G.A.; Iacobucci, D. *Marketing Research: Methodological Foundations*; Dryden Press: New York, NY, USA, 2006; ISBN 0030314720.
80. Comrey, A.L.; Lee, H.B. *A First Course in Factor Analysis*, 2nd ed.; Lawrence Erlbaum Associates, Inc.: Hillsdale, NJ, USA, 1992; ISBN 0-8058-1062-5.
81. Aitken, R.; Watkins, L.; Williams, J.; Kean, A. The positive role of labelling on consumers' perceived behavioural control and intention to purchase organic food. *J. Clean Prod.* **2020**, *255*, 120334. [CrossRef]
82. Zafar, M.Z.; Hashim, N.A.; Halim, F.B.; Attique, S. Factors Affecting on Healthy Package Food Selection; The Impact of Personality Traits. *Abasyn Univ. J. Soc. Sci.* **2020**, *13*, 169–193. [CrossRef]
83. Malhotra, N.K.; Kim, S.S.; Patil, A. Common Method Variance in IS Research: A Comparison of Alternative Approaches and a Reanalysis of Past Research. *Manag. Sci.* **2006**, *52*, 1865–1883. [CrossRef]
84. Ali, S.; Ullah, H.; Akbar, M.; Akhtar, W.; Zahid, H. Determinants of Consumer Intentions to Purchase Energy-Saving Household Products in Pakistan. *Sustainability* **2019**, *11*, 1462. [CrossRef]
85. Ali, S.; Danish, M.; Khuwaja, F.M.; Sajjad, M.S. The Intention to Adopt Green IT Products in Pakistan: Driven by the Modified Theory of Consumption Values. *Environments* **2019**, *6*, 53. [CrossRef]
86. Hair, J.F.; Ringle, C.M.; Sarstedt, M. PLS-SEM: Indeed a Silver Bullet PLS-SEM: Indeed a Silver Bullet. *J. Mark. Theory Pract.* **2011**, *19*, 37–41. [CrossRef]
87. Ramli, N.A.; Latan, H.; Solovida, G.T. Determinants of Capital Structure and Firm Financial Performance—A PLS-SEM Approach: Evidence from Malaysia and Indonesia. *Q. Rev. Econ. Financ.* **2018**, *71*, 148–160. [CrossRef]
88. Anderson, J.C.; Gerbing, D.W. Structural Equation Modeling in Practice: A Review and Recommended Two-Step Approach. *Psychological. Bull.* **1988**, *103*, 411–423. [CrossRef]
89. Danish, M.; Ali, S.; Ahmad, M.A.; Zahid, H. The Influencing Factors on Choice Behavior Regarding Green Electronic Products: Based on the Green Perceived Value Model. *Economies* **2019**, *7*, 99. [CrossRef]
90. Tabachnick, B.G.; Fidell, L.S. Multivariate analysis of variance and covariance. *Using Multivar. Multivar. Stat.* **2007**, *3*, 402–407.
91. Hair, J.F.; Hult, G.T.M.; Ringle, C.M.; Sarstedt, M. *A Primer on Partial Least Squares Structural Equation Modeling (PLS-SEM)*; Sage Publications: Thousand Oaks, CA, USA, 2016; Volume 18.
92. Fornell, C.; Larcker, D.F. Evaluating Structural Equation Models with Unobservable Variables and Measurement Error. *J. Mark. Res.* **1981**, *18*, 39–50. [CrossRef]
93. Cohen, J. *Statistical Power Analysis for the Behavioral Sciences*, 2nd ed.; Routledge: London, UK, 1988.
94. Akbar, A.; Ali, S.; Ahmad, M.A.; Akbar, M.; Danish, M. Understanding the Antecedents of Organic Food Consumption in Pakistan: Moderating Role of Food Neophobia. *Int. J. Environ. Res. Public Health* **2019**, *16*, 4043. [CrossRef] [PubMed]
95. Grunert, K.G.; Fernández-Celemín, L.; Wills, J.M.; Storcksdieck Genannt Bonsmann, S.; Nureeva, L. Use and understanding of nutrition information on food labels in six European countries. *J. Public Health* **2010**, *18*, 261–277. [CrossRef] [PubMed]
96. Silayoi, P.; Speece, M. The importance of packaging attributes: A conjoint analysis approach. *Eur. J. Mark.* **2007**, *41*, 1495–1517. [CrossRef]
97. Cha, E.; Kim, K.H.; Lerner, H.M.; Dawkins, C.R.; Bello, M.K.; Umpierrez, G.; Dunbar, S.B. Health Literacy, Self-efficacy, Food Label Use, and Diet in Young Adults. *Am. J. Health Behav.* **2014**, *38*, 331–339. [CrossRef]
98. Li, F.; Miniard, P.W.; Barone, M.J. The Facilitating Influence of Consumer Knowledge on the Effectiveness of Daily Value Reference Information. *J. Acad. Mark. Sci.* **2000**, *28*, 425. [CrossRef]
99. Becker, M.W.; Bello, N.M.; Sundar, R.P.; Peltier, C.; Bix, L. Front of pack labels enhance attention to nutrition information in novel and commercial brands. *Food Policy* **2015**, *56*, 76–86. [CrossRef]

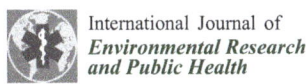

Review

A Thematic Review on Using Food Delivery Services during the Pandemic: Insights for the Post-COVID-19 Era

Yezheng Li [1], Pinyi Yao [2,*], Syuhaily Osman [2], Norzalina Zainudin [2] and Mohamad Fazli Sabri [2]

1 Business School, Guilin University of Technology, Guilin 541004, China
2 Faculty of Human Ecology, Universiti Putra Malaysia, Serdang 43400, Malaysia
* Correspondence: pinyi_y@foxmail.com

Abstract: The food delivery service is the most typical and visible example of online-to-offline (O2O) commerce. More consumers are using food delivery services for various reasons during the COVID-19 pandemic, making this business model viral worldwide. In the post-pandemic era, offering food delivery services will become the new normal for restaurants. Although a growing number of publications have focused on consumer behavior in this issue, no review paper has addressed current research and industry trends. Thus, this paper aims to review the literature published from 2020 to the present (October 2022) on consumers' use of food delivery services during the pandemic. A thematic review was conducted, with 40 articles searched from Scopus and Web of Science being included. Quantitative findings showed current research trends, and thematic analyses formed eight themes of factors influencing consumer behavior: (1) technical and utilitarian factors, (2) system-related attributes, (3) emotional and hedonic factors, (4) individual characteristics, (5) service quality, (6) risk-related factors, (7) social factors, and (8) food-related attributes. The paper also emphasizes COVID-19-related influences and suggests promising future research directions. The results offer insights into industry practices and starting points for future research.

Keywords: food delivery app; online food delivery; online-to-offline (O2O); consumer behavior; COVID-19; post-pandemic; thematic review

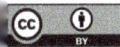

1. Introduction

The rapid expansion of electronic commerce (e-commerce) or mobile commerce (m-commerce) is changing people's food consumption patterns, with more and more consumers considering purchasing food online. They generally purchase food online in business-to-consumer (B2C) and online-to-offline (O2O) models. B2C is a traditional e-commerce model where consumers purchase food from B2C platforms (e.g., China's JD.com and USA's Amazon.com) and receive the parcel in approximately 3–10 days, while O2O is a new e-commerce model focused on local business where consumers order online and then consume offline [1]. In the O2O model, consumers can visit the offline store or use the home delivery service. The former is called to-shop O2O, while the latter is known as to-home O2O [2]. Food delivery is the most obvious and widely discussed O2O market segment, in which restaurants work with third-party O2O platforms, i.e., online food delivery platforms, to offer delivery of ready-to-eat food [3]. Consumers can easily find nearby restaurants through the food delivery app, accessing the convenience and diversity of food delivery services. Although the food delivery market has continued to expand since the emergence of the O2O concept, its growth was uneventful [3] until the outbreak of coronavirus disease 2019 (COVID-19).

COVID-19 is an infectious disease caused by the severe acute respiratory syndrome coronavirus 2 (SARS-CoV-2) [4]. The World Health Organization (WHO) declared its outbreak in January 2020 and subsequently called it a pandemic in March 2020. During the pandemic, the WHO strongly advises that people wear masks in public places, maintain social distancing, self-isolate, and take other self-protective actions to avoid contracting COVID-19 [5,6]. In the early stages of the pandemic, many countries worldwide adopted strict measures such as lockdowns, quarantine, and movement control to reduce the risk of COVID-19 spread. Industries around the world, especially the food and restaurant industries, have been severely impacted as a result because consumers use fewer public services or dine less in public places [7,8].

The COVID-19 pandemic has significantly changed consumer behavior, with more and more people purchasing food online due to social distancing policies or fear of infection. Since food is a daily necessity for individuals, buying food through to-home O2O (i.e., instant food delivery) seems to meet consumer needs better than B2C and is more popular. To sustain the business, many restaurants started to access online platforms offering food delivery services to meet consumers' demands [7,9]. According to statistics, the COVID-19 pandemic led to unprecedented growth in food delivery services, with restaurant food delivery growing 47% worldwide in 2020; more than 1.6 billion people globally used some form of online food delivery service in 2021 [10,11]. In a way, the COVID-19 pandemic has accelerated the digitalization of numerous industries, including the restaurant industry [6,12,13]. On the other hand, the pandemic disrupted the pre-existing food delivery market, with users more cautious in their decision to continue using the food delivery service due to concerns about the safety of the delivered food [14,15].

Previous studies have investigated the factors influencing consumer behavior in the context of online food delivery service from different perspectives, such as technology adoption [16–18], service quality [19,20], food choice motives [1,21], etc. However, research has shown that many aspects of consumer expectations during the pandemic differ from normal times [9] and that consumer purchasing behavior during the crisis is unusual [22]. Consumers' thinking and behavior are being reshaped by COVID-19 [9,23,24]. This means that new factors may influence consumer behavior, while the identified factors may work in different ways. In fact, many studies have focused on using food delivery services during the COVID-19 pandemic. However, no review paper has attempted to explore the research and industry trends of food delivery in the (post-) pandemic era. Accordingly, this paper aims to identify these trends by reviewing the current literature.

In the post-pandemic era, continued research on consumer behavior regarding food delivery services is necessary for the following reasons: First, consumers will adapt to the new normal situation, and some behavioral changes resulting from the pandemic might continue. Consumer behavior is generally highly predictable; nonetheless, many aspects of the COVID-19 pandemic increase prediction uncertainty [25]. Second, food deliveries will be the new normal for restaurants and diners in the foreseeable future [26,27], and a comprehensive understanding of consumer behavior can help businesses remain resilient in their business. Lastly, food delivery as a segment of O2O commerce is not restricted to delivering ready-to-eat food [2,28]. The combined effect of innovation and COVID-19 has given rise to many new business models. This is an effort by restaurants and food delivery platforms to sustain their business, which may become the new fashion after the pandemic fades. New insights and marketing strategies are hence needed in the post-pandemic era. Therefore, another objective of this paper is to identify literature gaps to offer a starting point for future research.

2. Materials and Methods

This paper collected literature from dominant online databases and used a non-systematic approach to review. Most systematic reviews aim to measure the effectiveness of prior studies rigorously and scientifically to reveal whether their findings are consistent across studies [29]. In contrast, non-systematic reviews seek to identify what the literature says about a particular issue and where effective research should be conducted [29]. In this paper, the non-systematic approach was adopted based on the research objectives: identifying research and industry trends regarding food delivery services use in the COVID-19 pandemic and offering future research directions. Furthermore, a systematic review would not be particularly useful or effective if only a limited number of published studies were published in a given field [29]. Since the COVID-19 pandemic began in 2020, it can be expected that there are not many relevant studies. For example, studies involving the relationship between perceived risk from COVID-19 and consumers' use of food delivery apps might be limited. Hence, the non-systematic review approach was more appropriate for this paper. Specifically, a thematic analysis procedure was used, which is a typical design for non-systematic reviews [30].

However, the non-systematic review does not mean it is not rigorous and scientific. In fact, any non-systematic review must be systematic to some extent to ensure its credibility [29]. Thus, this paper adopted Zairul's [31–33] thematic review method and conducted a thematic review following the steps suggested by Greetham [29].

2.1. Formulating the Research Question

The research questions can help a researcher judge what is relevant to their topic, providing clarity, cohesion, and direction to their work. In this paper, we follow the research questions to gather, structure, and analyze the literature in the following steps. Therefore, we proposed the following research questions:

- RQ1: What are the current trends of the food delivery service discussed in the literature related to consumer behavior during the COVID-19 pandemic?
- RQ2: What factors influence consumer behavior in using food delivery services during the COVID-19 pandemic?
- RQ3: What are the characteristics or changes in consumer behavior using food delivery services during the COVID-19 pandemic?

2.2. Literature Screening

In order to determine which article should be reviewed, we developed explicit inclusion and exclusion criteria. First, we determined "food delivery" and "COVID-19" as the core keywords after a preliminary study of industry reports and previous literature. The title of the article to be reviewed must simultaneously include these two core keywords or their synonyms. Second, we only selected peer-reviewed journal articles to ensure the quality of the research to be reviewed. However, review articles were excluded because of the contradiction with the objective of our paper. Third, we only considered articles written in English. Fourth, the articles to be included must focus on consumers' use of food delivery services during the COVID-19 pandemic. Last, studies must involve the influence of the COVID-19 pandemic on consumer behavior rather than simply using it as a writing background.

2.3. Searching the Literature

We chose two prevailing citation databases, namely the Scopus and the Web of Science (WOS) core collection, from which to search articles. We searched and selected the literature according to the inclusion and exclusion criteria as mentioned previously, with the procedure shown in Figure 1. All authors searched and assessed articles from the two databases separately, following the same procedure. We discussed the respective search results and repeated the above procedure until the results were consistent. Given that "food delivery" may have many synonyms in different contexts, we changed the keywords to search again to avoid missing valuable articles. In addition, those articles with repeated content using the same data were excluded. Ultimately, 40 articles that met the criteria published from 2020 to the present (updated on 15 October 2022) were included in this review, as shown in Table A1 of Appendix A.

2.4. Data Extraction and Synthesis

Following Zairul's [31–33] method, we used the ATLAS.ti 9 software (ATLAS.ti GmbH, Berlin, Germany) to extract and synthesize data, importing documents into the software for further thematic review. Specifically, we read the articles thoroughly and performed a thematic analysis procedure to construct the themes, which were identified by an iterative process of comparing similarities and differences between the reviewed subjects to achieve consistency. The bibliometric information and other directly identifiable metadata from the reviewed articles were extracted for descriptive quantitative analysis. Subsequently, we used a coding method similar to the qualitative study to conduct the thematic analysis. We coded the influencing factors of consumer behavior in using food delivery services during the COVID-19 pandemic and categorized them into several themes after several rounds of recoding and merging codes.

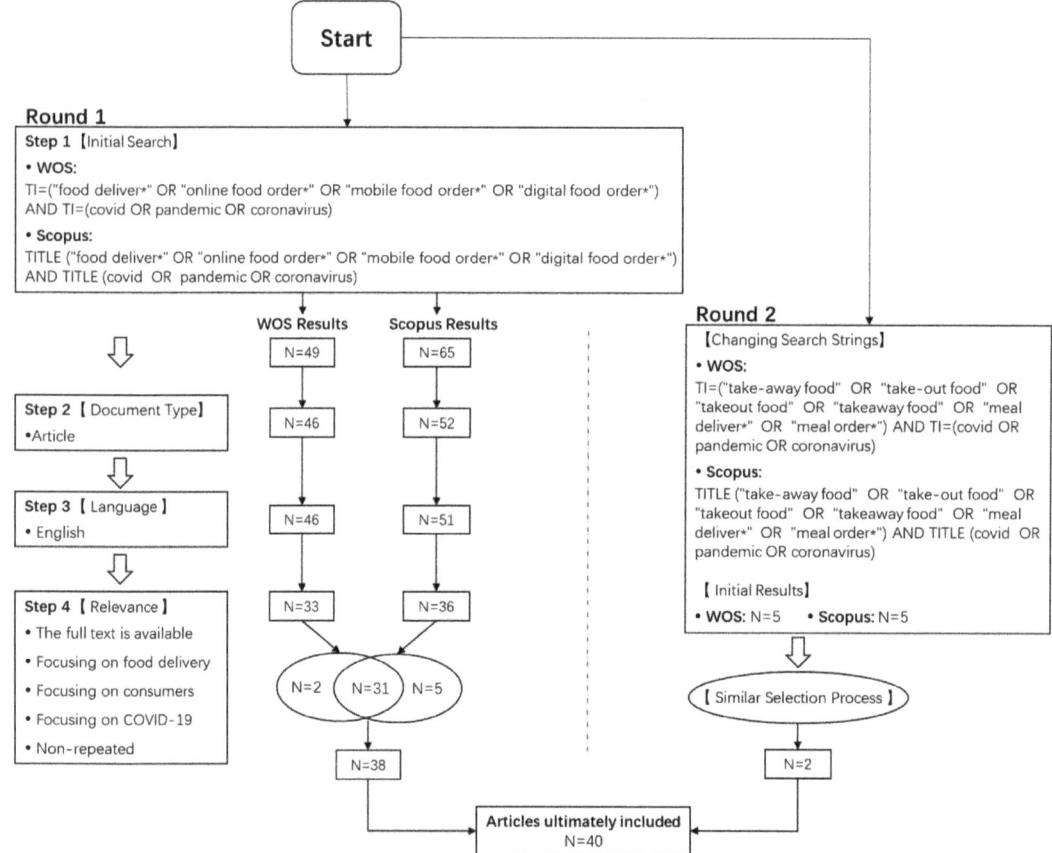

Figure 1. Literature searching process.

3. Results and Discussion

The results were classified into quantitative findings and qualitative findings. The former was mainly used to answer RQ1, while the latter addressed RQ2 and RQ3. The discussion in each subsection may involve literature outside of the reviewed articles for illustrative purposes.

3.1. Quantitative Results

Research trends were examined by general bibliometric information and directly identifiable metadata, including the year of publication and data collection, source of publication, study site, and key dependent variables or research focuses. First, as shown in Figure 2, the earliest studies appeared in 2020 because that is when the COVID-19 pandemic began. We checked the time of data collection for each study and marked it as

Not Applicable (N/A) when it could not be identified or inferred. Figure 2 shows that most of the studies collected data in 2020, of which six (i.e., [34–39]) collected data before and after 2020 for comparative analysis. In addition, Meena and Kumar [9] analyzed what consumers posted online in 2020 and 2021 and showed that consumers' net sentiment (positive-negative) during the second wave of COVID-19 was significantly higher than that during the first wave, which may be due to consumers psychologically adapting to the new normal. Therefore, consumers' behavioral characteristics or changes regarding the use of using food delivery services in the post-pandemic era are worth investigating. However, even in the articles published in 2022, few studies used data from 2021 and beyond. One possible reason is that the articles in question have not yet been officially published.

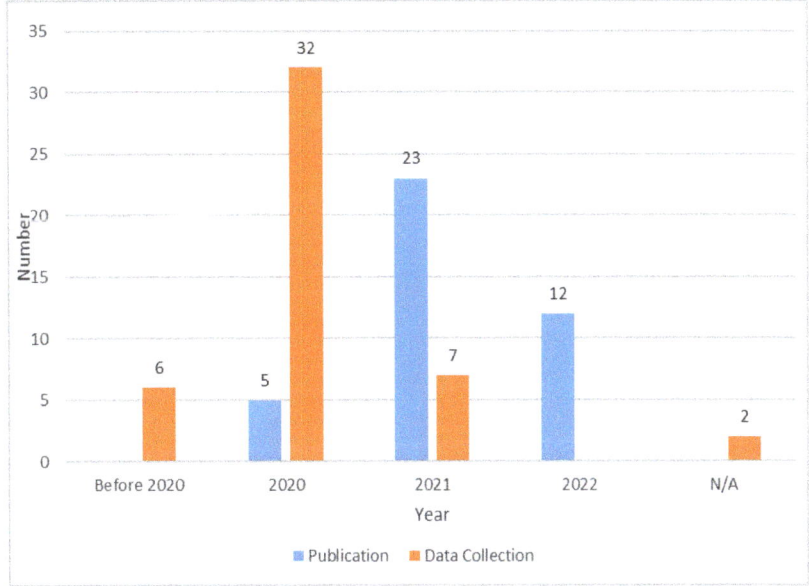

Figure 2. The year of publication and data collection.

Second, 40 articles were published in 25 different journals, as shown in Table A1 in Appendix A, indicating that consumers using food delivery services during the COVID-19 overhaul is an interdisciplinary and widely discussed issue. Regarding the study site, we were interested in where the study was conducted and where the researcher focused. This is because economic and cultural contexts are important aspects of understanding consumer behavior. As can be seen from Table 1, studies involved 17 countries or regions with different cultures and continents, suggesting that the issue is a globally widespread phenomenon.

Table 1. Countries or regions of research by the year of publication.

No.	Countries or Regions	2020	2021	2022	Count *	References
1	Bangladesh		2		2	[12,40]
2	Brazil		1	1	2	[41,42]
3	China's mainland	1	2	3	6	[6,43–47]
4	Ecuador		1		1	[48]
5	India		4	2	6	[7,9,14,15,49,50]
6	Indonesia		1		1	[51]
7	Macau			1	1	[24]
8	Malaysia			1	1	[52]
9	Mexico			1	1	[53]

Table 1. Cont.

No.	Countries or Regions	2020	2021	2022	Count *	References
10	Pakistan	1			1	[23]
11	Romania			1	1	[54]
12	South Korea	2	3		5	[34,37–39,55]
13	Spain		1		1	[28]
14	Thailand		3		3	[13,35,56]
15	Turkey		1		1	[57]
16	USA	1	3	3	7	[9,26,27,36,58–60]
17	Vietnam		1		1	[61]

* Some studies were cross-country

We also examined key dependent variables or research focuses of articles reviewed to identify the scope of consumer behavior and present the research trends. As presented in Figure 3, consumer behavior mainly involved use intention, continuance intention, satisfaction, actual use, loyalty, etc. Some articles involved several keywords and vice versa. In addition, some studies have analyzed online comments [9,24,27,47] or conducted general behavioral surveys [41,45] to understand consumer behavior towards using food delivery services during the pandemic. Previous studies argued that the use of food delivery services may be associated with some outcome phenomena, such as sedentary lifestyles [62] or environmental pollution issues [63]. However, in the articles reviewed, no studies focused on outcome phenomena related to the use of food delivery services, except for Sharma et al. [50] investigating consumers' over-ordering phenomenon.

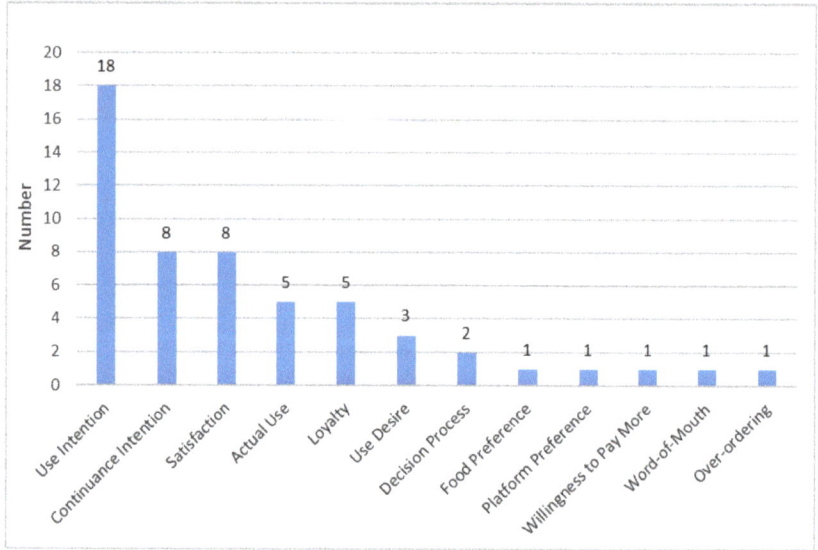

Figure 3. Key dependent variables.

In summary, this section answers research question 1, in which research trends reflected the industry trends to some degree.

3.2. Qualitative Results

We thoroughly read all the articles and coded consumer behavior and its influencing factors. Several rounds of recoding, merging, and categorization was conducted on the initial codes. Since we are concerned with factors that are broadly considered and validated by researchers, the codes that were not used frequently and could not be categorized as any theme were excluded, as well as non-significant results. Specifically, we first coded the factors that directly or indirectly influence consumer behavior in terms of using food delivery services, generating eight main themes (see Figure 4 and Section 3.2.1). Subsequently, COVID-19-related influences were highlighted (see Section 3.2.2).

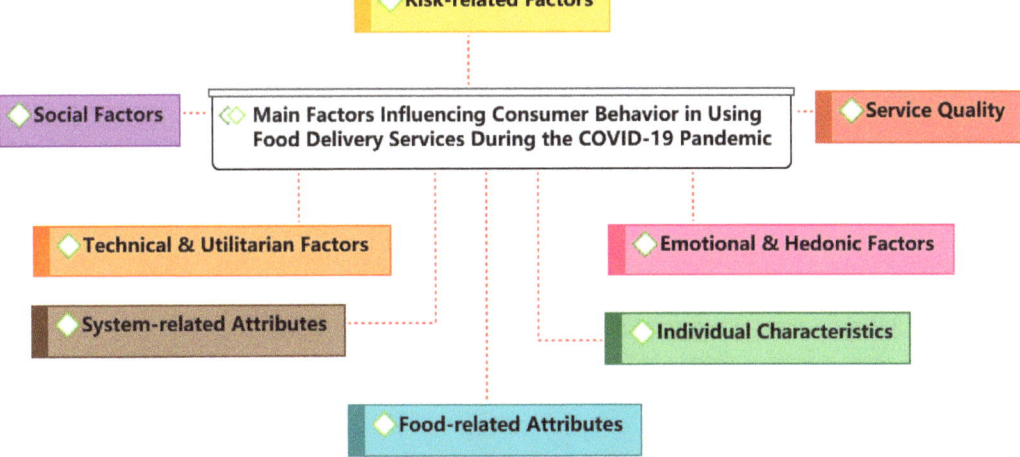

Figure 4. Main factors influencing consumer behavior.

3.2.1. General Themes

The first theme is the technical and utilitarian factors, as shown in Figure 5. The popularity of food delivery services cannot be separated from the development of e-commerce and mobile internet. As a result, the discussion always centers on the technological aspect, whether before or during the COVID-19 pandemic. Consistent with the e-commerce literature, social psychology-based technology adoption theories were often used to explain consumer behavior in the context of food delivery services, such as the technology acceptance model (TAM) [64,65] and the unified theory of acceptance and use of technology (UTAUT) [66,67]. Perceived usefulness, perceived ease of use, and their synonyms constituted the main aspects of the theme. This means that consumers are more likely to use a food delivery app if they find it useful and easy to use. Such technical attributes highlight the extrinsic (utilitarian) motivation of consumers' technology usage. Extrinsic motivation is also expressed in terms of perceived benefits, convenience, functional aspects, etc. In addition, UTAUT suggested that facilitating conditions or compatibility is also a key factor in determining consumer use of a particular technology.

The second theme is the system-related attributes, as shown in Figure 6. Consumers use food delivery services typically through mobile apps, so many studies have focused on the influence of the quality of information systems on consumer behavior. System-related attributes focused on the specific functional aspect of the food delivery app. According to the information systems success model (ISSM) [68,69], a successful information system involves three main exogenous factors: system quality, information quality, and service quality. This theme was mainly concerned with the first two factors, while service quality was discussed separately in Theme 5 because it includes not only the online part (i.e., the system aspect) but also the offline part in the context of food delivery. System-related attributes often indirectly influence consumer behavior and decision-making processes. For example, information quality and system quality may contribute to perceived usefulness [12] (see Theme 1); visual design (facility aesthetics) may evoke consumers' emotions such as dominance and pleasure [7] (see Theme 3).

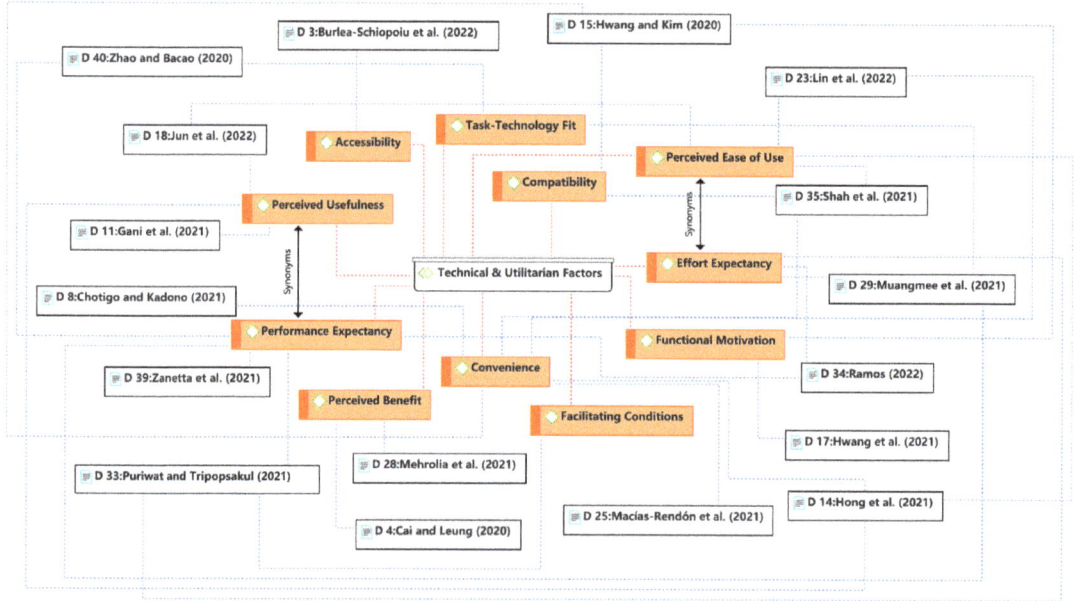

Figure 5. Theme 1: technical and utilitarian factors [6,12,13,15,26,35–37,42,44,46,48,53–56,58].

The third theme is the emotional and hedonic factors, as shown in Figure 7. Apart from cognitive-based extrinsic (utilitarian) factors (see Theme 1), emotional-based hedonic motivations are also key factors influencing consumers' technology use [67]. However, with increasing experience, the novelty contributing to hedonic motivation become less attractive [67]. Furthermore, researchers should be cautious in using hedonic motivation as a predictor in the context of focusing on utilitarian aspects (e.g., food delivery service). Previous research has shown a non-significant result of hedonic motivation [17]. Surprisingly, this review found a number of studies that reported significant effects of hedonic motivation. One possible explanation is that food delivery services may be novel to specific communities, such as new users, or that the study is on a new food delivery business model, such as drone food delivery [37]. On the other hand, the fun may not come from the use of technology but from other aspects. For example, people had limited outdoor recreation during the COVID-19 pandemic, making online ordering a meal potentially fun. The other emotional aspects have also been the focus of many studies. During the pandemic, food delivery services helped restaurants maintain their businesses, provided jobs to the unemployed, and delivered food and medicine to consumers, which enhanced the emotional connection between people and food delivery platforms [7]. In addition, consumers who used food delivery services during the COVID-19 pandemic were more likely to have positive emotions because they were more easily able to access food than non-users [70].

The fourth theme is the individual characteristics, as shown in Figure 8. In line with e-commerce literature, individual characteristics were also found to be a popular aspect influencing consumer behavior, with the most discussed being attitude and trust. Attitude is one of the core constructs of behavioral theories, such as the theory of reasoned action (TRA) [71] and the theory of planned behavior (TPB) [72]. Attitude as an individual characteristic has been broadly used in the e-commerce literature [73]. In general, consumers with positive attitudes toward information technology are more likely to use food delivery services. The role of trust has also been discussed in depth due to the uncertainty implicit in e-commerce [74–76]. In the context of food delivery, the trust may influence consumer perceptions of food quality or restaurant reputation (see Theme 8), which in turn affects the consumer decision-making process. TPB's perceived behavioral control is similar to self-efficacy from social cognitive theory (SCT) [77], which were both viewed as individual characteristics in this theme, they are the extent to which individuals believe they can master a skill. During the pandemic, self-efficacy may refer to individuals' belief that they can overcome COVID-19-related difficulties. Other individual characteristics discussed were culture (i.e., collectivism and individualism), risk propensity, personal traits (e.g., optimism), and sense of self, which may influence consumers' use of food delivery services in different ways (directly or indirectly).

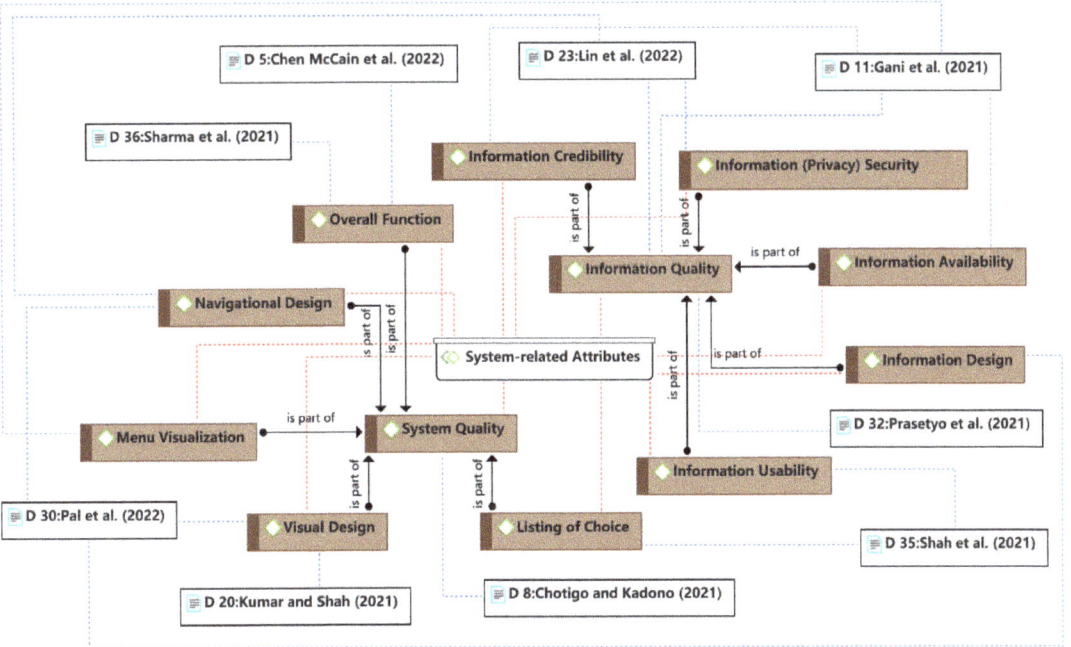

Figure 6. Theme 2: system-related attributes [7,12,27,35,44,46,49–51].

The fifth theme is the service quality, as shown in Figure 9. In the traditional marketing literature, service quality was usually used as an antecedent of satisfaction to influence consumers' purchase intention [78–80]. Similar to most O2O services, food delivery services involve both online and offline service quality [2]. Online service quality is achieved through e-service quality and platform interactivity, which are part of system service quality (see Theme 2). Offline service quality in the context of food delivery is mainly involved in delivery quality, including delivery time, order correctness, personal aspects of delivery workers, etc. Safety measures and hygiene issues of restaurants and delivery workers are new concerns of consumers caused by the COVID-19 pandemic. In addition, Cheong and Law [24] and Yang et al. [47] found that the interaction quality between restaurants and customers plays an influential role, especially during the pandemic. Such interaction can be online or offline, and the interaction with delivery workers is the most direct and most influential to the consumer's perceived service quality. Macías-Rendón et al. [48] observed that consumers provide positive comments to delivery workers during the pandemic due to empathy (see Theme 7). Nevertheless, the literature showed that consumers may complain about delivery workers for a variety of reasons [81,82].

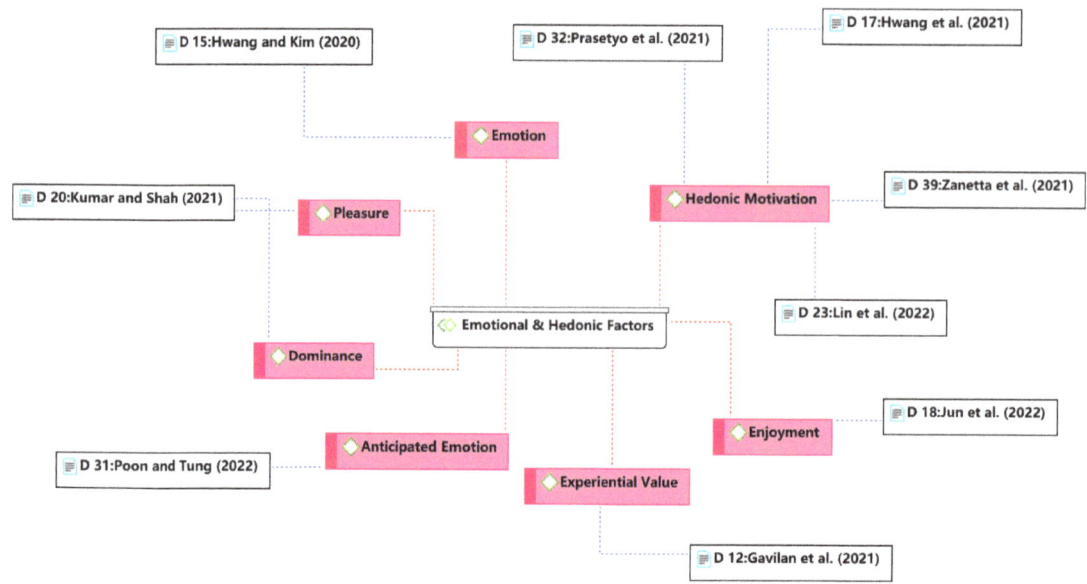

Figure 7. Theme 3: emotional and hedonic factors [7,28,37,42,44,51,52,55,58].

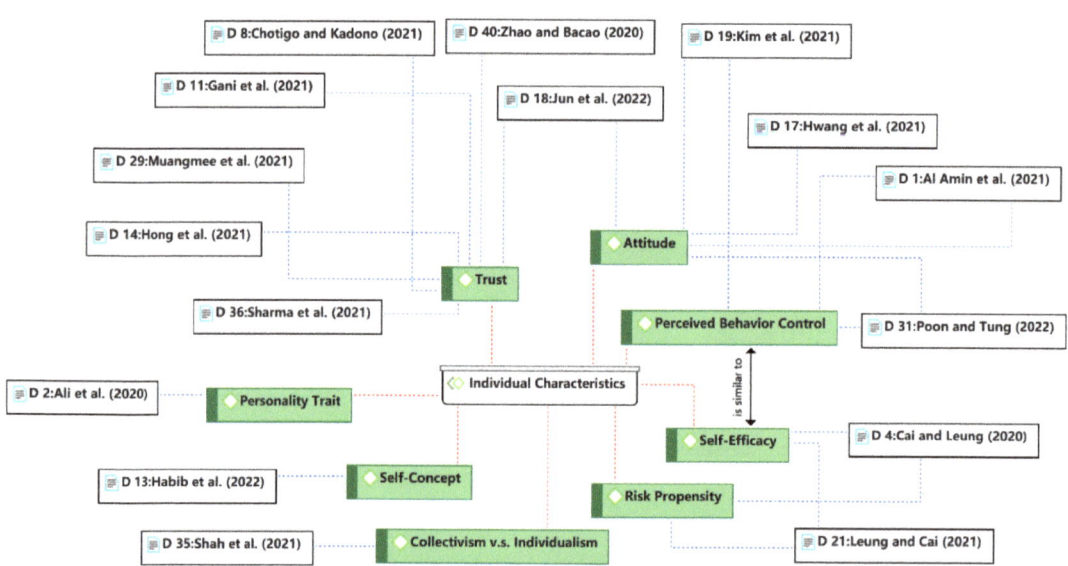

Figure 8. Theme 4: individual characteristics [6,12,23,26,35–37,39,40,43,46,50,52,56,58,59].

The sixth theme is the risk-related factors, as shown in Figure 10. As with trust discussed in Theme 5, perceived risk is widely studied in the e-commerce literature due to the uncertainty implied of the online environment. Risk-related factors formed the theme because of the increase in its discussion during the COVID-19 pandemic. Previous research has shown that perceived risk in the online environment involves many dimensions, such as performance risk, financial risk, time risk, privacy risk, and psychological risk [83]. In the reviewed studies, researchers focused on COVID-19-related risks in addition to discussing the traditional risk dimensions. Perceived risk usually negatively influences consumers' behavioral intention or attitude; however, fear of COVID-19 [13] and perceived severity [44] were found to positively influence consumers' intention to use food delivery services. This is because researchers viewed the perceived COVID-19-related risks from different perspectives (see Section 3.2.2). In addition, researchers focused more on COVID-19-related moderating effects, such as fear of COVID-19 [28], before and during the pandemic [35], severe and mild regions [26], and two COVID-19 waves [9]. COVID-19-related situations were observed to influence the consumer decision-making process in various ways.

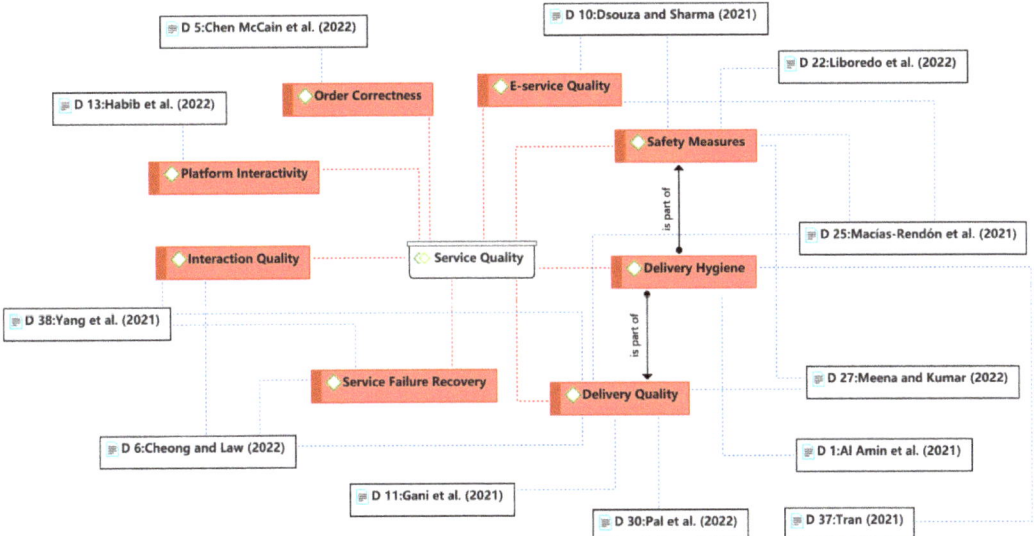

Figure 9. Theme 5: service quality [9,12,14,24,27,40,41,43,47–49,61].

The seventh theme is the social factors, as shown in Figure 11. Social factors are an essential aspect in both traditional behavioral theories (e.g., TRA and TPB) and technology use theories (e.g., UTAUUT). The subjective norm and social influence were found to be the most widely used constructs in the theme, which refer to the extent to which consumer behavior is influenced by others [66,67]. Consumer behavior in using food delivery services may be influenced by subjective norms or social pressures, as non-users (e.g., the elderly) may be socially excluded during the COVID-19 pandemic [84]. Social value is the perceived enhancement of the consumer's self-concept or social prestige by using a certain food delivery service, such as using contactless food delivery during the pandemic. Consumer social responsibility is another aspect of social factors, which has been found to influence consumer behavior during the COVID-19 pandemic, mainly in the form of support or empathy for restaurants and delivery personnel affected by the crisis. Consumers' complaints or other behaviors may make delivery workers' livelihoods precarious [81,82]. However, during the pandemic, some consumers may increase their use of food delivery services or tip delivery workers due to social responsibility or empathy. In addition, social isolation was included in the theme as it relates to compliance with social norms or social responsibility regarding public policies during the pandemic.

The eighth theme is the food-related attributes, as shown in Figure 12. The previous themes discussed why consumers use food delivery services. However, using the service is just a means for consumers to achieve their fundamental goals, namely, to purchase food. Previous studies have shown that food choice motives involve many aspects, such as health, taste, food quality, food safety, price, convenience, familiarity, etc. [21,85]. In this theme, price-related factors were the most discussed. No studies reported non-significant results for the price-related factors, except for Chotigo and Kadono [35], finding that the

COVID-19 pandemic moderated the effect of price on satisfaction. Food quality, safety, and hygiene are also of concern to consumers and researchers during the pandemic. In addition, the restaurant reputation and taste aspects remain prominent in the customer experience [24,47]. However, health factors as an important aspect of food choice motives were not discussed in the reviewed articles. One possible explanation is that dietary health was not a major concern during the pandemic compared with fundamental food needs.

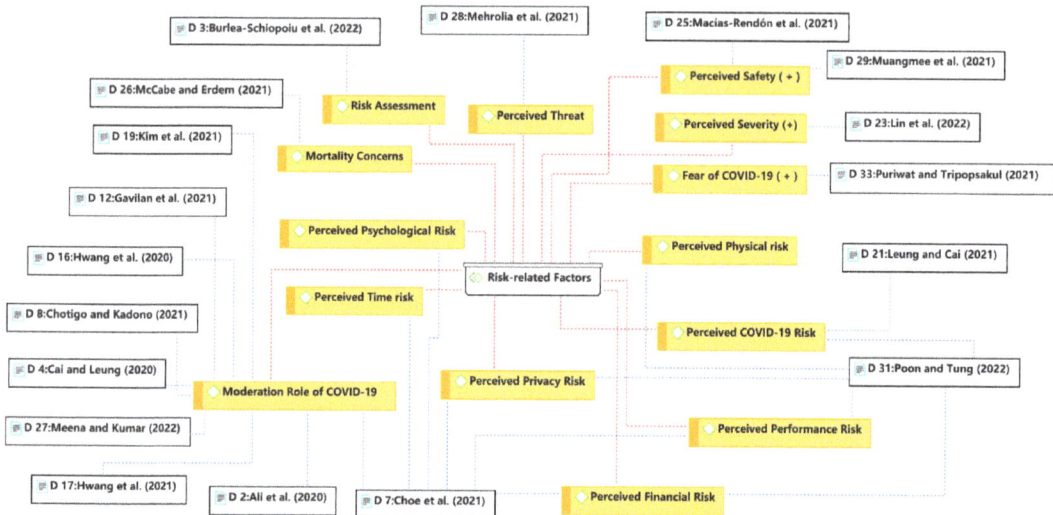

Figure 10. Theme 6: risk-related factors [9,13,15,23,26,28,34,35,37–39,44,48,52,54,56,59,60].

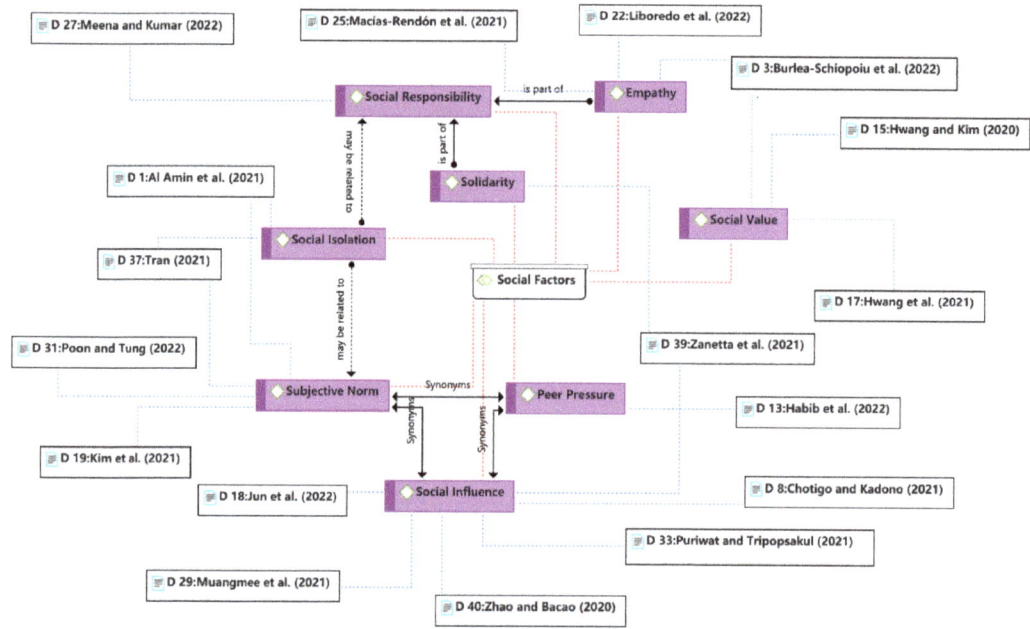

Figure 11. Theme 7: social factors [6,9,13,23,35,37,39,41–43,48,52,54–56,58,61].

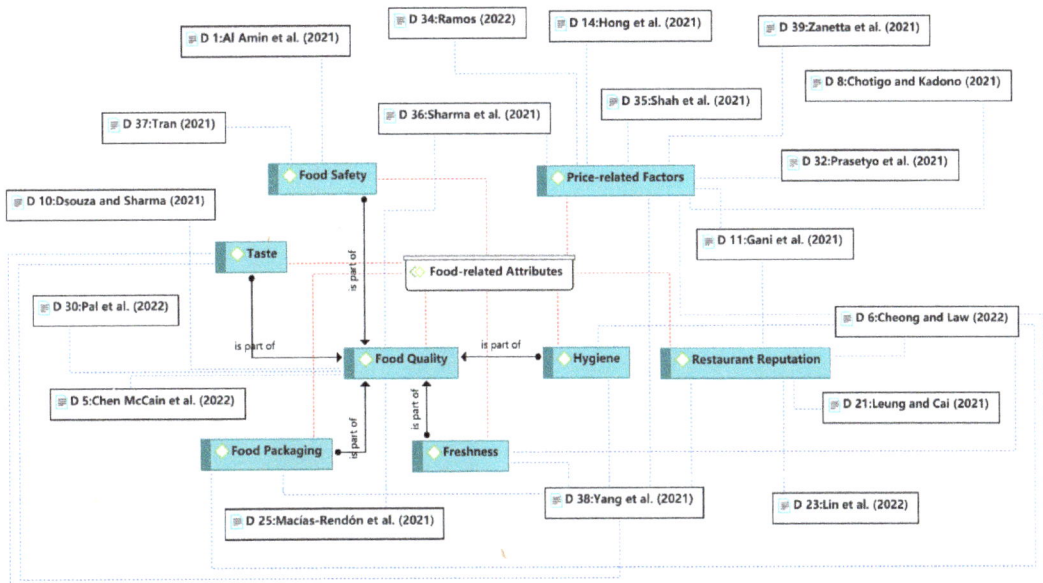

Figure 12. Theme 8: food-related attributes [12,14,24,27,35,36,40,42,44,46–51,53,59,61].

In addition to the eight themes identified, several codes that could not contribute to any themes nevertheless deserve attention, such as habit [35,42], use frequency [15,42,48], product involvement [15], consumer engagement [43], etc. Previous studies have demonstrated that habit is a key predictor of technology use [16,67]. Consumer involvement and online engagement mean more frequent use [86,87], which is related to habit formation. In fact, we are more interested in the antecedents of the habit. In other words, researchers should focus on what fosters or breaks consumers' habits in the post-pandemic era.

In summary, this section addresses research question 2, generating eight themes pertinent to the factors influencing consumers' use of food delivery services during the COVID-19 pandemic. The results are basically similar to the previous e-commerce literature [2,73], suggesting that these factors have been extensively discussed and examined in different literature. However, the elements and mechanisms of these themes may differ from those of normal times. The COVID-19-related elements are presented separately in Section 3.2.2.

3.2.2. COVID-19-Related Themes

Although conventional factors and theories can explain consumer behavior in using food delivery services during the pandemic, several new factors caused by COVID-19 have caused concern among researchers. Figure 13 presents an overview of the COVID-19-related factors. Among these, the mechanisms by which COVID-19-related risks influence consumer behavior were observed to be different. When the perceived COVID-19 risk is from online channels (i.e., delivery workers, food packaging, etc.), it negatively affects consumer behavior or behavioral intention to use food delivery services. Conversely, consumers are more likely to use online channels to purchase food if their fear is from offline channels (i.e., in-person offline purchases). Similarly, the roles of the perceived threat and perceived severity are different. Social responsibility is another topic of interest. A study found that corporate social responsibility is an important expectation of consumers during the pandemic [9]. Correspondingly, consumer social responsibility is one of the factors influencing their use of food delivery services, mainly expressed in terms of support and empathy for restaurants and delivery workers. In addition, social isolation was found to positively influence consumers' use behavior or intention, possibly due to fear of COVID-19 or social responsibility to comply with public policies. Regarding safety measures, many restaurants or platforms implemented sanitization, contactless delivery, and other measures during the pandemic to respond to consumer concerns.

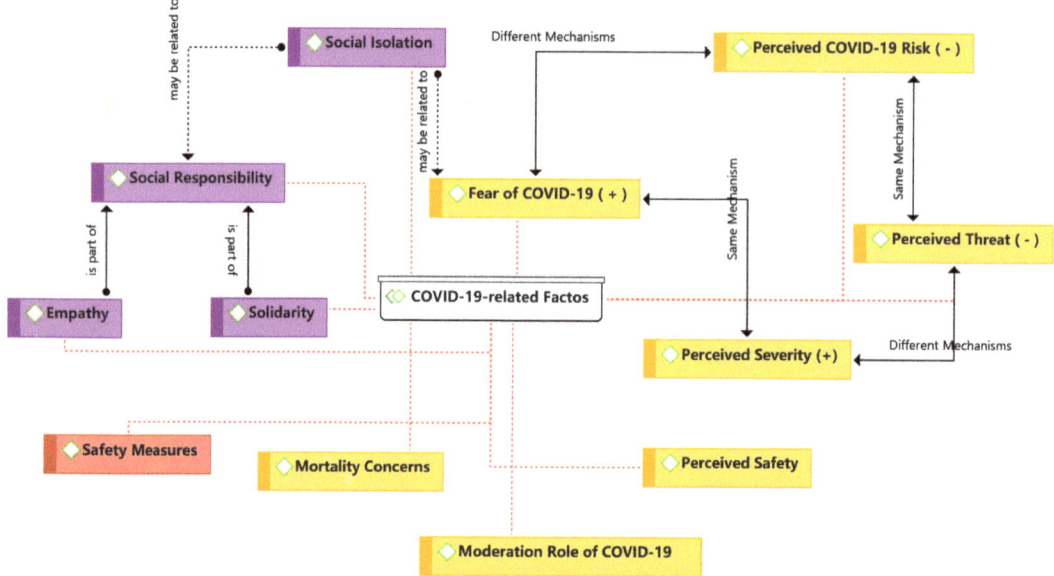

Figure 13. COVID-19-related factors.

The COVID-19 pandemic has significantly changed people's lifestyles and behaviors [23,24,39]. Several studies observed changes in consumer behavior in terms of using food delivery services during the pandemic, as shown in Figure 14. In line with most industry reports on food delivery services, Chotigo and Kadono [35] and Hong et al. [36] observed an increase in the frequency of use or number of new users. However, some studies observed a decrease in use [15,41,45]. One of the possible reasons for the inconsistency is the different mechanisms of consumers' perceived COVID-19-related risks, as mentioned previously. Other reasons may come from differences in sample, culture, policy, etc. For example, students use fewer food delivery services when they study at home and live with their parents during the pandemic [45]; some users clean food packaging or reheat delivered food before consumption for various reasons [41]. Additionally, previous studies have shown that people aware of health risks may change their behavior in a preventive way [88–90]. This means that more new users may use the food delivery service, while existing ones may be more cautious.

During the COVID-19 pandemic, consumers were more concerned about safety measures and social responsibility than the usual expectations (e.g., prompt service and good taste). The pandemic may also influence consumers' food choice preferences. Consumers may prefer food from their own culture because people counteract the psychological threat of death by supporting positive evaluations of their own cultural products [60]. On the other hand, the COVID-19 pandemic has had positive consequences in terms of technological advances and business model innovation. Consumers began to experiment with new technologies, such as drone delivery [39]; restaurants began to offer new services, such as Home Chef and DIY meal kits [28].

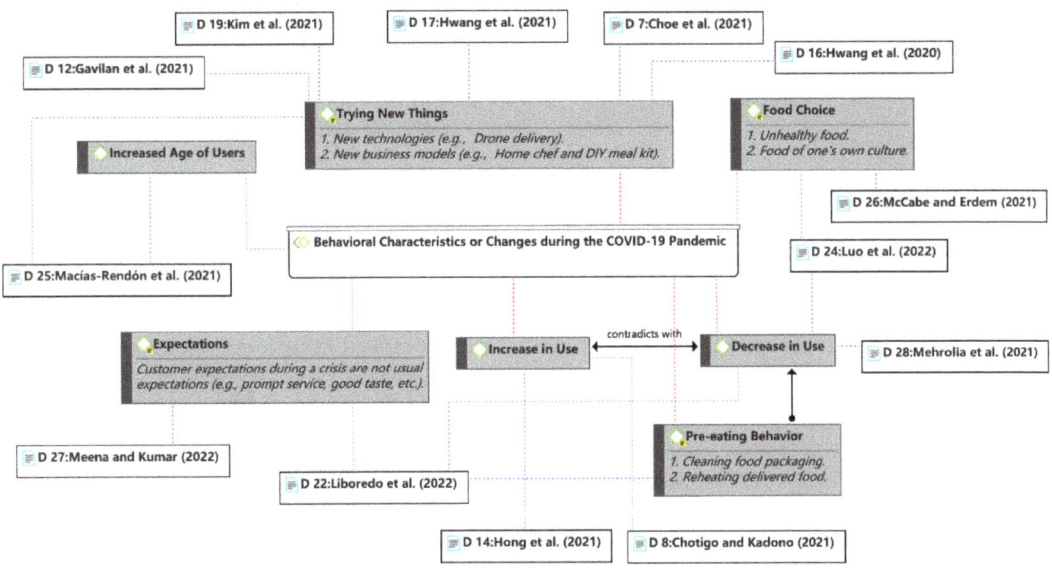

Figure 14. Observed behavioral characteristics or changes [9,15,28,34–39,41,45,48,60].

A study found that younger consumers are more likely to use food delivery services than older generations [36]. In fact, the respondents mentioned in most of the studies reviewed the young generations were predominant (i.e., Generation Y and Z). Nonetheless, the average age of users was observed to be significantly higher compared with that before the COVID-19 pandemic [48]. In addition, although an increase in the consumption of unhealthy foods was observed [45], the relationship between the use of food delivery services and unhealthy lifestyles during the pandemic has not been discussed.

To summarize, this section answers research question 3, partially presenting the influence of the COVID-19 pandemic on consumers in terms of using food delivery services.

3.3. Future Research Directions

As discussed in Section 1, it is necessary to continue studying consumer behavior in food delivery services in the post-pandemic era. Several future research directions are suggested based on our results.

3.3.1. Dependent Variables or Outcome Phenomena

Firstly, since relatively few studies have focused on consumer behavior in the post-COVID-19 era, it is unclear whether consumers will continue to use food delivery services as frequently as they did during the pandemic. Consequently, consumers' continued use intention or behavior can be one of the future research directions.

Secondly, overusing food delivery services may be associated with unhealthy lifestyles or negative outcomes. The use of food delivery services may contribute to a sedentary lifestyle, increasing the risk of adverse health outcomes [62]. Food safety and health issues have raised people's concerns [91,92]; however, online food delivery platforms always seem to promote unhealthy food [93]. During the pandemic, people's diets changed, especially as unhealthy diets increased [45,93,94]. Although Sharma et al. [50] investigated the over-ordering of food delivery service users, the discussion of the negative outcomes is not enough. Therefore, exploring the relationship between the use of food delivery services and unhealthy lifestyles or negative outcomes is suggested as a future research direction.

Thirdly, consumers' green consumption behavior is another outcome phenomenon that needs to be concerned. Although green consumer behavior has long been discussed [95,96], it seems to be ignored in the food delivery industry, especially during the pandemic when people suffer from COVID-19. A large number of food delivery orders means massive amounts of packaging materials, typically non-biodegradable and challenging to recycle, leading to serious environmental problems [63]. Thus, future research should pay attention to green consumption issues in the food delivery industry.

3.3.2. Independent Variables or Factors

The development of new habits or the disappearance of old ones depends on many aspects, such as individual social context changes, technological advances, public policies, natural disasters, etc. [25]. Future research can examine potential interventions to foster or break habits of using food delivery services. Furthermore, despite the efforts of restaurants and food delivery platforms to adopt various measures to encourage consumer purchases during the pandemic, the continued effectiveness of such marketing strategies is unclear. Maintaining these marketing efforts can challenge small and medium-sized restaurants or companies [14]. Therefore, it makes sense to continue studying the factors influencing consumer behavior (i.e., existing marketing strategies) in the post-pandemic era to develop new marketing strategies.

New factors are also worth being investigated. First, although consumer involvement and online engagement do not form any themes, they should continue to be studied. They mean more frequent use and may be related to habit formation. Second, consumer social responsibility is another future research direction. While existing studies have discussed the influences of consumer responsibility on the use of food delivery services during a pandemic, many other dimensions of consumer responsibility have received little attention, such as environmental responsibility.

3.3.3. Research Contexts

The food delivery service is a broad category not only limited to ready-to-eat food delivery, which we can call O2O delivery service or to-home O2O business model. The COVID-19 pandemic has spawned many new business models, and more new ones will emerge as technology develops. For example, the concept of "food delivery" in China is constantly being broadened, with the rapid development of instant delivery services represented by fresh food and medicine [97]; drone delivery service in Korea is favored for its novelty and contactless delivery [39]; restaurants in Spain offer standard delivery services as well as experiential services such as Home Chef and DIY meal kits [28]. Future research can therefore focus on new research contexts, i.e., new business models.

In addition, the elderly suffered from increased social exclusion during the COVID-19 pandemic due to their inability to access food and necessities through food delivery platforms [84]. Technology acceptance and use among the elderly should be of concern to researchers. However, existing studies mainly investigated the younger generations of O2O delivery service users rather than the older ones. Therefore, future research can focus on the acceptance of technology or business models in the context of the elderly.

4. Conclusions

The popularity of e-commerce and mobile internet allows consumers to purchase food online through B2C or O2O models. The COVID-19 pandemic has accelerated the development of these business models, especially the to-home O2O, namely the food delivery service business. The provision or use of food delivery services is expected to become a new normal in the post-pandemic era. However, the discussion on consumer behavior toward food delivery services will continue. Therefore, the purpose of this paper was to review the literature on consumers' use of food delivery services during the COVID-19 pandemic to offer a foundation and insights for future research.

A thematic review was conducted in this paper, with 40 articles published from 2020 to the present being reviewed. The quantitative results showed the current research trends and, to some extent, reflect the industry trends. The qualitative results mainly generated eight themes regarding the factors that influence consumer behavior in using food delivery services: (1) technical and utilitarian factors, (2) system-related attributes, (3) emotional and hedonic factors, (4) individual characteristics, (5) service quality, (6) risk-related factors, (7) social factors, and (8) food-related attributes. The influence of COVID-19 was subsequently highlighted. Based on the results, future research directions were suggested in three aspects: (1) dependent variables or outcome phenomena, (2) independent variables or factors, and (3) research contexts.

4.1. Contributions

This paper brings contributions in several aspects. First of all, this paper presents an overview to policymakers regarding consumer behavior in certain aspects in times of crisis. Meanwhile, this paper offers starting points for future research. It is comprehensive enough to help scholars understand how themes are formed and detailed enough to allow many different sub-themes to be focused on.

This paper also provides beneficial insights for marketers and managers in food-related industries. First, despite the similarity of the eight themes identified to previous marketing literature, their composition and the way they work may be different. Marketers and managers can gain a more comprehensive understanding of consumer behavior from this paper to reconsider their marketing strategies. Second, consumers may have different expectations in times of crisis than in normal times, for example, they may place more value on corporate social responsibility. Lastly, restaurants and food delivery platforms should manage human resources well in terms of delivery workers. Delivery is an essential part of the industry, and the delivery worker's performance can directly influence the customer experience. Consumer behavior may, in turn, lead to precariousness among food delivery workers.

4.2. Limitations

A number of limitations need to be noted regarding this review paper. First, although we developed a detailed and comprehensive literature search strategy, it is possible to miss some valuable articles. Second, while the most difficult period of the COVID-19 pandemic has passed, relevant studies may be in the process of being published, resulting in not being included in this review. Lastly, the thematic review approach cannot examine the effectiveness of previous studies. Notwithstanding these limitations, this review benefits the industry practice and future research of O2O food delivery services.

Author Contributions: Conceptualization, Y.L. and P.Y.; methodology, P.Y. and S.O.; investigation, Y.L., P.Y., S.O. and N.Z.; formal analysis, Y.L., P.Y., S.O., N.Z. and M.F.S.; writing—original draft preparation, P.Y.; writing—review and editing, S.O., N.Z. and M.F.S.; visualization, P.Y.; supervision, P.Y. All authors have read and agreed to the published version of the manuscript.

Funding: This research received no external funding.

Institutional Review Board Statement: Not applicable.

Informed Consent Statement: Not applicable.

Data Availability Statement: Not applicable.

Conflicts of Interest: The authors declare no conflict of interest.

Appendix A

Table A1. A list of articles included in the review.

No.	Articles	Journals
1	Al Amin et al. (2021) [40]	*Journal of Food Products Marketing*
2	Ali et al. (2020) [23]	*Journal of Open Innovation: Technology, Market, and Complexity*

Table A1. Cont.

No.	Articles	Journals
3	Burlea-Schiopoiu et al. (2022) [54]	Socio-Economic Planning Sciences
4	Cai and Leung (2020) [26]	International Journal of Hospitality Management
5	Chen McCain et al. (2022) [27]	British Food Journal
6	Cheong and Law (2022) [24]	International Journal of Environmental Research and Public Health
7	Choe et al. (2021) [34]	International Journal of Contemporary Hospitality Management
8	Chotigo and Kadono (2021) [35]	Sustainability
9	Dirsehan and Cankat (2021) [57]	Journal of Retailing and Consumer Services
10	Dsouza and Sharma (2021) [14]	International Journal of Innovation Science
11	Gani et al. (2021) * [12]	Journal of Foodservice Business Research
12	Gavilan et al. (2021) [28]	International Journal of Gastronomy and Food Science
13	Habib et al. (2022) [43]	Future Business Journal
14	Hong et al. (2021) [36]	Journal of Hospitality and Tourism Management
15	Hwang and Kim (2020) [55]	Sustainability
16	Hwang et al. (2020) [38]	International Journal of Environmental Research and Public Health
17	Hwang et al. (2021) [37]	Journal of Travel and Tourism Marketing
18	Jun et al. (2022) [58]	Foods
19	Kim et al. (2021) [39]	International Journal of Hospitality Management
20	Kumar and Shah (2021) [7]	Journal of Retailing and Consumer Services
21	Leung and Cai (2021) [59]	Journal of Hospitality and Tourism Management
22	Liboredo et al. (2022) * [41]	Nutrition & Food Science
23	Lin et al. (2022) [44]	Sustainability
24	Luo et al. (2022) [45]	European Journal of Nutrition
25	Macías-Rendón et al. (2021) [48]	Estudios Gerenciales
26	McCabe and Erdem (2021) [60]	Journal of Applied Social Psychology
27	Meena and Kumar (2022) [9]	Journal of Retailing and Consumer Services
28	Mehrolia et al. (2021) [15]	International Journal of Consumer Studies
29	Muangmee et al. (2021) [56]	Journal of Theoretical and Applied Electronic Commerce Research
30	Pal et al. (2022) [49]	Journal of Foodservice Business Research
31	Poon and Tung (2022) * [52]	European Journal of Management and Business Economics
32	Prasetyo et al. (2021) [51]	Journal of Open Innovation: Technology, Market, and Complexity
33	Puriwat and Tripopsakul (2021) [13]	Emerging Science Journal
34	Ramos (2022) [53]	British Food Journal
35	Shah et al. (2021) * [46]	British Food Journal
36	Sharma et al. (2021) [50]	International Journal of Hospitality Management
37	Tran (2021) [61]	Sustainability
38	Yang et al. (2021) [47]	International Journal of Hospitality Management
39	Zanetta et al. (2021) [42]	Food Research International
40	Zhao and Bacao (2020) [6]	International Journal of Hospitality Management

* Article in press (early access).

References

1. Wang, O.; Somogyi, S.; Charlebois, S. Food Choice in the E-Commerce Era: A Comparison between Business-to-Consumer (B2C), Online-to-Offline (O2O) and New Retail. *Br. Food J.* **2020**, *122*, 1215–1237. [CrossRef]
2. Yao, P.; Osman, S.; Sabri, M.F.; Zainudin, N. Consumer Behavior in Online-to-Offline (O2O) Commerce: A Thematic Review. *Sustainability* **2022**, *14*, 7842. [CrossRef]
3. Talwar, S.; Dhir, A.; Scuotto, V.; Kaur, P. Barriers and Paradoxical Recommendation Behaviour in Online to Offline (O2O) Services. A Convergent Mixed-Method Study. *J. Bus. Res.* **2021**, *131*, 25–39. [CrossRef]
4. World Health Organization. Coronavirus Disease (COVID-19). Available online: https://www.who.int/health-topics/coronavirus (accessed on 24 October 2022).
5. World Health Organization. Advice for the Public on COVID-19–World Health Organization. Available online: https://www.who.int/emergencies/diseases/novel-coronavirus-2019/advice-for-public (accessed on 23 October 2022).
6. Zhao, Y.; Bacao, F. What Factors Determining Customer Continuingly Using Food Delivery Apps during 2019 Novel Coronavirus Pandemic Period? *Int. J. Hosp. Manag.* **2020**, *91*, 102683. [CrossRef]
7. Kumar, S.; Shah, A. Revisiting Food Delivery Apps during COVID-19 Pandemic? Investigating the Role of Emotions. *J. Retail. Consum. Serv.* **2021**, *62*, 102595. [CrossRef]
8. Statista. Year-Over-Year Daily Change in Seated Restaurant Diners due to the Coronavirus (COVID-19) Pandemic Worldwide from 24 February 2020 to 1 August 2022. Available online: https://www.statista.com/statistics/1103928/coronavirus-restaurant-visitation-impact/ (accessed on 22 October 2022).

9. Meena, P.; Kumar, G. Online Food Delivery Companies' Performance and Consumers Expectations during COIVD-19: An Investigation Using Machine Learning Approach. *J. Retail. Consum. Serv.* **2022**, *68*, 103052. [CrossRef]
10. Statista. Number of Users of the Online Food Delivery Market Worldwide from 2017 to 2026. Available online: https://www.statista.com/forecasts/891088/online-food-delivery-users-by-segment-worldwide (accessed on 18 October 2022).
11. Statista. Restaurant Food Delivery Growth in Selected Countries Worldwide between 2019 and 2020. Available online: https://www.statista.com/statistics/1238889/restaurant-food-delivery-growth-in-selected-countries-worldwide/ (accessed on 18 October 2022).
12. Gani, M.O.; Faroque, A.R.; Muzareba, A.M.; Amin, S.; Rahman, M. An Integrated Model to Decipher Online Food Delivery App Adoption Behavior in the COVID-19 Pandemic. *J. Foodserv. Bus. Res.* **2021**; *ahead-of-print*. [CrossRef]
13. Puriwat, W.; Tripopsakul, S. Understanding Food Delivery Mobile Application Technology Adoption: A UTAUT Model Integrating Perceived Fear of COVID-19. *Emerg. Sci. J.* **2021**, *5*, 94–104. [CrossRef]
14. Dsouza, D.; Sharma, D. Online Food Delivery Portals during COVID-19 Times: An Analysis of Changing Consumer Behavior and Expectations. *Int. J. Innov. Sci.* **2021**, *13*, 218–232. [CrossRef]
15. Mehrolia, S.; Alagarsamy, S.; Solaikutty, V.M. Customers Response to Online Food Delivery Services during COVID-19 Outbreak Using Binary Logistic Regression. *Int. J. Consum. Stud.* **2021**, *45*, 396–408. [CrossRef]
16. Alalwan, A.A. Mobile Food Ordering Apps: An Empirical Study of the Factors Affecting Customer e-Satisfaction and Continued Intention to Reuse. *Int. J. Inf. Manag.* **2020**, *50*, 28–44. [CrossRef]
17. Lee, S.W.; Sung, H.J.; Jeon, H.M. Determinants of Continuous Intention on Food Delivery Apps: Extending UTAUT2 with Information Quality. *Sustainability* **2019**, *11*, 3141. [CrossRef]
18. Roh, M.; Park, K. Adoption of O2O Food Delivery Services in South Korea: The Moderating Role of Moral Obligation in Meal Preparation. *Int. J. Inf. Manag.* **2019**, *47*, 262–273. [CrossRef]
19. Choi, Y.; Zhang, L.; Debbarma, J.; Lee, H. Sustainable Management of Online to Offline Delivery Apps for Consumers' Reuse Intention: Focused on the Meituan Apps. *Sustainability* **2021**, *13*, 3593. [CrossRef]
20. Zhang, Y.-B.; Kim, H.-K. A Study on the Factors Affecting Satisfaction and Reuse Intention among Customers Using O2O Delivery Platform in China. *J. Syst. Manag. Sci.* **2021**, *11*, 58–74. [CrossRef]
21. Wang, O.; Scrimgeour, F. Consumer Adoption of Online-to-Offline Food Delivery Services in China and New Zealand. *Br. Food J.* **2021**, *124*, 1590–1608. [CrossRef]
22. Laato, S.; Islam, A.K.M.N.; Farooq, A.; Dhir, A. Unusual Purchasing Behavior during the Early Stages of the COVID-19 Pandemic: The Stimulus-Organism-Response Approach. *J. Retail. Consum. Serv.* **2020**, *57*, 102224. [CrossRef]
23. Ali, S.; Khalid, N.; Javed, H.M.U.; Islam, D.M.Z. Consumer Adoption of Online Food Delivery Ordering (OFDO) Services in Pakistan: The Impact of the COVID-19 Pandemic Situation. *J. Open Innov. Technol. Mark. Complex.* **2020**, *7*, 10. [CrossRef]
24. Cheong, F.; Law, R. Will Macau's Restaurants Survive or Thrive after Entering the O2O Food Delivery Platform in the COVID-19 Pandemic? *Int. J. Environ. Res. Public. Health* **2022**, *19*, 5100. [CrossRef]
25. Sheth, J. Impact of COVID-19 on Consumer Behavior: Will the Old Habits Return or Die? *J. Bus. Res.* **2020**, *117*, 280–283. [CrossRef]
26. Cai, R.; Leung, X.Y. Mindset Matters in Purchasing Online Food Deliveries during the Pandemic: The Application of Construal Level and Regulatory Focus Theories. *Int. J. Hosp. Manag.* **2020**, *91*, 102677. [CrossRef]
27. Chen McCain, S.-L.; Lolli, J.; Liu, E.; Lin, L.-C. An Analysis of a Third-Party Food Delivery App during the COVID-19 Pandemic. *Br. Food J.* **2022**, *124*, 3032–3052. [CrossRef]
28. Gavilan, D.; Balderas-Cejudo, A.; Fernández-Lores, S.; Martinez-Navarro, G. Innovation in Online Food Delivery: Learnings from COVID-19. *Int. J. Gastron. Food Sci.* **2021**, *24*, 100330. [CrossRef] [PubMed]
29. Greetham, B. *How to Write Your Literature Review*; Red Global Press: London, UK, 2020; ISBN 978-1-352-01104-3.
30. Cook, D.A. Narrowing the Focus and Broadening Horizons: Complementary Roles for Systematic and Nonsystematic Reviews. *Adv. Health Sci. Educ.* **2008**, *13*, 391–395. [CrossRef] [PubMed]
31. Zairul, M. A Thematic Review on Student-Centred Learning in the Studio Education. *J. Crit. Rev.* **2020**, *7*, 504–511. [CrossRef]
32. Zairul, M. A Thematic Review on Industrialised Building System (IBS) Publications from 2015–2019: Analysis of Patterns and Trends for Future Studies of Ibs in Malaysia. *Pertanika J. Soc. Sci. Humanit.* **2021**, *29*, 635–652. [CrossRef]
33. Zairul, M. Opening the Pandora's Box of Issues in the Industrialised Building System (IBS) in Malaysia: A Thematic Review. *J. Appl. Sci. Eng.* **2022**, *25*, 297–310. [CrossRef]
34. Choe, J.Y.; Kim, J.J.; Hwang, J. Perceived Risks from Drone Food Delivery Services before and after COVID-19. *Int. J. Contemp. Hosp. Manag.* **2021**, *33*, 1276–1296. [CrossRef]
35. Chotigo, J.; Kadono, Y. Comparative Analysis of Key Factors Encouraging Food Delivery App Adoption Before and During the COVID-19 Pandemic in Thailand. *Sustainability* **2021**, *13*, 4088. [CrossRef]
36. Hong, C.; Choi, H.; Choi, E.-K.; Joung, H.-W. Factors Affecting Customer Intention to Use Online Food Delivery Services before and during the COVID-19 Pandemic. *J. Hosp. Tour. Manag.* **2021**, *48*, 509–518. [CrossRef]
37. Hwang, J.; Choe, J.Y.; Choi, Y.G.; Kim, J.J. A Comparative Study on the Motivated Consumer Innovativeness of Drone Food Delivery Services before and after the Outbreak of COVID-19. *J. Travel Tour. Mark.* **2021**, *38*, 368–382. [CrossRef]
38. Hwang, J.; Kim, D.; Kim, J.J. How to Form Behavioral Intentions in the Field of Drone Food Delivery Services: The Moderating Role of the COVID-19 Outbreak. *Int. J. Environ. Res. Public. Health* **2020**, *17*, 9117. [CrossRef] [PubMed]

39. Kim, J.J.; Kim, I.; Hwang, J. A Change of Perceived Innovativeness for Contactless Food Delivery Services Using Drones after the Outbreak of COVID-19. *Int. J. Hosp. Manag.* **2021**, *93*, 102758. [CrossRef]
40. Al Amin, M.; Arefin, M.S.; Alam, M.R.; Ahammad, T.; Hoque, M.R. Using Mobile Food Delivery Applications during COVID-19 Pandemic: An Extended Model of Planned Behavior. *J. Food Prod. Mark.* **2021**, *27*, 105–126. [CrossRef]
41. Liboredo, J.C.; Amaral, C.A.A.; Carvalho, N.C. Food Delivery before and during the COVID-19 Pandemic in Brazil. *Nutr. Food Sci.* 2022; ahead-of-print. [CrossRef]
42. Zanetta, L.D.; Hakim, M.P.; Gastaldi, G.B.; Seabra, L.M.J.; Rolim, P.M.; Nascimento, L.G.P.; Medeiros, C.O.; da Cunha, D.T. The Use of Food Delivery Apps during the COVID-19 Pandemic in Brazil: The Role of Solidarity, Perceived Risk, and Regional Aspects. *Food Res. Int.* **2021**, *149*, 110671. [CrossRef] [PubMed]
43. Habib, A.; Irfan, M.; Shahzad, M. Modeling the Enablers of Online Consumer Engagement and Platform Preference in Online Food Delivery Platforms during COVID-19. *Future Bus. J.* **2022**, *8*, 6. [CrossRef]
44. Lin, Y.; Marjerison, R.K.; Choi, J.; Chae, C. Supply Chain Sustainability during COVID-19: Last Mile Food Delivery in China. *Sustainability* **2022**, *14*, 1484. [CrossRef]
45. Luo, M.; Wang, Q.; Yang, S.; Jia, P. Changes in Patterns of Take-Away Food Ordering among Youths before and after COVID-19 Lockdown in China: The COVID-19 Impact on Lifestyle Change Survey (COINLICS). *Eur. J. Nutr.* **2022**, *61*, 1121–1131. [CrossRef] [PubMed]
46. Shah, A.M.; Yan, X.; Qayyum, A. Adoption of Mobile Food Ordering Apps for O2O Food Delivery Services during the COVID-19 Outbreak. *Br. Food J.* **2022**, *124*, 3368–3395. [CrossRef]
47. Yang, F.X.; Li, X.; Lau, V.M.-C.; Zhu, V.Z. To Survive or to Thrive? China's Luxury Hotel Restaurants Entering O2O Food Delivery Platforms amid the COVID-19 Crisis. *Int. J. Hosp. Manag.* **2021**, *94*, 102855. [CrossRef]
48. Macías-Rendón, W.; Rodríguez-Morales, K.; Barriga-Medina, H.R. COVID-19 Lockdown and the Satisfaction with Online Food Delivery Providers. *Estud. Gerenciales* **2021**, *37*, 200–209. [CrossRef]
49. Pal, D.; Funilkul, S.; Eamsinvattana, W.; Siyal, S. Using Online Food Delivery Applications during the COVID-19 Lockdown Period: What Drives University Students' Satisfaction and Loyalty? *J. Foodserv. Bus. Res.* **2022**, *25*, 561–605. [CrossRef]
50. Sharma, R.; Dhir, A.; Talwar, S.; Kaur, P. Over-Ordering and Food Waste: The Use of Food Delivery Apps during a Pandemic. *Int. J. Hosp. Manag.* **2021**, *96*, 102977. [CrossRef]
51. Prasetyo, Y.T.; Tanto, H.; Mariyanto, M.; Hanjaya, C.; Young, M.N.; Persada, S.F.; Miraja, B.A.; Redi, A.A.N.P. Factors Affecting Customer Satisfaction and Loyalty in Online Food Delivery Service during the COVID-19 Pandemic: Its Relation with Open Innovation. *J. Open Innov. Technol. Mark. Complex.* **2021**, *7*, 76. [CrossRef]
52. Poon, W.C.; Tung, S.E.H. The Rise of Online Food Delivery Culture during the COVID-19 Pandemic: An Analysis of Intention and Its Associated Risk. *Eur. J. Manag. Bus. Econ.* 2022; ahead-of-print. [CrossRef]
53. Ramos, K. Factors Influencing Customers' Continuance Usage Intention of Food Delivery Apps during COVID-19 Quarantine in Mexico. *Br. Food J.* **2022**, *124*, 833–852. [CrossRef]
54. Burlea-Schiopoiu, A.; Puiu, S.; Dinu, A. The Impact of Food Delivery Applications on Romanian Consumers' Behaviour during the COVID-19 Pandemic. *Socioecon. Plann. Sci.* **2022**, *82*, 101220. [CrossRef]
55. Hwang, J.; Kim, H. The Effects of Expected Benefits on Image, Desire, and Behavioral Intentions in the Field of Drone Food Delivery Services after the Outbreak of COVID-19. *Sustainability* **2020**, *13*, 117. [CrossRef]
56. Muangmee, C.; Kot, S.; Meekaewkunchorn, N.; Kassakorn, N.; Khalid, B. Factors Determining the Behavioral Intention of Using Food Delivery Apps during COVID-19 Pandemics. *J. Theor. Appl. Electron. Commer. Res.* **2021**, *16*, 1297–1310. [CrossRef]
57. Dirsehan, T.; Cankat, E. Role of Mobile Food-Ordering Applications in Developing Restaurants' Brand Satisfaction and Loyalty in the Pandemic Period. *J. Retail. Consum. Serv.* **2021**, *62*, 102608. [CrossRef]
58. Jun, K.; Yoon, B.; Lee, S.; Lee, D.-S. Factors Influencing Customer Decisions to Use Online Food Delivery Service during the Covid-19 Pandemic. *Foods* **2022**, *11*, 64. [CrossRef]
59. Leung, X.Y.; Cai, R. How Pandemic Severity Moderates Digital Food Ordering Risks during COVID-19: An Application of Prospect Theory and Risk Perception Framework. *J. Hosp. Tour. Manag.* **2021**, *47*, 497–505. [CrossRef]
60. McCabe, S.; Erdem, S. The Influence of Mortality Reminders on Cultural In-group versus Out-group Takeaway Food Safety Perceptions during the COVID-19 Pandemic. *J. Appl. Soc. Psychol.* **2021**, *51*, 363–369. [CrossRef] [PubMed]
61. Tran, V.D. Using Mobile Food Delivery Applications during the Covid-19 Pandemic: Applying the Theory of Planned Behavior to Examine Continuance Behavior. *Sustainability* **2021**, *13*, 12066. [CrossRef]
62. Li, L.; Wang, D. Do Neighborhood Food Environments Matter for Eating through Online-to-Offline Food Delivery Services? *Appl. Geogr.* **2022**, *138*, 102620. [CrossRef]
63. Pan, C.; Lei, Y.; Wu, J.; Wang, Y. The Influence of Green Packaging on Consumers' Green Purchase Intention in the Context of Online-to-Offline Commerce. *J. Syst. Inf. Technol.* **2021**, *23*, 133–153. [CrossRef]
64. Davis, F.D. Perceived Usefulness, Perceived Ease of Use, and User Acceptance of Information Technology. *MIS Q.* **1989**, *13*, 319. [CrossRef]
65. Davis, F.D.; Bagozzi, R.P.; Warshaw, P.R. User Acceptance of Computer Technology: A Comparison of Two Theoretical Models. *Manag. Sci.* **1989**, *35*, 982–1003. [CrossRef]
66. Venkatesh, V.; Morris, M.G.; Davis, G.B.; Davis, F.D. User Acceptance of Information Technology: Toward a Unified View. *MIS Q.* **2003**, *27*, 425. [CrossRef]

67. Venkatesh, V.; Thong, J.Y.L.; Xu, X. Consumer Acceptance and Use of Information Technology: Extending the Unified Theory of Acceptance and Use of Technology. *MIS Q.* **2012**, *36*, 157. [CrossRef]
68. DeLone, W.H.; McLean, E.R. Information Systems Success: The Quest for the Dependent Variable. *Inf. Syst. Res.* **1992**, *3*, 60–95. [CrossRef]
69. DeLone, W.H.; McLean, E.R. The DeLone and McLean Model of Information Systems Success: A Ten-Year Update. *J. Manag. Inf. Syst.* **2003**, *19*, 9–30. [CrossRef]
70. Liu, Q.; Liu, Z.; Lin, S.; Zhao, P. Perceived Accessibility and Mental Health Consequences of COVID-19 Containment Policies. *J. Transp. Health* **2022**, *25*, 101354. [CrossRef] [PubMed]
71. Fishbein, M.; Ajzen, I. *Belief, Attitude, Intention, and Behavior: An Introduction to Theory and Research*; Addison-Wesley Series in Social Psychology; Addison-Wesley: Reading, MA, USA, 1975; ISBN 978-0-201-02089-2.
72. Ajzen, I. The Theory of Planned Behavior. *Organ. Behav. Hum. Decis. Process.* **1991**, *50*, 179–211. [CrossRef]
73. Haryanti, T.; Subriadi, A.P. Factors and Theories for E-Commerce Adoption: A Literature Review. *Int. J. Electron. Commer. Stud.* **2020**, *11*, 87–105. [CrossRef]
74. Gefen; Karahanna; Straub Trust and TAM in Online Shopping: An Integrated Model. *MIS Q.* **2003**, *27*, 51. [CrossRef]
75. McKnight, D.H.; Chervany, N.L. What Trust Means in E-Commerce Customer Relationships: An Interdisciplinary Conceptual Typology. *Int. J. Electron. Commer.* **2001**, *6*, 35–59. [CrossRef]
76. Pavlou, P.A. Consumer Acceptance of Electronic Commerce: Integrating Trust and Risk with the Technology Acceptance Model. *Int. J. Electron. Commer.* **2003**, *7*, 101–134. [CrossRef]
77. Bandura, A. *Social Foundations of Thought and Action: A Social Cognitive Theory*; Prentice-Hall: Englewood Cliffs, NJ, USA, 1986; ISBN 978-0-13-815614-5.
78. Brady, M.K.; Cronin, J.J.; Brand, R.R. Performance-Only Measurement of Service Quality: A Replication and Extension. *J. Bus. Res.* **2002**, *55*, 17–31. [CrossRef]
79. Cronin, J.J.; Taylor, S.A. Servperf Versus Servqual: Reconciling Performance-Based and Perceptions-Minus-Expectations Measurement of Service Quality. *J. Mark.* **1994**, *58*, 125–131. [CrossRef]
80. Parasuraman, A.; Zeithaml, V.A.; Berry, L.L. SERVQUAL: A Multiple-Item Scale for Measuring Consumer Perceptions of Service Quality. *J. Retail.* **1988**, *64*, 12–40.
81. Leung, L.Y.M. 'No South Asian Riders, Please': The Politics of Visibilisation in Platformed Food Delivery Work during the COVID-19 Pandemic in Hong Kong. *Crit. Sociol.* **2022**, *48*, 1189–1203. [CrossRef]
82. Parwez, S.; Ranjan, R. The Platform Economy and the Precarisation of Food Delivery Work in the COVID-19 Pandemic: Evidence from India. *Work Organ. Labour Glob.* **2021**, *15*, 11–30. [CrossRef]
83. Featherman, M.S.; Pavlou, P.A. Predicting E-Services Adoption: A Perceived Risk Facets Perspective. *Int. J. Hum.-Comput. Stud.* **2003**, *59*, 451–474. [CrossRef]
84. Liu, Q.; Liu, Y.; Zhang, C.; An, Z.; Zhao, P. Elderly Mobility during the COVID-19 Pandemic: A Qualitative Exploration in Kunming, China. *J. Transp. Geogr.* **2021**, *96*, 103176. [CrossRef] [PubMed]
85. Steptoe, A.; Pollard, T.M.; Wardle, J. Development of a Measure of the Motives Underlying the Selection of Food: The Food Choice Questionnaire. *Appetite* **1995**, *25*, 267–284. [CrossRef]
86. Leong, M.K.; Osman, S.; Paim, L.; Sabri, M.F. Enhancing Consumer Online Engagement through Consumer Involvement: A Case of Airline and Hospitality Services in Malaysia. *Manag. Sci. Lett.* **2019**, *9*, 795–808. [CrossRef]
87. O'Brien, H.L.; Toms, E.G. What Is User Engagement? A Conceptual Framework for Defining User Engagement with Technology. *J. Am. Soc. Inf. Sci. Technol.* **2008**, *59*, 938–955. [CrossRef]
88. Ali, F.; Harris, K.J.; Ryu, K. Consumers' Return Intentions towards a Restaurant with Foodborne Illness Outbreaks: Differences across Restaurant Type and Consumers' Dining Frequency. *Food Control* **2019**, *98*, 424–430. [CrossRef]
89. Cahyanto, I.; Wiblishauser, M.; Pennington-Gray, L.; Schroeder, A. The Dynamics of Travel Avoidance: The Case of Ebola in the U.S. *Tour. Manag. Perspect.* **2016**, *20*, 195–203. [CrossRef]
90. Fenichel, E.P.; Kuminoff, N.V.; Chowell, G. Skip the Trip: Air Travelers' Behavioral Responses to Pandemic Influenza. *PLoS ONE* **2013**, *8*, e58249. [CrossRef]
91. Ahmad, N.S.S.; Sulaiman, N.; Sabri, M.F. Food Insecurity: Is It a Threat to University Students' Well-Being and Success? *Int. J. Environ. Res. Public. Health* **2021**, *18*, 5627. [CrossRef]
92. Fusté-Forné, F.; Filimon, N. Using Social Media to Preserve Consumers' Awareness on Food Identity in Times of Crisis: The Case of Bakeries. *Int. J. Environ. Res. Public. Health* **2021**, *18*, 6251. [CrossRef] [PubMed]
93. Horta, P.M.; Matos, J.D.P.; Mendes, L.L. Food Promoted on an Online Food Delivery Platform in a Brazilian Metropolis during the Coronavirus Disease (COVID-19) Pandemic: A Longitudinal Analysis. *Public Health Nutr.* **2022**, *25*, 1336–1345. [CrossRef] [PubMed]
94. Aguilar-Martínez, A.; Bosque-Prous, M.; González-Casals, H.; Colillas-Malet, E.; Puigcorbé, S.; Esquius, L.; Espelt, A. Social Inequalities in Changes in Diet in Adolescents during Confinement Due to COVID-19 in Spain: The DESKcohort Project. *Nutrients* **2021**, *13*, 1577. [CrossRef] [PubMed]
95. Noguer-Juncà, E.; Fusté-Forné, F. Marketing Environmental Responsibility through "Green" Menus. *J. Foodserv. Bus. Res.* **2022**; ahead-of-print. [CrossRef]

96. Wijekoon, R.; Sabri, M.F. Determinants That Influence Green Product Purchase Intention and Behavior: A Literature Review and Guiding Framework. *Sustainability* **2021**, *13*, 6219. [CrossRef]
97. China Internet Network Information Center. The 48th Statistical Report on China's Internet Development. Available online: http://www.cnnic.com.cn/IDR/ReportDownloads/202111/P020211119394556095096.pdf. (accessed on 1 October 2022).

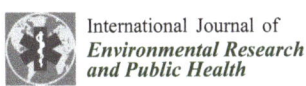

Article

Culinary Solitude in the Diet of People with Functional Diversity

Carmen Cipriano-Crespo [1], Francesc-Xavier Medina [2,*] and Lorenzo Mariano-Juárez [3]

1. Faculty of Health Sciences, University of Castilla La Mancha, 45600 Talavera de la Reina, Spain; mariacarmen.cipriano@uclm.es
2. Faculty of Health Sciences/Foodlab & Unesco Chair on Food, Culture, and Development, Universitat Oberta de Catalunya (UOC), 08018 Barcelona, Spain
3. Faculty of Nursing and Occupational Therapy, University of Extremadura, 10003 Caceres, Spain; lorenmariano@unex.es
* Correspondence: fxmedina@uoc.edu

Abstract: This qualitative ethnographic study identifies how problems in the feeding process of a group of people with functional diversity influence different eating situations. The study, which was carried out in the Autonomous Community of Castilla La Mancha, Spain, is based on interviews conducted at the headquarters of the different participating associations for functionally diverse people, at the participants' homes, and in public spaces. The study included 27 subjects aged between 18–75 years. Their functional diversity had caused significant changes in their sociability, particularly in contexts associated with food consumption. The analysis identified three main themes: social ghettoisation and culinary loneliness; stigma, shame, feeling like a burden, and loneliness; and exclusion or self-exclusion at the dining table. Our participants' narratives underscored the importance of acknowledging the significance of changes in eating-related sociability due to functional diversity. For the study subjects, grief, loneliness, and shame contributed to disassociating food consumption from social celebrations, withdrawing from restaurant meals, or conversations while eating to avoid other people's stares.

Keywords: functional diversity; commensality; self-esteem; shame; loneliness

Citation: Cipriano-Crespo, C.; Medina, F.-X.; Mariano-Juárez, L. Culinary Solitude in the Diet of People with Functional Diversity. *Int. J. Environ. Res. Public Health* **2022**, *19*, 3624. https://doi.org/10.3390/ijerph19063624

Academic Editor: Paul B. Tchounwou

Received: 7 February 2022
Accepted: 17 March 2022
Published: 18 March 2022

Publisher's Note: MDPI stays neutral with regard to jurisdictional claims in published maps and institutional affiliations.

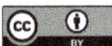

Copyright: © 2022 by the authors. Licensee MDPI, Basel, Switzerland. This article is an open access article distributed under the terms and conditions of the Creative Commons Attribution (CC BY) license (https://creativecommons.org/licenses/by/4.0/).

1. Introduction

Eating is an essential aspect of life—a basic component of the daily activities of social groups, and a cornerstone of the biological, psychological, and cultural characterization of human beings [1]. From the viewpoint of anthropology, eating is a key dimension of social relationships—encompassing much more than the consumption a certain number of nutrients based on biological or dietary considerations [2]. As Contreras [3] notes, eating is a social act and a key aspect for the creation of cultural identities. Eating together involves participating in a social activity where attitudes, protocols, behaviors, and situations are shared with others [3]. It is an emotional act that allows us to draw symbolic nourishment from the values represented by different foods [4], and it is closely intertwined with personal well-being and the happiness derived from sitting at a table with others. As Spanish chef Carme Ruscalleda notes: *"Cooking is like embracing someone: it creates happiness"* [5].

As eating is crucial for our physical and social development, eating in the company of others is an essential aspect of creating and maintaining a sense of community. When food is consumed with others, the personal, intimate act of eating is transformed into a shared experience—a collective experience. Thus, the dining table can be perceived as a scenario in which the relationships—kinship, friendship—between those sitting together are reproduced, and common traditions, tastes, and pleasures are displayed [6,7].

As a result, the practice of eating together is a basic component of our social nature. [8]. As Medina [7] has suggested, commensality is more than sharing food and spending time together—its final goal is the preservation of the social structure of a group. Flandrin and Montanari [9] suggest that the difference between human beings' culinary behavior and animal eating practices lies in culture, the methods of food preparation, and the social role of food consumption.

As Levi-Strauss [10] notes, food is closely intertwined with social relationships—not only does it provide nourishment, it also allows us to transmit emotions and feelings. While we share food with others, we communicate, and we reminisce about the past. While we eat, we converse, get closer to others, and establish bonds. Indeed, as Maffesoli [11] suggests, "most of the time, human beings prefer to eat in the company of others—conveying feelings and thoughts and communicating problems and different kinds of situations".

Eating together creates a spatial and temporal convergence among individuals who share a common bond. Commensality requires interaction among the members of a group—to gather in a specific place at a particular time to eat together, thus engaging in a shared practice. This reinforces the symbolic feeling of belonging to the group that the table is shared with [12]. At the same time, the practice of eating together can have different meanings for the people involved, depending on their gender, age, their role within the social group, and their social and cultural position. For some, it might be just one of their day-to-day obligations—they might sit at the table while watching television, oblivious to the social dimensions of commensality [13].

Functional diversity is an alternative term for "disability" that aims to avoid the negative connotations of this concept. To acknowledge each individual's diversity fosters a richer society—one that recognizes that this is an inherent dimension of the human condition and that, indeed, each individual can be considered functionally diverse [14]. However, functional diversity can substantially impact different spheres of life, including nutrition. Grignon described a "segregative commensality", with eating and drinking as a way of reinforcing and/or rejecting the social group. Accordingly, those who are perceived as alien or different because of their eating practices might experience social distancing. Our study explored the major difficulties experienced by our participants in the eating process—difficulties that affected these situations of social commensality and caused social distancing and eating in situations of loneliness.

Rather than enduring those uncomfortable situations, our participants opted for social (self) isolation—a progressive distancing from social situations involving food consumption such as restaurants and other social events—as they felt that functional diversity prevented them from performing adequately. As a result, they preferred to eat alone, out of sight from others. Although eating alone is often associated with a reduced enjoyment of life, for those experiencing eating difficulties, it was a better alternative [15]. At the same time, these situations of isolation they lived with, the feeling of being deprived when compared to others, increased their feelings of loneliness—as often happens to people with functional diversity, who feel their personal situation is somehow deficient [16]. This has been noticed often in people with dysphagia, who experience social limitations during mealtimes due to difficulties swallowing and maintaining conversations while eating. In these situations, eating with their families can be an element of friction rather than the source of social pleasure that commensality is supposed to be [15].

From childhood to adulthood, human beings are influenced in their eating habits by their surrounding society. Other people's behavior provides guidelines for our own—making us act, at the very least, in the most appropriate way according to the social rules within a given group [17]. For instance, although food consumption always has a social dimension—the dining table being, by definition, a space for social interaction—this is more important than ever in exceptional situations of commensality that include extended family or friends. Eating is an act that allows us to integrate into society: "we eat according to certain standards that translate into permissions and prohibitions regarding times, places, and table manners; and we invite others to our table to share, negotiate, flaunt, or dominate" [18].

In this sense, eating incorporates a series of material or immaterial dimensions closely associated with the participants themselves, including following a certain number of explicit or implicit rules [8]. However, many people experiencing eating problems due to functional diversity are unable to comply with these rules and find themselves rejected by individuals who do not experience these problems, eventually deciding to eat alone.

This study proposes an ethnographic approach to the eating experience of a group of people with different types of functional diversity that caused eating difficulties. These problems sometimes made them feel that they did not belong within the group on which they had built their social identity. Although eating before functional diversity was a source of enjoyment, the difficulties it entailed in their present situation contributed to their perceiving food as a stress factor—an activity that required extra effort and where social and sensorial satisfaction was denied. The experience becomes incomplete because neither food nor the experience of food consumption is shared with others. On the contrary, the relationship between food and functional diversity only led to the emergence of feelings of shame and loneliness.

2. Materials and Methods

This is a qualitative ethnographic study of subjective experiences of commensality among a group of functionally diverse people. Data collection and analysis followed an inductive approach [19–21]. Several categories were established from the analysis of the empirical materials, based on constant comparison and grounded theory methods [22,23]. This provided a better understanding of our participants' experiences of challenges associated with food consumption [23,24].

On the other hand, this study was conceived from the viewpoint of the anthropology of food, whose methods have their own characteristics, perspectives, and applications [25–28].

2.1. Participants

This study included a total of 27 participants, aged between 18 and 75 years. All were functionally diverse people, with different functional deficiencies—total or partial—that caused challenges related to eating and drinking—i.e., cancer, spinal cord injuries, Niemann–Pick disease, duchenne muscular dystrophy, multiple sclerosis, amyotrophic lateral sclerosis, ictus, or acquired brain damage (Table 1). The main factor behind the selection of each participant was, above all, the researchers' accessibility to the field.

Table 1. Participants' profiles and types of disability.

	Count (*n*)
Gender	
Female	6
Male	21
Disability	
Brain injury	6
Spinal cord injury	5
Cancer	10
Amyotrophic lateral sclerosis	1
Multiple sclerosis	2
Muscular dystrophy	2
Niemann–Pick disease	1

Additionally, all participants experienced eating difficulties due to the presence of functional diversity. Some of our participants presented with difficulties chewing or swallowing food, whereas others struggled to use the implements necessary to feed themselves. Consent for the interviews being audio-recorded and signing the informed consent form were essential prerequisites for participation in the study. Individuals with dementia and/or severe cognitive impairment, those who did not provide informed consent, or those who refused to have their interviews audio-recorded were excluded from the study.

Potential participants were approached through different channels. The project was introduced to the heads of different associations for functionally diverse people, who recommended suitable participants who were experiencing eating difficulties. We also contacted occupational therapy professionals at the National Hospital for Paraplegics (Toledo, Spain) who, after obtaining approval from the head of the department, facilitated contact details of patients with eating problems.

2.2. Data Collection

Data were collected through semi-structured, in-depth interviews that followed a pre-established guide (Table 2). This allowed new themes to emerge and be explored during the course of the interviews [29,30]. All the interviews were audio-recorded.

Table 2. In-depth interview guide: categories and questions.

Biography
Medical history, social and economic profile
Food and feeding
Feelings and emotions
Food and social activities
Acceptance of changes
Community and personal relationships
Successes, failures, exclusion
Friendship loss

Most of the interviews were conducted in designated areas at the headquarters of different associations for functionally diverse people, although some took place at the participants' homes or in public spaces. Empirical data were also collected through participant observation in settings such as kitchens or canteens. Ensuring the participants' comfort and privacy during the interviews was always a priority. To guarantee privacy, each audio recording was assigned a coded name, and any personal data revealing the participants' identity has been removed from this article. The names used in the text are fictitious; they have been added to make the text easier to read and humanize the context. The original recordings were destroyed once the interviews were transcribed. All interviews were conducted by the three members of the team, all of whom had extensive experience in qualitative research. Interviews had durations of between 60–120 min.

2.3. Data Analysis

The interviews were transcribed verbatim by the researcher who conducted them. Data analysis used Microsoft Access and was performed by two experienced qualitative researchers, who worked independently. The results were shared and discussed once their analyses were completed. The participants' responses were used to create a thematic map with different themes and subthemes.

Each participant received an alphanumeric code that was used for logging data and creating categories, and as a reference for literal quotations extracted from the participants' interviews.

The study followed the items defined in the COREQ checklist for reporting qualitative research [31] and Lincoln and Guba's quality criteria framework [32].

2.4. Ethical Considerations

The study was approved by the Clinical Research Ethical Committee of the Talavera de la Reina Integrated Management Area (CEIm del AGI de Talavera de la Reina, Spain, Hospital Nuestra Señora del Prado, ref: 18/2014). The study was conducted in accordance with ethical principles outlined in the Declaration of Helsinki and the Belmont Report. Data were treated in line with current guidelines on the ethical implications of research. Data were used with the utmost confidentiality, and remain protected under the Law 15/1999, of December 13, on Protection of Personal Data.

3. Results

Functional diversity causes significant challenges and transformations in the life situations of the people affected at very different levels—physical, social, and emotional. It also creates challenges related to eating—with changes in the way food is consumed affecting commensality and sociability.

The analysis of empirical materials revealed three recurrent themes that highlight the importance of commensality for people with functional diversity.

3.1. Social Ghettoisation and Culinary Loneliness

Some of the participants in our study mentioned withdrawing or being socially excluded by people without eating problems, thus triggering feelings of "culinary loneliness". In a way, this exclusion provided a certain sense of comfort that was impossible when eating while being subjected to other people's scrutiny. In their accounts, our participants mentioned avoiding eating out in restaurants or deciding to eat on their own—without being stared at, but also without other people's company. Eventually, this fostered a process of culinary ghettoization and a withdrawal from public spaces—the visible space, without culinary limitations, that used to be enjoyed in restaurants. One participant, Paloma, who lived in a care home for older adults due to limitations caused by amyotrophic lateral sclerosis, noted that she often asked assistants to place her with her back to other residents during special celebrations such as birthdays or Christmas.

> "[. . .] leave me in my little corner so I can eat a bit of cake on my own, with nobody looking at me in disgust."

Social exclusion and isolation due to problems in the eating process are not an issue when food and drink are consumed within a social environment in which our participants feel included—i.e., when eating with people with similar difficulties and who belong to the same associations as them. This helps normalize their experience and increases the opportunities to re-establish lost relationships based on sociability and commensality. In these environments, their experiences are normalized, and they do not feel questioned in their social interactions. One subject, Fernando, described his experience:

> "When I go out with friends I feel embarrassed that I will spill food down the sides, because people stare at me; but when I attend the meals organised by the association, which I love doing—I do not mind if one of my buddies asks me to wipe something that I've dropped, he has been through the same as me, and I do not need to justify anything."

Isaac, another participant, decided to go out less often due to his increasing difficulties eating and speaking, caused by multiple sclerosis. Before that, he enjoyed meeting friends for lunch or dinner, since it was a perfect excuse to catch up with them. Now, however, he did not attend these meetings. Instead, he ate with his parents—but only because he had no other option, always keeping the television on to avoid interacting with them.

> "I have nothing to talk about; before, there were plenty of subjects, but now everything revolves around my illness, and I rather not speak."

Our participants tended to look for people experiencing similar challenges to theirs, so they could feel understood in what they were going through. They needed to share their feelings, emotions, and experiences, instead of feeling rejected due to their problems. A small number of participants admitted sometimes eating alone, in quiet corners in restaurants, looking at a television, and withdrawing from social conventions and contact with others—thus breaking implicit rules of social communication. On the other hand, when people eat alone, what they eat is of less consequence—they can eat whatever is there. Additionally, the amount of time devoted to eating also decreases. The practice of eating loses its social dimension and is reduced to satiating a physical need, which only takes a few minutes. However, eating alone and in such a short amount of time is another way of breaking with normality.

3.2. Burden, Shame, and Loneliness

To eat in society necessarily implies a certain degree of interaction with other people—mutually passing each other food, serving beverages, sharing an experience. Each of those attending a family or work meal are crucial threads of the social mechanism that contributes to creating pleasure and enjoyment for themselves and other people.

Our participants, by contrast, described feeling like a burden, a nuisance that got in the way of the logical order of things. Gradually, certain thoughts, feelings, and ways of acting emerged, reflecting the social isolation and monotony that, they felt, had been imposed upon them.

This feeling of being a burden was clearly associated with the shame experienced during social interaction in food-related contexts. For instance, those participants who had undergone a laryngectomy reported drastically reducing their participation in collective gatherings that involved food being served and consumed, due to their feeling shame and being a hindrance to everybody else.

Paloma understood very well this feeling of being ashamed. In the care home where she lives, she eats in a room on her own, at a different time from other residents, with only the company of the assistant who helps her.

> "Initially, I used to eat with everybody else, but while I eat, I drop a lot of food, and once I heard a man saying aloud that it was disgusting, and he turned his back on me so he would not see me. Since that day, I prefer to eat when I am alone."

Paloma described feeling ashamed of eating in front of other people, facing their looks and comments. Consequently, she made a decision that also implied giving up on certain things—for instance, due to her difficulties swallowing, her food always cooled down, and she had to eat it like that.

> "Since the kitchen is too far from the room where we eat, they do not warm [the food] to avoid wasting time, and when I have asked for a microwave to be brought close by they've said that this was not a dining room—so it is either eating cold food or going back to eating with the others, and I do not want to go through that again."

The feeling of shame could also be triggered by sharing a table with people who were not familiar with the difficulties they were currently experiencing. For example, María, who has muscular dystrophy, felt ashamed of not being able to eat as before with those who were part of her life back when she did not need any help to eat, and who still remembered her as she used to be. They were aware that she had a neurodegenerative disorder, but they had not seen its actual impact on her.

> "[...] I remember the day I met for dinner with a childhood friend, I felt like a stranger by her side despite her being aware of my illness because we had lived together—it was like going back in time and being compared with my younger self. With the people I see on a day-to-day basis, everything is normalised, there is feedback, so often I do not need to ask for anything—with a look or even my posture they know whether or not I want a drink, or a bite of some of the food at the table. They have assumed this gradual neurodegenerative process as naturally as I have. However, I find it a bit harder with those who were part of my life when I was better, it triggers these internal emotions."

Another participant, Isaac, with multiple sclerosis, also mentioned feeling ashamed when he spilt the food he was eating. His frustration over this made him eat less, particularly those foods that required using a spoon—which used to be his favorite. He used thick straws to eat soup without spilling it, but only at home—he was ashamed of being seen eating like a small child.

Progressively, this feeling of shame acquires new layers of meaning, eventually causing them to make difficult decisions—such as not serving or eating food in any celebration.

This, however, causes further distancing and isolation from the people who do. Javier, who underwent a laryngectomy due to laryngeal cancer, told us that his eating difficulties had changed everything.

> "Because of my issues, we do not celebrate anything, only my children's birthdays. We do not celebrate anymore because everybody knows that not being able to eat like them pains me, so to avoid it we do not celebrate with food, which is what we used to do in my family—like almost everybody else does, this is Spain! And here we like to eat and drink well."

The social stigma attached to people with functional diversity disrupts the consumption of food with other people in public spaces. The stares, the rejection, and sometimes even being denied service at certain restaurants make it almost impossible to share a table with others. As a result of these experiences, they feel lonely in their daily routines. This loneliness, however, might be perceived rather than real. This was the case with one of our participants, Isaac. His subjective perception was that he was lonely, despite being surrounded by people who cared about him. His parents and friends constantly knocked at his door to ask how he was feeling, to make him feel supported in this process he had to live with. However, he could not—or did not want to—feel comforted by this. Isaac admitted that his behavior towards others changed when he faced the unstoppable advance of his illness, and that this might have been the reason why his relationship with his wife soured.

> "My wife and I started bickering a lot because she did not understand what I was going through—she did not understand that I felt lonely despite her being with me, until one day she left me. It's just that this that I have—it is only half a life, and badly lived at it."

The negative experiences cause grief and yearning for their former selves, feeding the stigma attached to the new culinary situation of those who bring functional diversity to the dining table.

3.3. Exclusion or Self-Exclusion from the Table

When sitting around a table laden with food, we express our internal self, concerns, and differences with those with whom we share the table. In this context, those obstacles that might challenge or disrupt commensality quickly become apparent. In our study, these were associated with our participants' new dietary needs and how they consumed food or drink now—challenges caused by an illness or injury, which turned people with functional diversity into *outsiders* at the table.

For this reason, sometimes, they choose to withdraw from these situations—for fear that their presence will subvert the unspoken hygiene rules that guide table manners, that dictate that food has to be attractive and people have to enjoy each other's company.

For instance, regarding social conventions and habits established around communal dining, several participants with cancer noted that they could not follow the normal rhythm of food consumption or conversation—since they needed to eat slowly and concentrate on chewing to avoid choking. Fear of receiving puzzled stares, of the noises they might make, or of expelling tracheal mucus while eating were some of the reasons expressed to justify their feeling excluded or their decision to withdraw from such events. One participant, Leoncio, expressed it thus.

> "I do not want to eat out with friends or relatives, food dribbles down my sides, and I notice people staring at the hole in my throat—I feel ashamed of what I have—and when I do not eat out, I do not suffer."

Another participant, Florencio, mentioned eating out with friends occasionally but always in quiet places because otherwise he had to remain silent—since it upset him if nobody could understand what he was saying. Indeed, he did not often feel like eating out with large groups of people. He self-excluded because he felt different—always making demands that were not necessary for others, but they felt obliged to comply with.

"Besides, sometimes in the heat of the moment everybody raises their voices too much and drown my own, so I have to remain silent and just listen for the rest of the meal."

Both of these participants pointed out that the negative feelings they experienced made them withdraw from sitting at a table and sharing food with people who did not have any problems. In many cases, in the absence of individual or collective mechanisms specifically focused on their needs, people with functional diversity end up eating alone—a clear sign of social exclusion. As Jesús, with laryngeal cancer, pointed out: *"This is an illness that excludes you from society"*.

For people with functional diversity, self-imposed exclusion at mealtimes is primarily due to the stares they receive from others. Israel, with Duchenne muscular dystrophy, gradually severed his relationships with others as his illness progressed. His eating habits were gradually modified to adapt to the loss of manual dexterity in both hands. However, these new habits were not socially accepted by people *on the other side* of the functional diversity divide. Thus, he preferred to consume food in private—in the intimate environment of his dining room.

"People are surprised when they see me eating—I get very close to the plate and sometimes food dribbles down the sides; eventually my mother has to feed me and, at my age, I do not like people seeing me as a small child."

María also decided to exclude herself from situations in which she had to eat with other people because of her eating difficulties. Recently, attending the wedding of a close relative, she asked to be served food on her own, before other guests arrived at the restaurant—protected from prying eyes but consequently excluded from social engagement. This self-imposed exclusion meant giving up on exchanging opinions on the food served—flavors, textures, and recipes in which, as a cook, she was particularly interested. Instead, she chose to contemplate others while they enjoyed the flavors, textures, and presentation of the different dishes, finding comfort in not being scrutinized because of the way she ate.

Self-exclusion might also be caused by experiencing dysphagia problems, as was the case of Benito as a consequence of laryngeal cancer. He minimized his attendance at family birthday celebrations, despite his wife always carrying in her bag some fluid thickener to add to his drink. However, the constant coughing caused by drinking made him stop attending celebrations that involved food consumption.

"It looks like I am going to die, I get very red and cough a lot, scaring everyone around me. Besides, sometimes I dribble down the sides when I am drinking, and I get covered in stains, and people notice and give me weird looks."

Again, other people's stares made our participants want to *hide* when they were eating.

3.4. Condemned to Distance, Loneliness, and Ugliness

Some of the study participants had to be tube-fed, and their perception of their situation was even more dramatic. As Jesús described, *"I thought that I was going to die—that I was at the end"*.

For the people needing feeding tubes, the self-perception of their physical integrity is impaired. An exploration of tube-fed patients noted that some of them felt ugly [33]—despite most patients admitting that they were necessary, tubes were perceived as a negative element that disrupted the "normal" aesthetic image of an individual.

Most of our tube-fed participants reported experiencing a certain degree of rejection. As Isaac noted, *"When something like this happens that is forever, people turn their backs on you—they do not want to know much about the course of the illness, they run away from grief"*.

These feelings of loneliness are closely related to sadness at being distanced from a world that once included them, leaving a gap that is sometimes filled with people with similar experiences to theirs—the only ones who could understand what they were going through. For instance, Samuel had a rare disease. His mother, Isabel, faced a lack of understanding from people unaware of the amount of suffering that an eventual diagnosis and the progression of the disease could cause. With a voice tinged with sadness, she told us:

> "We gave our everything to the association—in there, there were no excuses and no lies, we all felt abandoned by the healthy ones and understood that they could not cope with the disease—people don't want grief."

There was no need to explain anything in the association she became a member of. Sooner or later, everybody went through the same experiences, which made them all equal despite their individualities. She felt it was important to give visibility and create social awareness of her son's disease, and she did this with the association's support—without it, she would not have been strong enough.

Initially, friends and relatives visit the person with functional diversity regularly. However, as time goes on, visits become less and less frequent. Isabel remembers that her friends stopped calling because they could not endure the image of her son, sitting in his chair, absently watching cartoons. *"At first, they used to phone me and say, 'I could not cope with what you are going through!' But eventually, the phone calls became few and far between, until one day the phone stopped ringing."*

Those participants who moved back permanently to their homes after a period at a hospital soon had to face a new reality: other people had busy lives. As a result, their opportunities for social engagement were often sharply reduced—since they depended on others to go out for walks or eat out in restaurants. Arturo, who has a spinal cord injury, told us that *"My friends are keeping an eye on me, they are shocked by what happened to me—they have to come and pick me up, take me places, and sometimes they are not available when I would like them to, but until I get a license and I can drive myself I have no choice but to rely on them"*.

This constant reliance on others to participate in gatherings or special meals dramatically increases the plight of people with functional diversity and their relatives. It makes them even more aware of everything that has changed and what they have lost due to their new life situation.

The realization that these new circumstances are permanent, as was the case of the study participants, might make them feel condemned to loneliness—a feeling that they attributed to their weakness and the grief caused by their inability to cope with their difficulties, which affected their self-esteem. Indeed, some of the participants clearly stated that their withdrawal from food-related events was due to their eating difficulties—so they did not make food *ugly*. They preferred not to display their challenges to those they shared the table with and assume the price to be paid for this—an increasingly reduced sociability. This not only affects them but also, indirectly, their closest relatives—who sometimes are unable to participate in social events either as a result. That was the case with Oliva, Paco's wife. Paco had acquired brain damage, which caused difficulties in eating without spilling food and swallowing without choking. Oliva felt she had been forced into culinary loneliness due to his decision to reduce his participation in situations of commensality. With tears in her eyes, she described that because of Paco's eating and communication problems, her only social interaction was with their son and with the healthcare assistant who helped them at home. *"I am having to pay the price—because he does not want to go out anywhere, I am doomed to stay at home all day—it's like being locked for life, just because he is ashamed of eating in front of others."*

However, there are also situations in which feelings of anxiety and fear are counterbalanced by the willingness to experience the pleasure of social engagement. That was the case of Javier who, despite requiring artificial feeding, fought his fears to be able to enjoy participating in situations of sociability. *"I play a round of cards with my friends and, very slowly, I drink a shot of gin—real slow, it can last me the whole afternoon. All of my friends were drinking and I could not stand it anymore. I felt like a third wheel."*

The loss of independence and intimacy gives rise to a whole host of new emotions—due to the shame of not being the same as they used to be before, and other people noticing the difficulties they experienced in conducting simple, day-to-day tasks. This process made them feel lonely, despite the support and involvement of relatives and professionals in important moments of their lives.

4. Discussion

Our analysis revealed the importance of loss of food-related sociability for people with functional diversity due to the eating challenges they experience. These challenges impacted our participants' self-esteem, as they equated the loss of their physical abilities with their bodies losing their value. Their bodies were different from before, no longer fit for purpose. They were no longer legitimate, productive, independent bodies. Instead, they were *disabled bodies* [34]—which, for our participants, meant the loss of their symbolic capital. The increasing limitations in their manual dexterity were translated into the loss of their ability to engage with other people through food consumption.

As noted in previous studies [35,36], the loss of social interaction in this kind of context is a frequently mentioned issue. People with functional diversity are aware that the experience of culinary loneliness will be there for the rest of their lives, which is detrimental to their mental health [37].

For our participants, functional diversity meant losing opportunities to derive pleasure from situations of commensality that were a source of enjoyment before—as experiences shared with their loved ones. This loss affects not only the people with functional diversity, but also those who share their lives—in many cases, through self-imposed exclusion, due to their perceived inadequacy when eating in front of others in work or family social gatherings. Studies such as those of Winkler have pointed out that human interactions help define personal identities [38,39]. For people with functional diversity experiencing eating and drinking challenges, spaces and opportunities for sociability are reduced, thus affecting their personal identity.

Most people feel the importance of belonging to a wider social sphere—a group, a family—and to be recognized as individual members of their community. The practice of eating together as a group has a normative dimension—there are some common rules and expectations from those participating in a situation of commensality, and those who do not abide by them are excluded [40]. However, as described above, our participants experienced difficulties maintaining these standards due to their new life situation. This disrupted the balance required to follow the internal rules guiding the social groups to which they belong. To help maintain a harmonious environment where they could feel comfortable, people with functional diversity tend to withdraw and exclude themselves. Consequently, they deny themselves the right to participate and derive enjoyment from previously pleasurable situations of commensality. When they eat, it is out of necessity—to receive nourishment. Their functional diversity does not allow them to experience enjoyment in relation to food. Instead, food is perceived as a requirement, something that has to be consumed to reach specific dietary goals without providing any pleasure [41]. As a result of subjective perceptions of external attitudes, our participants consider themselves useless—a burden, an affront to others—and choose instead to withdraw [42].

The results of this study have relevance for clinical practice. In general, intervention models related to food and drink intake for people with functional diversity who experience eating difficulties tend to focus on the nutritional aspects of the process. However, the stories analyzed in this study underline the importance attributed to the social and symbolic dimensions of the eating process. At the same time, the study provides a detailed examination of the consequences of the new food situation on contextual relationships and culinary loneliness, all of which can be detrimental to mental health [37].

This study has suggested a possible approach to explore the experiences of people with functional diversity. However, an important limitation is that the participants presented very different kinds and levels of functional diversity, caused by a wide range of pathologies.

Another potential limitation is that the study did not assess how age and gender affected these experiences. Our main aim was to explore the impact of different types of functional diversity on eating practices and how this was perceived. However, a gender-based approach could help explore whether these situations were differentially experienced and assess possible male/female variations in meaning.

Finally, it would also be interesting to explore how cooking and eating aid equipment—e.g., cutlery with special handles, etc.—can mediate these subjective experiences.

5. Conclusions

Ethnographic evidence gathered in our study revealed how functionally diverse people progressively reduced their participation in situations of social commensality—either attending fewer events or reducing the number of people present at a time—thus modifying conditions to access and derive pleasure from food consumption. Our study also revealed the importance of food for the construction of society—particularly the emotional and social relationships established around shared food consumption. The evidence emerging from the exploration of culinary sociability suggests that the loss of physiological function has a direct impact on the loss of the social value attached to food and food consumption.

Spinal cord injuries, the progress of neurodegenerative disorders, or the consequences of laryngeal cancer, among others, are factors that prevented our participants from enjoying eating and drinking together with other people—which eventually led them to perceive food only as a dietary requirement.

In contexts involving people other than their closest personal relationships, most of our participants expressed feeling ashamed of the difficulties they experienced or the way in which they now had to eat or drink. To avoid experiencing more grief regarding their personal situation, they placed limitations on the number of people they felt comfortable sharing situations of commensality with. This resulted in a gradual reduction in their sociability, and that of their closest relatives—whose opportunities to derive pleasure from social engagements were also altered and diminished.

Author Contributions: Conceptualization, C.C.-C. and L.M.-J.; methodology, C.C.-C., F.-X.M. and L.M.-J.; software, C.C.-C., F.-X.M. and L.M.-J.; validation, C.C.-C., F.-X.M. and L.M.-J.; formal analysis, C.C.-C., F.-X.M. and L.M.-J.; investigation, C.C.-C. and L.M.-J.; writing—original draft preparation, C.C.-C., F.-X.M. and L.M.-J.; writing—review and editing, C.C.-C. and L.M.-J.; visualization, C.C.-C., F.-X.M. and L.M.-J.; supervision, C.C.-C., F.-X.M. and L.M.-J. All authors have read and agreed to the published version of the manuscript.

Funding: This research received no external funding.

Institutional Review Board Statement: The study was conducted according to the guidelines of the Declaration of Helsinki and approved by the Clinical Research Ethical Committee of the Talavera de la Reina Integrated Management Area (CEIm del AGI de Talavera de la Reina in Spain, Nuestra Señora del Prado Hospital (ref: 18/2014) 18 March 2014).

Informed Consent Statement: Informed consent was obtained from all subjects involved in the study.

Data Availability Statement: The data presented in this study, except those protected under confidentiality agreements with participants, are available on request from the corresponding author.

Conflicts of Interest: The authors declare no conflict of interest.

References

1. Gracia Arnaiz, M.I. ¿Somos lo que comemos? Alimentos, Significados e Identidades. *Aliment. Hoy.* **2011**, *20*, 3–5.
2. Aguirre, P. Qué Puede Decirnos una Antropóloga sobre Alimentación. Hablando sobre Gustos. In *Cuerpos, Mercados y Genes Instituto de Altos Estudios Sociales*; Universidad Nacional de San Martín: Buenos Aires, Argentina, 2007. Available online: http://www.fac.org.ar/qcvc/llave/c027e/aguirrep.php (accessed on 10 March 2022).
3. Contreras, J. *Alimentación y Cultura: Necesidades, Gustos y Costumbres*; Edicions Universitat Barcelona: Barcelona, Spain, 1995.
4. Dos Santos, C.R. A alimentação e seu lugar na história: Os tempos da memória gustativa. *História Questões Debates* **2005**, *42*, 11–31. [CrossRef]
5. Rodriguez Hernández, A. *Gastronomía para Aprender a ser Feliz (Serendipity)*; Desclee De Brouwer: Bilbao, Spain, 2015; Available online: https://es1lib.org/book/11905900/c342f8 (accessed on 20 January 2022).

6. Lozano, M.O. *El acto de Comer en el Arte: Del Eat Art a Ferran Adrià en la Documenta 12*; Universidad Complutense de Madrid: Madrid, Spain, 2013; Available online: http://purl.org/dc/dcmitype/Text (accessed on 20 January 2022).
7. Medina, F.-X. Looking for Commensality: On Culture, Health, Heritage, and the Mediterranean Diet. *Int. J. Environ. Res. Public Health* **2021**, *18*, 2605. [CrossRef]
8. Jönsson, H.; Michaud, M.; Neuman, N. What Is Commensality? A Critical Discussion of an Expanding Research Field. *Int. J. Environ. Res. Public Health* **2021**, *18*, 6235. [CrossRef]
9. Sonnenfeld, A.; Flandrin, J.-L.; Montanari, M. *Food: A Culinary History from Antiquity to the Present*; Columbia University Press: New York, NY, USA, 2013; 624p.
10. Levi-Strauss, C. Lo crudo y lo cocido. *Rev. Univ. Nac. 1944—1992* **1971**, *9*, 119–157.
11. Maffesoli, M. *El Tiempo de las Tribus: El Declive del Individualismo en las Sociedades de Masas*; Siglo XXI: Mérida, Spain, 2004; Available online: https://www.casadellibro.com/libro-el-tiempo-de-las-tribus-el-declive-del-individualismo-en-las-soc-iedades-de-masa/9789682325298/1139471 (accessed on 20 January 2022).
12. Giacoman, C. The dimensions and role of commensality: A theoretical model drawn from the significance of communal eating among adults in Santiago, Chile. *Appetite* **2016**, *107*, 460–470. [CrossRef]
13. Le Moal, F.; Michaud, M.; Hartwick-Pflaum, C.A.; Middleton, G.; Mallon, I.; Coveney, J. Beyond the Normative Family Meal Promotion: A Narrative Review of Qualitative Results about Ordinary Domestic Commensality. *Int. J. Environ. Res. Public Health* **2021**, *18*, 3186. [CrossRef]
14. Romanach, J.; Palacios, A. El modelo de la diversidad: Una nueva visión de la bioética desde la perspectiva de las personas con diversidad funcional (discapacidad). *Intersticios Rev. Sociológica De Pensam. Crítico* **2008**, *2*, 37–47. Available online: http://www.intersticios.es/article/view/2712 (accessed on 17 June 2018).
15. Adolfsson, P.; Mattsson Sydner, Y.; Fjellström, C. Social aspects of eating events among people with intellectual disability in community living. *J. Intellect Dev. Disabil.* **2010**, *35*, 259–267. [CrossRef]
16. Bogaerts, S.; Vanheule, S.; Desmet, M. Feelings of subjective emotional loneliness: An exploration of attachment. *Soc. Behav. Personal. Int. J.* **2006**, *34*, 797–812. [CrossRef]
17. Higgs, S.; Thomas, J. Social influences on eating. *Curr. Opin. Behav. Sci.* **2016**, *9*, 1–6. [CrossRef]
18. Hernández, H.M. Deleites y sinsabores de la comida y el comer: Situando el tema. *Atenea (Concepción)* **2007**, *496*, 41–54. [CrossRef]
19. Catoni, M.I.; Salas, S.P.; Roessler, E.; Valdivieso, A.; Vukusich, A.; Rivera, M.S. Toma de decisiones en hemodiálisis crónica: Estudio cualitativo en adultos mayores. *Rev. Médica Chile.* **2020**, *148*, 281–287. [CrossRef]
20. Einarsson, S.; Laurell, G.; Tiblom Ehrsson, Y. Experiences and coping strategies related to food and eating up to two years after the termination of treatment in patients with head and neck cancer. *Eur. J. Cancer Care* **2019**, *28*, e12964. [CrossRef]
21. San Martín Cantero, D. Teoría fundamentada y Atlas.ti: Recursos metodológicos para la investigación educativa. *Rev. Electrónica Investig. Educ.* **2014**, *16*, 104–122.
22. Bovio, G.; Bettaglio, R.; Bonetti, G.; Miotti, D.; Verni, P. Evaluation of nutritional status and dietary intake in patients with advanced cancer on palliative care. *Minerva Gastroenterol. Dietol.* **2008**, *54*, 243–250.
23. Corbin, J.; Strauss, A. *Basics of Qualitative Research: Techniques and Procedures for Developing Grounded Theory*, 3rd ed.; Sage Publications, Inc.: Thousand Oaks, CA, USA, 2008; 379p.
24. Larsson, M.; Hedelin, B.; Athlin, E. Lived experiences of eating problems for patients with head and neck cancer during radiotherapy. *J. Clin. Nurs.* **2003**, *12*, 562–570. [CrossRef]
25. Macbeth, H.; MacClancy, J. *Researching Food Habits: Methods and Problems*; Berghahn: Oxford, UK, 2004; Available online: https://www.berghahnbooks.com/title/MacbethResearching (accessed on 21 January 2022).
26. Medina, F.X. Methodological Notes on the Interaction between Researcher and Informants in the Anthropology of Food. In *Researching Food Habits: Methods and Problems*; Berghahn Books: New York, NY, USA, 2004; pp. 307–310.
27. Medina, F.X. Food culture: Anthropology of food and nutrition. In *Encyclopedia of Food Security and Sustainability*; Elsevier: Amsterdam, The Netherlands, 2019; pp. 307–310. Available online: https://www.elsevier.com/books/encyclopedia-of-food-security-and-sustainability/ferranti/978-0-12-812687-5 (accessed on 21 January 2022).
28. Messer, E. Revitalising the food systems perspective in the study of food-based identity. In *Researching Food Habits: Methods and Problems*; Berghahn Books: New York, NY, USA, 2004; pp. 181–192.
29. Carpenter, C.M.; Suto, M. *Qualitative Research for Occupational and Physical Therapists: A Practical Guide*; Wiley: Hoboken, NJ, USA, 2008; Available online: https://pureportal.coventry.ac.uk/en/publications/qualitative-research-for-occupational-and-physical-therapists-a-p-2 (accessed on 1 April 2021).
30. Newman, G. El razonamiento inductivo y deductivo dentro del proceso investigativo en ciencias experimentales y sociales. *Laurus* **2006**, *12*, 180–205.
31. Tong, A.; Sainsbury, P.; Craig, J. Consolidated criteria for reporting qualitative research (COREQ): A 32-item checklist for interviews and focus groups. *Int. J. Qual. Health Care* **2007**, *19*, 349–357. [CrossRef]
32. Lincoln, Y.S.; Guba, E.G. But is it Rigorous? Trustworthiness and Authenticity in Naturalistic Evaluation. *New Dir. Program Eval.* **1986**, *30*, 73–84. [CrossRef]
33. Guimarães, J. O que pensam os pacientes sobre o uso de sondas para se alimentar [¿Qué piensan los pacientes sobre el uso de sondas para alimentarse?]. *Rev. Tecer. Belo. Horiz.* **2010**, *3*, 30–37.

34. Ferrante, C. Cuerpo, discapacidad y violencia simbólica. Un acercamiento a la experiencia de la discapacidad motriz como relación de dominación encarnada. *Bol. Onteaiken.* **2014**, *8*, 17–34.
35. Malmström, M.; Ivarsson, B.; Johansson, J.; Klefsgard, R. Long-term experiences after oesophagectomy/gastrectomy for cancer-A focus group study. *Int. J. Nurs. Stud.* **2013**, *50*, 44–52. [CrossRef]
36. McQuestion, M.; Fitch, M.; Howell, D. The changed meaning of food: Physical, social and emotional loss for patients having received radiation treatment for head and neck cancer. *Eur. J. Oncol. Nurs.* **2011**, *15*, 145–151. [CrossRef]
37. Boesveldt, S.; Postma, E.M.; Boak, D.; Welge-Luessen, A.; Schöpf, V.; Mainland, J.D.; Martens, J.; Ngai, J.; Duffy, V.B. Anosmia—A Clinical Review. *Chem. Senses* **2017**, *42*, 513–523. [CrossRef]
38. Röing, M.; Hirsch, J.-M.; Holmström, I. The uncanny mouth—A phenomenological approach to oral cancer. *Patient Educ. Couns.* **2007**, *67*, 301–306. [CrossRef]
39. Winkler, M.F. 2009 Lenna Frances Cooper Memorial Lecture: Living with Enteral and Parenteral Nutrition: How Food and Eating Contribute to Quality of Life. *J. Am. Diet. Assoc.* **2010**, *110*, 169–177. [CrossRef]
40. Grignon, C. *Commensality and Social Morphology: An Essay of Typology*; Berg Publishers: New York, NY, USA, 2001; Available online: https://hal.inrae.fr/hal-02834203 (accessed on 22 January 2020).
41. Cipriano-Crespo, C.; Rivero-Jiménez, B.; Conde-Caballero, D.; Medina, F.X.; Mariano-Juárez, L. The Denied Pleasure of Eating: A Qualitative Study with Functionally Diverse People in Spain. *Foods* **2021**, *10*, 628. [CrossRef]
42. Venturiello, M.P. Los cuerpos con discapacidad en los diferentes ámbitos sociales: Espacios físicos e interacciones sociales. In *VII Jornadas de Jóvenes Investigadores*; Instituto de Investigaciones Gino Germani, Facultad de Ciencias Sociales, Universidad de Buenos Aires: Buenos Aires, Argentina, 2013.

Article

Are Spanish Surveys Ready to Detect the Social Factors of Obesity?

Cecilia Díaz-Méndez, Sonia Otero-Estévez * and Sandra Sánchez-Sánchez

Department of Sociology, University of Oviedo, 33006 Oviedo, Spain
* Correspondence: uo221461@uniovi.es

Abstract: The social origins of obesity are now recognised: a problem that is initially biological is today a public health problem with a social origin. This paper raises the question of whether the official statistical sources used to understand changes in diet are able to detect this shift in analysis. After reviewing the social factors that explain obesity, we examine the official Spanish statistics that can inform about dietary changes: the ENS National Health Survey, the EPF Family Budget Survey, and the EET Time Use Survey, all carried out by the Spanish Statistical Office. All of them include socio-demographic variables and some locational variables. However, the lack of health variables in the economic survey and the lack of social variables in the health survey prevent the gathering of reliable scientific evidence to offer solid support in stopping the obesity epidemic. Food has become particularly important as one of the main areas where unhealthy decisions and choices involve high risk; the situation also demonstrates the relationship between social inequality and obesity. Obesity is now understood in a radically different way and the origin of the problem lies in social and cultural factors. The current surveys do not provide the resources to capture the social causality of obesity, but slight modifications would help expand their capabilities and offer reliable scientific evidence to stop the obesity epidemic.

Keywords: food surveys; food change; food policies; sociology of food; obesity

1. Introduction

In recent years, obesity figures have become alarming, both in Spain and elsewhere. Obesity has increased in countries without food shortages, but also in poor countries, where it coexists with hunger [1–4]. Concern about its spread has prompted in-depth study of its causes from a variety of perspectives, revealing the social origins of a problem that initially seemed strictly biological and individual; these social roots are no longer questioned [5]. Therefore, research into the social factors linked to obesity is a constant in the academic literature, especially since the appearance of Wilkinson and Marmot's work *Social Determinants of Health* in 1998 [6] and following the World Health Organisation's report on obesity and overweight as a public health problem [7].

Since the beginning of the 21st century, researchers in the fields of both public health and social science have begun to address this issue and offer explanations about the origins and/or consequences of a problem associated with changes in eating habits and the social transformations of modern life [8–12].

Spain is no stranger to the problem of obesity and, according to the National Health Survey, the proportion of obese adults rose from 2.4% of the population in 1987 to 17.4% in 2017 [13]. Studies showing the social factors linked to obesity point to multiple causes, although they focus on different causal factors. The majority of them associate obesity with the types of products consumed, i.e., obesity is attributed to the poor composition of the diet, and social factors influence the food choices that lead to obesity. Obesity is considered to be caused by dietary choices that take individuals away from healthy eating patterns, and socio-demographic variables explain these choices. This has been confirmed in both older and more recent studies [14,15]. For some, inappropriate choices are prompted by the consumer's economic means, preventing them from choosing the healthiest products, something that has been observed in a variety of contexts and at different historical moments [16–18]; others claim that these incorrect choices are made because some social groups are insufficiently educated about nutrition [19,20]. Many of these studies focus on food spending, an explanation initiated by Drewnoswski and Darmon [21] and today continued in studies on poverty and food [22–24].

It is increasingly common to associate obesity with physical activity—or lack of it—and to incorporate this as a variable in analysis [25]. Although the data are not always conclusive and it is not clear that physical exercise reduces obesity in the same way that dietary control does [26], a more sedentary lifestyle has been observed among the obese population; this is the case in Spain, and socio-demographic variables continue to influence this behaviour [15]. Studies have been extended to include so-called obesogenic environments, understood as those that promote unhealthy lifestyles, and they incorporate locational variables into the analysis of obesity [27,28].

There is also a group of studies dedicated to exploring the effects of the pressure exerted by society on individuals to adopt behaviours and roles that condition their eating habits. Behind these explanations are variables relating to motivation: attitudes, perceptions, beliefs, the meaning attributed to food, and the pressure on people to conform to a body model. They also explain the effect that women's role in looking after others in the home has on their own eating behaviours and those of their families [29,30]. It has been confirmed that beliefs about health and food, or the significance attributed to foods, determine whether they are included in or excluded from the diet, which may then lead to obesity [8,31,32]. The importance of social relationships connected with food as mediating factors in beliefs and the meanings attributed should also be noted, given that eating is essentially an act of social relationship [33–35]. The body shows a person's social position and their lifestyle, as well as their cultural and economic resources and how they project themselves in terms of health [35].

All the empirical studies reviewed adopt a social conception of obesity, distanced from theoretical biomedical approaches, which view obesity or being overweight as a disease and analyse it as a risk factor for other diseases. However, within a social conception of the problem, obesity marks a body and affects a person's social image in terms of first impressions [36]. When adopting a social perspective, the analysis should not only be framed from descriptive research that shows the social groups in which obesity occurs, but should also include the conditioning factors of the actions, the secondary factors that come into play, the consequences for overweight or obese individuals, as well as the cultural resources that they have to deal with the problem [37].

The causal explanations of obesity reviewed here can be grouped into four areas: first come those that link socio-economic variables with obesity, which detect in particular the social groups most affected, according to gender, education, age, or income [14–26]. Secondly, other studies attribute this problem mainly to the creation of obesogenic contexts and they give special relevance to location as a determining factor in the dietary pattern [27,28]. Thirdly, other studies consider that food choices are explained through the subjective interpretation of reality, emphasising the way in which individuals attribute meanings or interpret food and its characteristics or the effects of ingestion on the body, which guides their choices in the purchase and preparation of food [8,30–32]. Fourthly, there are studies that associate eating behaviour and obesity in particular with relationships with other people and the social links established around food [3,29,30,34,35].

This paper asks, as a research question, what the gaps are in official Spanish surveys that hinder analysis of the social determinants of obesity. The aim is to make proposals to improve the instruments in order to facilitate public intervention in the epidemic.

Several researchers have examined the surveys critically in relation to obesity and have raised questions about their limitations. These existing studies consider that measurement needs to be improved: for some, it is necessary to revise the weight and height registers;

others suggest a need to modify the list of foods that are asked about; all of them call for agreement between professionals to reach a consensus on the methods for measuring overweight and obesity. Furthermore, the three existing studies coincide in adopting a nutritional approach [38–40]. There are no other studies in Spain that address the measurement of social factors influencing obesity, despite the general consensus that these are the main determinants of the increase in overweight and obesity and that, therefore, intervening here is what can help to curb their rise.

The contribution of the present work is the consideration of sources that do not explore strictly nutritional factors but can be used to capture changes in diet over time. Hence, not only is attention paid to the outcome (obesity), but the processes leading to it are included (dietary change) and thus the social determinants of overweight and obesity.

2. Materials and Methods

To describe and explain dietary changes, the official European statistical agencies use three surveys, which in the case of the Spanish Statistical Office (hereafter INE) are: the Spanish Health Survey (hereafter ENS until 2006, and ENSE from 2011–2012 onwards) [41]; the Household Budget Survey (hereafter EPF) [42]; and the Time Use Survey (hereafter EET) [43]. All three are standardised with the European surveys of the European statistical office EUROSTAT [44]. None of them were designed to examine food alone, but all are the reference resources for national and European research in this area.

There are two other Spanish surveys that study food that are conducted somewhat irregularly: the Food Consumption Panel of the Ministry of Agriculture [45] and the Aladdin Study on childhood obesity promoted by the Ministry of Health, which has now been conducted four times (2011, 2013, 2015, and 2019) [46]. Unlike the three mentioned above, these surveys are not integrated into the National Statistical Plan (Royal Decree-Law 410/2016), so the agencies responsible are not obliged to make the data they collect publicly available and the databases are not public either. Nor do they have direct equivalents in other European countries to enable comparison, as with the statistics of the s Spanish Statistical Office, which we analyse below.

In order to carry out the analysis of the three INE surveys, their methodological files have each been examined and three areas have been analysed: the questionnaires' objectives, their design, and their variables, in terms of the concepts behind them and their characteristics [47–54].

The ENS National Health Survey has a section on 'Social determinants' which asks about food. It enables researchers to describe eating habits based on the frequency of consumption of a short list of foods. It also asks about weight and height, and includes some data to calculate how autonomous the elderly are in their own food care (buying, preparing, and eating). This survey has an extensive list of socio-demographic variables. Its most significant shortcoming is the lack of references to the organisation of daily food and household roles (data on preparation, purchase, and day-to-day organisation), and there is no information on what motivates consumption behaviour.

This survey has undergone some notable changes with respect to our purposes. In the surveys of 2003–2006, weight and height were requested, as in all of them, but only from 2011–2012 onwards was the calculation of the Body Mass Index explained, and this calculation was modified for minors in 2017. In 2003, we started to ask whether the respondent was dieting or followed a special diet, and the reason for this diet. This question was dropped in 2017, when the question about breakfast also disappeared from the adult questionnaire. There are some shifts of interest in the list of foods, with clarifications about the items regularly consumed in 2011–2012, and new categories appear: fast food, pre-meal and savoury snacks, and natural juices.

The EPF provides information on household expenditure. Group 1 is for food and non-alcoholic beverages and Group 11 asks about eating outside the home, currently labelled 'Restaurants and hotels'. The list of products is extensive and varied and it provides an overview of what is eaten through what is bought for cooking. It has a broad sample base and an exhaustive list of geographical variables, characteristics related to the household and its members. It serves as a basis for preparing important socio-economic indices (calculation of the Consumer Price Index, the list of goods and services that make up the shopping basket). This survey does not show aspects of food related to intake, nor is it linked to health parameters, although a nutritional survey (ENNA-3) directed by Varela Moreira was carried out three times in the 1990s [55]. The survey effectively equates expenditure with consumption and lacks data that would help to understand how this spending is managed within the household. It does not include any variable relating to health.

From 2011–2012 onwards, there have been some changes in the classification of cohabitation and work activity, but these are minimal in the case of spending on food. It is worth noting that in 2016 the 'Restaurants and hotels' section included holiday rentals, which further blurs the calculation of food expenditure outside the home.

The EET is oriented towards examining the organisation of time in daily life and has a specific section on how meals and shopping are organised. It records the times of meals, the time devoted to preparation and eating, where meals take place, and the people they are shared with, as well as any other activities engaged in at the same time. It provides information on the incidence of gender roles and inequality in the sharing of tasks both within and outside the home. It does not contain specific records on health, but it registers activities, so it notes if sport is done, if the person goes to the doctor, and any other health-related activity that requires time. Height and weight appear in both iterations.

Some changes occurred between the two iterations. There was a change in the way income was measured, with new bands and slight changes in the variables relating to work activity. The options with respect to occupational status, however, were reduced. The variable for nationality was expanded, asking in 2009–2010 not only whether the respondent was Spanish or foreign-born, but also from the EU or not, and what the country of birth was.

Under marital status, there was a new category of cohabitation (as a couple). The classifications of main and secondary meals were grouped under the same heading and there were slight changes in the classification of tasks involved in preparing meals. More detailed information on the characteristics of the three surveys can be found in the Annex (Supplementary Material Tables S1 and S2).

For a comparative analysis of the three surveys, four criteria have been used, based on the results of the social studies reviewed in the literature review. These studies consider four types of explanatory variables for obesity: those that consider the causes of obesity linked to socio-demographic variables; those that provide contextual explanations and consider variables in location; those that explain obesity on the basis of subjective motivations in the choice and preparation of food; and finally relational variables, associated with the social links between individuals.

3. Results

The four criteria used for the analysis of the surveys show the gaps common to all of them, as well as the characteristics that make them complementary. These are summarised in Table 1.

Table 1. Types of variables in the ENS National Health Survey, the EPF Household Budgeting Survey, and the EET Time Use Survey.

	Socio-Economic Variables	Locational Variables	Motivational Variables	Relational Variables	Weight and Height
ENS	X	X	X	X	X
EPF	X	X		X	
EET	X	X	X	X	X

Source: Authors.

It is, however, not only a question of considering whether the variables are present, but also of specifying in what way they are present, in order to determine their usefulness. To this end, it is possible to observe the way in which these variables are expressed and, in particular, the limitations of each of the surveys (Table 2).

Table 2. Capabilities and limitations of the National Health Survey (ENS), the Household Budget Survey (EPF), and the Time Use Survey (EET) for capturing the social factors involved in obesity.

	Capabilities	Limitations
ENS National Health Survey (from INE Methodology 2017)	Socio-economic and socio-demographic variables Extensive socio-economic information on household members Questionnaire about household, adults, and children Dietary parameters: frequency of food consumption Non-dietary parameters: health status, physical activity, sleep, smoking, alcohol, eating outside the home, sedentary leisure time Subjective perceptions: happiness and health Body mass index (weight and height)	No information on the amount of energy consumed No reference to preparation Lacks questions on motivation, beliefs, and values Lacks questions on nutritional and/or culinary knowledge Does not report on how food is shared in the household Does not report on household roles (who cooks/buys) Does not report on whether or not a diet is followed Self-classification of social class according to occupation Weight and height self-reported
EPF Household Budget Survey (from INE Methodology 2016)	Socio-economic and socio-demographic variables, and household characteristics Individual and household questionnaire Links food to the rest of the household budget Extensive list of food products Records quantities purchased Reports on how food is shared within the household	Purchase and consumption are equated Lacks questions on motivation, beliefs, and values Lacks questions on nutritional and/or culinary knowledge Does not report on household roles (who cooks/buys) Lacks variables associated with health and Body Mass Index (weight and height)
EET Time Use Survey (from INE Methodology 2011)	Socio-demographic and socio-economic variables relating to the individual and the household Reports on perceived health status Reports on physical activity Reports on activities associated with food and eating Reports on routines and their interaction Reports on social relationships connected with eating Calculates time spent on paid work and household work Reports on household roles (shopping, preparation, and eating) Shows social roles, eating and shopping routines, eating places	Individual questionnaire Does not include food eaten or bought Lacks questions on motivation, beliefs, and values Lacks questions on nutritional and/or culinary knowledge Lacks variables associated with health and Body Mass Index (weight and height).

Source: authors.

4. Discussion

The surveys examined offer information on the complexity of dietary change but do not have enough variables to provide the necessary detail on the social factors linked to obesity.

Socio-demographic variables. The ENS health surveys enable us to correlate obesity with socio-demographic variables, but this is not the case with the other two surveys. The EPF household survey does not provide information on obesity, although it does corroborate dietary inequalities, showing socio-economic differences and the dietary patterns followed by individuals or households according to socio-economic and demographic variables. It provides information on the relationship between economic status and diet through an extensive list of foods. From the EET on time use researchers can extract information about the timing of meals and the importance of different daily food-related activities (preparation and eating) as a function of socio-demographic variables: gender, income, education, and age. It offers information about eating outside the home and also portrays relationships, showing gender roles and social relations in connection with food.

Locational variables. The surveys have some variables associated with the environment, which could help to identify obesogenic contexts. The EET includes classification of province, municipality, and district, and also specifically asks where meals are eaten. The ENS has data by region (Autonomous Community) and considers the population size of communities, allowing differences between urban and rural areas to be captured. The EPF enables researchers to explore variations in food expenditure according to region and by population size or relative concentration. These territorial approaches make it possible to find areas where more or less is spent on fresh or processed products depending on the district (EPF) or the food patterns by region (Autonomous Community). All of this helps to identify variations by area or to determine whether there are food deserts in Spain [56], although only the ENS and the EET allow this information to be associated with obesity. The EPF also makes it possible to differentiate between food eaten at home and out.

Motivational variables. None of the three surveys analysed include any questions aimed at finding out behavioural motivations. It is recognised that healthy habits are helped or hindered by the objective conditions of social life, which allow more or less room for manoeuvre depending on a person's or family's social, economic, or cultural capital, in line with the theoretical model proposed by Bourdieu [57]. However, there is no plan for any subjective self-assessment that would provide insight into what incites (or restrains) behaviour, so that it is not possible to know to what extent values, attitudes, beliefs, or the meaning associated with food are related to dietary choices. There are, however, questions about motivation in relation to respondents' assessment of their own state of health in both the ENS and the EET surveys.

Relational variables. The survey that provides the best information on healthy eating and people's connections with others is the EET, as eating is associated with the time spent cooking and eating, and the relationship of these activities with other people (when and with whom), both inside and outside the home. The EPF, with its household questionnaires, reveals the collective activity involved in the purchase of food, as well as its quantification in terms of the members of the household. Although the relationships are not so evident in this case, a collective act of spending (and thus consumption) is reflected. These variables are not linked to obesity.

As for the ENS, it has no variables that bring us closer to the social relationships linked to food, except in the case of people over 65 who need care from others. It does, however, allow us to establish relationships between the activities carried out in daily life, such as the consumption of alcohol and tobacco, hours of sleep, or physical exercise, although only the EET confirms the daily routines and how much they fit in with those of other people. All the same, although it is complicated to estimate the importance that an individual or group gives to eating, the EET helps to quantify this through the time spent on eating and cooking.

5. Conclusions

It is evident that some of the social factors explaining dietary change can be corroborated with data from the three sources available from the National Institute of Statistics (INE), but this does not imply that it is equally possible to confirm the social factors explaining obesity.

These sources are complementary and their explanatory power would increase substantially with the inclusion of height and weight (for the calculation of the Body Mass Index) within the variables identifying the reporting person and the household members in the EPF.

Its interest is even greater if we bear in mind that this is the survey that incorporates the largest number of foods, which might facilitate the association between social variables and specific food consumption. This would make it possible to detect the relationship between changes in food consumption and the body changes associated with it (overweight and obesity), something of particular interest for analysing periods of crisis where the social context modifies purchasing habits, the effects of which manifest in the medium or long term.

Motivational variables are difficult to fit into a standardised questionnaire, although perhaps the use of Likert scales could facilitate this task without excessive complexity, as is done in national and European opinion barometers. Questions of an evaluative nature about eating habits and reasons for not eating healthily would introduce subjective assessment of interest. This would help substantially in interpreting statistical results, which often only provide figures that are of little use in curbing the epidemic.

The relationships are currently established through the different questionnaires—for the household, for children, and for the individual—and with data on household composition. However, the individualisation of eating leads to the loss of cultural transmission of dietary knowledge. In a context where more and more information is circulating about food in the media and social networks, not knowing how much is known and how people learn to eat and cook means remaining unaware of the reality of social groups with new culinary skills and new consumption practices. Points of reference concerning people's knowledge about healthy eating and how this knowledge is acquired would provide agencies with valuable information to guide nutritional information for groups at risk of food acculturation.

The incorporation of scales for social relations and motivations related to food in the ENS and the EPF would help to improve these statistical records. These changes would generate synergies that would greatly help to obtain a deeper understanding of the social causes of obesity and would make the current surveys extremely useful.

It is not, therefore, a question of creating new tools for obesity research, but of taking advantage of the capabilities of the INE's surveys to put rigorous and reliable data into shaping a food policy against a problem whose nature has changed radically.

Supplementary Materials: The following supporting information can be downloaded at: https://www.mdpi.com/article/10.3390/ijerph191811156/s1, Table S1: Principal methodological characteristics of the ENS, EPF, and EET surveys, Table S2: General modifications and, in detail, those related to food and eating in the ENS, EPF, and EET surveys in their different versions. References [48–55] are cited in the supplementary materials.

Author Contributions: Conceptualization, C.D.-M., S.O.-E. and S.S.-S.; Data curation, C.D.-M., S.O.-E. and S.S.-S.; Formal analysis, C.D.-M., S.O.-E. and S.S.-S.; Investigation, C.D.-M., S.O.-E. and S.S.-S.; Methodology, C.D.-M., S.O.-E. and S.S.-S.; Writing—original draft, C.D.-M., S.O.-E. and S.S.-S.; Writing—review & editing, C.D.-M., S.O.-E. and S.S.-S. All authors have read and agreed to the published version of the manuscript.

Funding: This research was funded by the Spanish National Research Plan (Project MINECO CSO2015-68434-R) and a grant of University of Oviedo (PAPI-18-PF-04).

Institutional Review Board Statement: Not applicable.

Informed Consent Statement: Not applicable.

Data Availability Statement: Spanish Statistical Office (INE). Encuesta de Presupuestos Familiares. Available online: https://www.ine.es/metodologia/t25/t2530p458.pdf (accessed on 23 November 2021). Spanish Statistical Office (INE). Encuesta de Empleo del Tiempo. Available online: https://www.ine.es/dyngs/INEbase/es/operacion.htm?c=Estadistica_C&cid=1254736176815&menu=metodologia&idp=1254735976608 (accessed on 23 November 2021). Spanish Statistical Office (INE). Encuesta Nacional de Salud. Available online: https://www.ine.es/dyngs/INEbase/es/operacion.htm?c=Estadistica_C&cid=1254736176783&menu=metodologia&idp=1254735573175 (accessed on 23 November 2021).

Conflicts of Interest: The authors declare no conflict of interest.

References

1. Devaux, M.; Sassi, F. Social inequalities in obesity and overweight in 11 OECD countries. *Eur. J. Public Health* **2013**, *23*, 464–469. [CrossRef]
2. Long, B.; Robertson, A. Obesity and inequities. In *Guidance for Addressing Inequities in Overweight and Obesity*; Word Health Organization: Geneva, Switzerland, 2014.
3. World Health Organization. *Global Status Report on Non-Communicable Diseases*; Word Health Organization: Geneva, Switzerland, 2014.
4. Food and Agriculture Organization of the United Nations; World Health Organization. Summary report. In Proceedings of the Second International Conference on Nutrition, ICN2, Rome, Italy, 19–21 November 2014.
5. Rutter, H. Where next for obesity? *Lancet* **2011**, *378*, 746–747. [CrossRef]

6. Wilkinson, R.G.; Marmot, M. (Eds.) *Social Determinants of Health: The Solid Facts*; World Health Organization: Geneva, Switzerland; Centre for Urban Health (Europe) and International Centre for Health and Society: Copenhagen, Denmark, 1998.
7. World Health Organization. *The World Health Report 2002: Reducing Risks, Promoting Healthy Life: Overview*; Word Health Organization: Geneva, Switzerland, 2002.
8. Aguirre, P. Aspectos socioantropológicos de la obesidad en la pobreza. In *La Obesidad en la Pobreza: Un Nuevo reto Para la Salud Pública*; Peña, M., Bacallao, J., Eds.; Organización Panamericana de la Salud: Washington, DC, USA, 2000; Volume 576, pp. 13–25.
9. Poulain, J.-P. *Sociologie de L'óbesité*; Presses Universitaires de France: Paris, France, 2002.
10. Murcott, A. Nutrition and inequalities: A note on sociological approaches. *Eur. J. Public Health* **2002**, *12*, 203–207. [CrossRef] [PubMed]
11. Díaz Méndez, C. El tratamiento institucional de la alimentación: Un análisis sobre la intervención contra la obesidad. *Pap. Rev. Sociol.* **2012**, *97*, 371–384. [CrossRef]
12. Guthman, J. Fatuous measures: The artifactual construction of the obesity epidemic. *Crit. Public Health.* **2013**, *23*, 263–273. [CrossRef]
13. Instituto Nacional de Estadística (España). *Encuesta Nacional de Salud*; Instituto Nacional de Estadística: Madrid, Spain, 2018.
14. Sobal, J.; Stunkard, A.J. Socioeconomic status and obesity: A review of the literature. *Psychol. Bull.* **1989**, *105*, 2603. [CrossRef]
15. Díaz-Méndez, C.; Garcia Espejo, I. Social inequalities in following official guidelines on healthy diet during the period of economic crisis in Spain. *Int. J. Health Serv.* **2019**, *49*, 582–605. [CrossRef]
16. Serra Majem Ll Ribas Barba, L.; Pérez Rodrigo, C.; Aranceta Bartrina, J. Dietary habits and food consumption in Spanish children and adolescents (1998–2000): Socioeconomic and demographic factors. *Med. Clínica* **2003**, *121*, 126–131. [CrossRef]
17. Kennedy, E.; Binder, G.; Humphries-Waa, K.; Tidhar, T.; Cini, K.; Comrie-Thomson, L.; Vaughan, C.; Francis, K.; Scott, N.; Wulan, N.; et al. Gender inequalities in health and well-being across the first two decades of life: An analysis of 40 low-income and middle-income countries in the Asia-Pacific region. *Lancet Glob. Health* **2020**, *8*, e1473–e1488. [CrossRef]
18. Orozco-Rocha, K.; González-González, C. Vulnerabilidad de salud y económica de los adultos mayores en México antes de la COVID-19. *Rev. Noved. Población* **2021**, *17*, 61–84.
19. Devaux, M.; Sassi, F.; Church, J.; Cecchini, M.; Borgonovi, F. Exploring the relationship between education and obesity. *OECD J. Econ. Stud.* **2011**, *5*, 121–159. [CrossRef]
20. Sagarra-Romero, L.; Gómez-Cabello, A.; Pedrero-Chamizo, R.; Vila-Maldonado, S.; Gusi-Fuertes, N.; Villa-Vicente, J.G.; Espino-Torón, L.; González-Gross, M.; Casajús-Mallén, J.A.; Vicente-Rodríguez, G.; et al. Relación entre el nivel educativo y la composición corporal en personas mayores no institucionalizadas: Proyecto Multi-céntrico EXERNET. *Rev. Esp. Salud Pública* **2017**, *91*, e201710041. [PubMed]
21. Drewnowski, A.; Darmon, N. Food choices and diet costs: An economic analysis. *J. Nutr.* **2005**, *135*, 900–904. [CrossRef]
22. Gracia Arnaiz, M.; Demonte, F.; Kraemer, F.B. Prevenir la obesidad en contextos de precarización: Respuestas locales a estrategias globales. *Salud Colect.* **2020**, *16*, e2838. [CrossRef]
23. Rasmusson, G.; Lydecker, J.A.; Coffino, J.A.; White, M.A.; Grilo, C.M. Household food insecurity is associated with binge-eating disorder and obesity. *Int. J. Eat. Disord.* **2019**, *52*, 28–35. [CrossRef]
24. Gracia-Arnaiz, M. Making measures in times of crisis: The political economy of obesity prevention in Spain. *Food Policy* **2017**, *68*, 65–76. [CrossRef]
25. Craigie, A.M.; Lake, A.A.; Kelly, S.A.; Adamson, A.J.; Mathers, J.C. Tracking of obesity-related behaviours from childhood to adulthood: A systematic review. *Maturitas* **2011**, *70*, 266–284. [CrossRef]
26. Bensimhon, D.R.; Kraus, W.E.; Donahue, M.P. Obesity and physical activity: A review. *Am. Heart J.* **2006**, *151*, 598–603. [CrossRef]
27. Burgoine, T.; Forouhi, N.G.; Griffin, S.J.; Brage, S.; Wareham, N.J.; Monsivais, P. Does neighborhood fast-food outlet exposure amplify inequalities in diet and obesity? A cross-sectional study. *Am. J. Clin. Nutr.* **2016**, *103*, 1540–1547. [CrossRef]
28. Orzanco-Garralda, M.; Guillén-Grima, F.; Sainz Suberviola, L.; Redín Areta, M.; de la Rosa Eduardo, R.; Aguinaga-Ontoso, I. Influencia de las características urbanísticas ambientales en el nivel de actividad física de la población de 18 a 65 años del área metropolitana de Pamplona. *Rev. Esp. Salud Pública* **2016**, *90*, e30002.
29. Lhuissier, A.; Regnier, F. Obesity and food in working classes: An approach to the female body. *INRA Sci. Soc.* **2005**, *910*, 2016–71797.
30. Martín Criado, E. Las grandes tallas perjudican seriamente la salud. La frágil legitimidad de las prácticas de adelgazamiento entre las madres de clases populares. *Rev. Int. Sociol.* **2010**, *68*, 349–373. [CrossRef]
31. Espeitx, E.; y Cáceres, J. Los comportamientos alimentarios de mujeres en precariedad económica: Entre la privación y el riesgo de malnutrición. *Zainak* **2011**, *34*, 127–146.
32. Garnweidner, L.M.; Terragni, L.; Pettersen, K.S.; Mosdøl, A. Perceptions of the host country's food culture among female immigrants from Africa and Asia: Aspects relevant for cultural sensitivity in nutrition communication. *J. Nutr. Educ. Behav.* **2012**, *44*, 335–342. [CrossRef]
33. Yates, L.; Warde, A. Eating together and eating alone: Meal arrangements in British households. *Br. J. Sociol.* **2017**, *68*, 97–118. [CrossRef]
34. Otero Estevez, S. La Obesidad Como Problema Social: Un Análisis de Las Prácticas Alimentarias y De Actividad Física en Hogares Con y sin Obesidad Infantil. Doctoral Thesis, Repositorio de la Universidad de Oviedo, Universidad de Oviedo, Asturias, Spain, 2021.

35. Gracía Arnáiz, M. (Des)encuentros entre comida, cuerpo y género. In *Cuerpo y Cultura*; Martínez Guirao, J.E., Téllez Infantes, A., Eds.; Icaria: Barcelona, Spain, 2010; pp. 79–107.
36. Bourdieu, P. Notas Provisionales sobre la percepción social del cuerpo. In *Materiales de Sociología Crítica*; La Piqueta: Madrid, Spain, 1986; pp. 183–194.
37. Cruz Sánchez, M.; Tuñón Pablos, E.; Villaseñor Farías, M.; Álvarez Gordillo, G.; Byron Nigh Nielsen, R. Sobrepeso y obesidad: Una propuesta de abordaje desde la sociología. *Reg. Soc.* **2013**, *57*, 165–202. [CrossRef]
38. Navarro, A.N.; Ortiz-Moncada, R.; Fernández-Sáez, J.; Álvarez-Dardet, C. Asociación entre la dieta y la presencia de sobrepeso y obesidad. Método de evaluación dietética de la Encuesta Nacional de Salud Española 2006. *Rev. Esp. Nutr. Hum. Dietética* **2013**, *17*, 102–109. [CrossRef]
39. Martínez Álvarez, J.R.; Villarino Marín, A.; García Alcón, R.M.; Calle Purón, M.E.; Marrodán Serrano, M.D. Obesidad infantil en España: Hasta qué punto es un problema de salud pública o sobre la fiabilidad de las encuestas. *Nutr. Clin. Diet. Hosp.* **2013**, *33*, 80–88.
40. Arija, V.; Abellana, R.; Ribot, B.; Ramón, J.M. Sesgos y ajustes en la valoración nutricional de las encuestas alimentarias. *Rev. Esp. Nutr. Comunitaria* **2015**, *21*, 112–117.
41. Instituto Nacional de Estadística (Spain). Encuesta Nacional de Salud. Available online: https://www.ine.es/dyngs/INEbase/es/operacion.htm?c=Estadistica_C&cid=1254736176783&menu=metodologia&idp=1254735573175 (accessed on 26 July 2022).
42. Instituto Nacional de Estadística (Spain). Encuesta de Presupuestos Familiares. Available online: https://www.ine.es/metodologia/t25/t2530p458.pdf (accessed on 26 July 2022).
43. Instituto Nacional de Estadística (Spain). Encuesta de Empleo del Tiempo. Available online: https://www.ine.es/dyngs/INEbase/es/operacion.htm?c=Estadistica_C&cid=1254736176815&menu=metodologia&idp=1254735976608 (accessed on 26 July 2022).
44. Eurostat (EU). Statistics; Office for Official Publications, European Union: Luxembourg. Available online: https://ec.europa.eu/eurostat/web/main/publications/all-publications (accessed on 23 November 2021).
45. Panel de Consumo Alimentario. Ministerio de Agricultura, Pesca y Alimentación. (In Spanish). Available online: https://www.mapa.gob.es/es/alimentacion/temas/consumo-tendencias/panel-de-consumo-alimentario/ultimos-datos/default.aspx (accessed on 23 November 2021).
46. García-Solano, M.; Gutiérrez-González, E.; López-Sobaler, A.M.; Saavedra, M.D.R.; de Dios, T.R.; Villar-Villalba, C.; Yusta-Boyo, M.J.; Pérez-Farinós, N. Situación ponderal de la población escolar de 6 a 9 años en España: Resultados del estudio ALADINO 2019. *Nutr. Hosp.* **2021**, *38*, 943–953. [CrossRef]
47. Instituto Nacional de Estadística (Spanish Statistical Office). *Encuesta Nacional de Salud 2003. Metodología*; Instituto Nacional de Estadística: Madrid, Spain, 2003.
48. Instituto Nacional de Estadística (Spanish Statistical Office). *Encuesta Nacional de Salud 2006. Metodología detallada*; Instituto Nacional de Estadística: Madrid, Spain, 2006.
49. Instituto Nacional de Estadística (Spanish Statistical Office). *Encuesta Nacional de Salud 2011–2012. Metodología*; Instituto Nacional de Estadística: Madrid, Spain, 2013.
50. Instituto Nacional de Estadística (Spanish Statistical Office). *Encuesta Nacional de Salud de España 2017. Metodología*; Instituto Nacional de Estadística: Madrid, Spain, 2017.
51. Instituto Nacional de Estadística (Spanish Statistical Office). *Encuesta de Presupuestos Familiares 2006. Metodología*; Instituto Nacional de Estadística: Madrid, Spain, 2006.
52. Instituto Nacional de Estadística (Spanish Statistical Office). *Encuesta de Presupuestos Familiares 2016. Metodología*; Instituto Nacional de Estadística: Madrid, Spain, 2016.
53. Instituto Nacional de Estadística (Spanish Statistical Office). *Encuesta de Empleo del Tiempo 2002–2003. Tomo I. Metodología y Resultados Nacionales*; Instituto Nacional de Estadística: Madrid, Spain, 2004.
54. Instituto Nacional de Estadística (Spanish Statistical Office). *Encuesta de Empleo del Tiempo 2009–2010. Metodología*; Instituto Nacional de Estadística: Madrid, Spain, 2011.
55. Varela, G.; Moreira, O.; Carbajal, A.; Campo, M. *Estudio ENNA-3. Estudio Nacional de Nutrición y Alimentación basado en la Encuesta de Presupuestos Familiares del Instituto Nacional de Estadística*; Departamento de Nutrición, Universidad Complutense: Madrid, Spain, 1991.
56. Ramos Truchero, G. El acceso a la alimentación: El debate sobre los desiertos alimentarios. *Investig. Desarro.* **2015**, *23*, 391–415. [CrossRef]
57. Bourdieu, P. *La Distinción*; Criterios y Bases Sociales del Gusto: Taurus, Mexico, 2002.

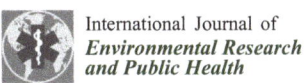

Article

Categorizations of Trust and Distrust in the Classifications and Social Representations of Food among Pregnant and Breastfeeding Women in Spain—Applying the Cultural Domains' Pile Sort Technique

Araceli Muñoz [1,2,3,*], Cristina Larrea-Killinger [3,4,5], Andrés Fontalba-Navas [3,6,7] and Miguel Company-Morales [3,8,9]

1. Training and Research Unit—School of Social Work, University of Barcelona, 08035 Barcelona, Spain
2. Research and Innovation Group in Social Work (GRITS), TRU—School of Social Work, University of Barcelona, 08035 Barcelona, Spain
3. "ToxicBody" Interdisciplinary Network, Department of Social Anthropology, University of Barcelona, 08001 Barcelona, Spain
4. Research Group "Anthropology of Crisis and Contemporary Transformations (CRITS)", Department of Social Anthropology, University of Barcelona, 08001 Barcelona, Spain
5. CIBER de Epidemiología y Salud Pública (CIBERESP), 28029 Madrid, Spain
6. Antequera Hospital, Northern Málaga Integrated Healthcare Area, 29200 Antequera, Spain
7. Department of Public Health and Psychiatry, University of Málaga, 29016 Málaga, Spain
8. Seron Primary Care Centre, Northern Almería Integrated Healthcare Area, 04600 Huercal-Overa, Spain
9. Department of Nursing, Physiotherapy and Medicine, University of Almería, 04120 La Cañada, Spain
* Correspondence: aracelimunoz67@ub.edu

Abstract: Food is fundamental in the decision making of pregnant and breastfeeding women to care for their own health and that of their child. In this paper, we explore some common food classification systems and certain attributes assigned to these categories, represented by values of trust and distrust. This study is based on an interdisciplinary research project in which we analysed discourses and practices regarding the dietary intake of pregnant and breastfeeding women in relation to the presence of chemical substances in foods. The results presented are part of the second phase of this research where we explored the results of our analysis of the pile sort technique based on an analysis of cultural domains in order to explore the categories and semantic relations among terms regarding trust and distrust in food. This technique was applied to the 62 pregnant and breastfeeding women of Catalonia and Andalusia. These women also participated in eight focus groups that provided information and narratives enabling us to analyse the meanings of the associative subdomains obtained in the pile sorts. They classified different foods and assigned certain attributes to them according to the level of trust and mistrust, providing a social representation of food risks. The mothers expressed great concern about the quality of the food they consume and about its possible effects on their own health and on that of their child. They perceive that an adequate diet is one based on the consumption of fruits and vegetables, preferably fresh. Fish and meat generate serious concern, as their properties are considered ambivalent depending on the food's origin and mode of production. These criteria are perceived by women as relevant to their food decisions and, therefore, emic knowledge should be taken into account when developing food safety programmes and planning actions aimed at pregnant and breastfeeding women.

Keywords: cultural domains; pile sorts; food risk; trust; distrust; pregnancy; breastfeeding

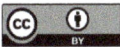

1. Introduction

This article is based on an exploratory study of the food classification system and the values assigned to the resulting categories according to the criteria of trust and distrust by pregnant and breastfeeding women. Knowledge of how consumers perceive the differences between foods enriches our understanding of eating behaviours [1]. It is also important to be able to evaluate the risks present in food selection and consumption [2]. This includes both risks derived from habits and lifestyles [3] and those resulting from transformations in the food system for increased production, possibly involving manipulations that increase risks to health [4,5].

Cognitive models related to decision making in food choices include the attributes of trust–distrust which are, in turn, components of perceptions of food (in)security. Trust is an intangible construct with many definitions, ranging from the multidimensional encompassing principles such as competence, coherence and empathy tosociopsychological principles. The latter includes both the trust inspired by the institutional structures that regulate daily life and the calculating, rational and mediated by logic, assumptions and experience [6]. In any relationship, this trust is an essential component, albeit highly dynamic and fragile.

In such an important period of life as pregnancy and lactation, women need to feel sure that the food they eat is safe and accompanied by accurate information. This demand for assurance is all the stronger within the present global food system, which is complex and interconnected, and where it is difficult to trust the sources of food information [7]. The "nutritional cacophony" referred to by Fischler [8] is part of this globalised system and has an evident influence on food choices. Women's nutrition, before and during pregnancy, plays a key role in their own health and in that of their child, and is an important aspect in optimising pregnancy outcomes [9]. For this reason, the concepts of confidence in food, related to its safety and perceived risks, are of cardinal importance in dietary preferences during pregnancy and breastfeeding [10,11].

Another important consideration is that the medicalisation of pregnancy [12,13] and nutrition [14] in Western countries, together with the biomedical discourses received, subject pregnant and breastfeeding women to incessant control and surveillance. Furthermore, in order to safeguard the health of their child (before and after birth), mothers are under great pressure to self-regulate and self-care [15,16]. Pregnancy and lactation, thus, are vital but stressful stages during which the woman may view what is happening to her body with fear and distrust [17], especially when subjected to the discourse of risk. As a result, many women apply precaution as a strategy for managing uncertainty [18] and for protecting the child [19]. As a consequence, food-related discourses and practices are a vital consideration in women's attitudes towards their health.

In this fundamental place that food occupies in the decision making of pregnant and breastfeeding women for the care of their own health and the baby's [20,21], the criteria applied for food choice and consumption depend on various socioeconomic and cultural factors [18,22].

In this paper, we analyse food classification systems and certain attributes assigned to these categories, represented by values of trust and distrust. An analysis of cultural domains [23], an area of cognitive anthropology, brings us closer to how members of a society think about certain sets of items that have a joint presence in their culture or which are represented as being of the same type [24,25]. Analyses of cultural domains are commonly used in medical anthropology, and there exists an extensive bibliography regarding this type of research. In the field of food and nutrition, the pile sort technique is especially useful [26–34].

2. Materials and Methods

2.1. Study Design and Setting

This study, which was part of a broader interdisciplinary research project, was conducted to analyse discourses and practices on the dietary intake of pregnant and breastfeeding women in relation to the presence of chemical substances in foods [11,18,22,35–37]. The research was conducted in two phases, the first from 2015 to 2017 (Ref. CSO2014-58144-P) and the second from 2018 to 2021 (Ref. AP-0139-2017).

The field work was carried out at various health centres (hospitals and primary care centres) in the Spanish autonomous regions of Catalonia (Barcelona and its metropolitan area, Baix Llobregat, Tarragona and Ribera d'Ebre) and Andalusia (Granada and its surroundings, Valle del Almanzora, Antequera and Cabra).

2.2. Study Sample

The sample selection process was intentional or purposive, seeking the maximum variation, heterogeneity and intensity, whilst obtaining a balanced sample with similar representations of age, education, occupation and socioeconomic stratum. The following inclusion criteria were applied: women born in Spain, 20 weeks pregnant or more, or who had given birth during the last six months and were breastfeeding (exclusively or also using formula). The exclusion criteria were that the women must not have had any pathology that entailed a change in their diet. All participants were informed of the objectives and methods of the research and gave written consent to take part. Approval was also obtained from the corresponding ethics committees.

2.3. Data Collection and Analysis

In the first phase of the research (Figure 1), 111 semistructured interviews were conducted (with 62 pregnant women and 49 breastfeeding women) together with 4 focused ethnographies, 2 focus groups, 71 food diaries, 71 free listings and 12 interviews with health professionals (Table 1). In the second phase, eight focus groups and 62 pile sorts were conducted with 62 mothers (26 of whom were pregnant and 36 of whom were breastfeeding) (Table 2).

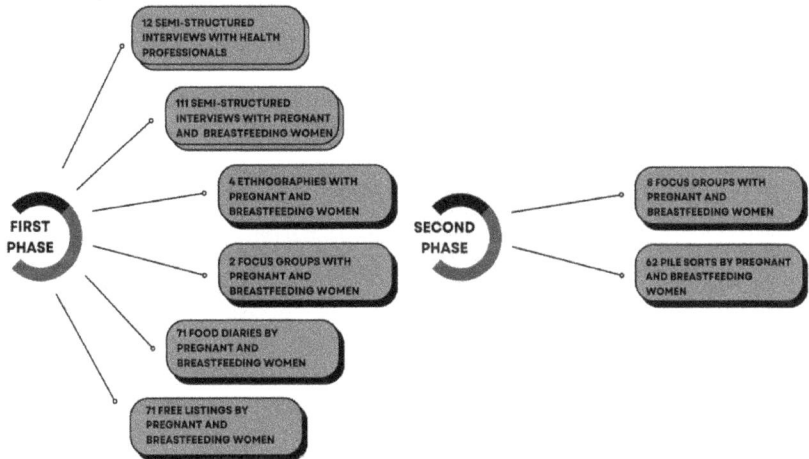

Figure 1. First and second phases. Data collection instruments.

In Muñoz et al. [36], we reported the results of our analysis of the data obtained from the free listings carried out in the first phase of the study, in which the mothers were urged to think about what types of food they saw as trustworthy and untrustworthy and to make lists of each type of food. In the article, we explained how the technique of free listings was applied to a group of pregnant and breastfeeding women to analyse the main shared items or elements regarding trust and distrust in food. This technique is based on an analysis of cultural domains [23], a method for analysing social meanings and shared knowledge [24], which enables us to understand how mothers assimilate different social meanings and to determine the most important categories used in talking about trust/distrust in relation to food.

Table 1. First phase. Sociodemographic characteristics of the participants.

		Pregnant Women	Breastfeeding Women
Age	20–29 years	3	2
	30–39 years	33	23
	40 years and over	4	6
Number of children	1	18	15
	2	18	12
	3 or more	4	4
Education level	Primary	3	0
	Secondary	11	8
	Higher	26	23
Place of residence	Catalonia	29	22
	Andalusia	11	9

Table 2. Second phase. Sociodemographic characteristics of the participants.

		Pregnant Women	Breastfeeding Women
Age	20–29 years	5	5
	30–39 years	22	27
	40 years and over	2	1
Number of children	1	16	28
	2	10	4
	3 or more	3	1
Education level	Primary	2	2
	Secondary	9	10
	Higher	18	21
Place of residence	Catalonia	7	19
	Andalusia	22	14

In this paper, we present the second phase of the study, in which we conducted a different technique that was also based on the analysis of cultural domains [23] in order to analyse categories and semantic relations among terms regarding trust and distrust in food [25]. This technique, pile sort, was applied to the 62 pregnant and breastfeeding women who participated in the eight focus groups. In this approach, free lists are usually followed by pile sorts [25] to identify the relations among terms within a given domain [38]. The basic aim of this technique is to formalise an associative cultural map for each of the indicated areas. Pile sorts are mainly used to obtain semblances between certain items in a cultural domain or attributes that are used to distinguish these items from the informants' criteria [39].

2.3.1. Items or Categories of Analysis from the Free Listings

The participants were instructed to group the main items/categories of food cited in the free listings obtained in phase one of the study, reflecting similarities or differences regarding their trust and distrust in each case. Thus, the food categories for trust ($n = 20$) and distrust ($n = 20$) used in the pile sorts were obtained from the free listings, i.e., the twenty most cited items in the free listings for trust and distrust, respectively (Table 3).

The mothers were asked to identify different types of food as trusted or distrusted and to attribute qualities and adjectives to each product together with the specific properties perceived and other relevant characteristics related to the origin, manipulation, processing and distribution of the product. Adjectives such as fresh, natural, organic, whole-grain, seasonal, local, from the garden, homemade, craft or washed are often associated with trust, while those termed as processed, industrial, precooked, prepared, packaged, canned, fried or foreign tend to be distrusted. It is important to note that some foods are mentioned several times, since distinctions are made depending on their handling.

Table 3. Food categories associated with trust (*n* = 20) and distrust (*n* = 20) in the pile sorts obtained from the free listings.

	Trust		Distrust
1.	Fruit	1.	Industrial pastries
2.	Vegetables	2.	Pre-cooked food
3.	Legumes	3.	Sausage products
4.	Fish	4.	Frozen food
5.	Meat	5.	Crisps
6.	Cereals	6.	Ready-made sauce
7.	Meal	7.	Frankfurters
8.	Nuts	8.	Fast food
9.	Bread	9.	Packaged meat
10.	Pasta	10.	Packaged juice
11.	Dairy products	11.	Packaged food
12.	Eggs	12.	Sweets
13.	Rice	13.	Processed meat
14.	Chicken	14.	Soft drinks
15.	Yoghurt	15.	Tuna
16.	Fresh fish	16.	Meat
17.	Organic meat	17.	Fish
18.	Organic products	18.	Canned food
19.	Fresh vegetables	19.	Supermarket meat
20.	Water	20.	Ready-to-eat meals

2.3.2. Item Sorts and Categories of Analysis

The pile sorts were obtained as follows: each participant was given two sets of cards, one with the names of types of food that generally inspire trust and the other with those associated with distrust [38]. Each set of cards was randomly shuffled, and the participants were instructed to group the cards by sorting them into piles with as many or as few cards as they wished. No specific criteria for doing so were mentioned [40]. However, the women were told they could not put all the cards in a single pile [38].

2.3.3. Analysing with ANTHROPAC and Nonmetric Multidimensional Scaling (nMDS)

The information from the pile sorts was classified and analysed using *ANTHROPAC* software (version 1.0.1.36, Software for Cultural Domain Analysis, Borgatti, SP.; Analytic Technologies: Natick, MA, USA, 2003), designed for the quantitative analysis of qualitative data and cultural domains [41]. From the *ANTHOPAC* findings, *nonmetric multidimensional scaling (nMDS)* was performed on the participants' trust and distrust in the food categories, to represent the pile sorts obtained that reflected the proximity/distance of each category in the mother's perceptive universe. *nMDS* provides a way to represent semantic proximities without requiring metric data [42], in which the distances between items reveal correlational, not metric distances [25]. The outcome of this process is a graphic display of the mothers' thought processes in creating the pile sorts [43].

2.3.4. Identifying Clusters or Dimensions

nMDS results may be interpreted by considering the items as dimensions or as clusters [25]. In our analysis, the associative subdomains in the women's perceptions were overlaid on the representation. The *nMDS* model enables various interpretations to be made, and so the item areas or dimensions proposed are tentative. Using the information obtained from the focus groups, we identified clusters or dimensions and decided which labels should be attached to each [29]. In the case in question, five clusters or dimensions in the *nMDS* were related to trust and another five to distrust (Table 4). The labels of these dimensions refer not only to different types of foods but also to the qualities and properties attributed to them, as well as other characteristics related to their origin, manipulation, processing and distribution.

Table 4. Clusters or dimensions in the *nMDS* related to trust (*n* = 5) and distrust (*n* = 5) in food items.

Trust	Distrust
1. Items inspiring confidence due to the nutritional properties of the food itself and/or its origin and manipulation.	1. Prepared or precooked products.
2. Items characterised by ambivalence regarding trust/distrust.	2. Processed basic foods.
	3. Highly artificial processed products with many added chemicals.
3. Cereals, legumes and nuts.	4. Items that are distrusted due to their origin, manipulation and/or distribution.
4. Eggs	5. Items that are distrusted due to worries about food preservation.
5. Dairy products	

2.3.5. Pile Sorts and Focus Groups' Narratives

The focus groups provided information and narratives enabling us to analyse the meanings of the associative subdomains obtained when the mothers constructed pile sorts. The focus groups also informed us about their sociocultural norms, attitudes and perceptions regarding interactions with the environment [44]. The participation of these women in the focus groups gave us a better understanding of the social contexts in which crucial decisions were made. These qualitative data were analysed following the strategies expressed in Grounded Theory [45,46] to identify, interpret and explain the core meaning of the data obtained from pregnant and breastfeeding women and thus to generate meaningful codes and categories. The study information was exhaustively systematised using *ATLAS-ti* qualitative analysis software (Version 8; ATLAS-ti Scientific Software Development GmbH: Berlin, Germany, 2019).

3. Results

We present the results obtained from analysing the pile sorting activity and the focus groups' contributions regarding associative subdomains for trust or distrust in different types of food. This analysis enabled us to distinguish similarities and differences in the categories generated by the focus group participants.

In these focus groups, the participants remarked on the complexity of determining which foods can be trusted and which cannot. In relation to food environments, for example, they reflect on how contamination may affect production and provoke distrust in the food consumed:

> "Absolutely. For me, this has a direct influence, because the plants, which rely on rain, on the water that falls, when they're in contaminated ground, this is where they feed. And the animals that eat contaminated grass, or that eat, well, everything ... the water, everything, the nitrates, everything that's in the soil, then everything ends up in the plant. And we eat all of that. So, yes, I do think it affects us".
>
> *(Tarragona focus group)*

They also note that distrust in some foods spurs a search for more information, which can then provoke even greater distrust in the products investigated:

> "Of course, you tend to distrust everything. Then again, if you have to look at what's in all the food, you wouldn't buy anything, you wouldn't eat anything. But finally, you end up eating it because you like it, full stop ... ".
>
> *(Tarragona focus group)*

The pregnant and breastfeeding mothers consulted expressed great concern about food quality and its potential effects on their health and that of their child, and emphasised the importance of knowing what they are eating, on reading the labels and on having good information about the composition of the products bought and consumed:

> "You try to take better care of yourself. Also, now that I've got over the gestational diabetes I had, well, I look at everything much more closely and now I'm looking

at the labels much more than I used to, I can see they add sugar to things, which I didn't know about before, I didn't ... For example. So, it's true that now, apart from being careful with freezing and washing food, and I don't know what else, when you start looking at the labels that's another question... In my case, due to my special circumstance, yes. When this is all over, sure, I won't look at them so carefully".

(Antequera focus group)

"Take fish, for example. Even if it's fresh today, I don't care. Even if it's fresh today, I won't eat it straight away. I always freeze it and eat it later, because once before, I was going to eat it on the same day and I found this little worm inside, the larva or whatever, though later I heard that you can't see anisakis, it's impossible. Well, I saw a worm, I don't know if it was anisakis or what it was, but from then on, I've always frozen everything".

(Tarragona focus group)

The women participating in the focus groups also argued that distrust is not incompatible with taste, since many of these foods are liked; nevertheless, they are avoided because they are not considered healthy. Distrust in itself does not prevent consumption. Some of the women acknowledged that you should not think too much about food because otherwise you would end up not eating anything. As some of the participants pointed out: "Everything creates distrust, but distrust doesn't stop you from eating" *(Tarragona focus group)*, or "We don't trust it, but we have to eat" *(Tíjola focus group)*.

Another idea that came out in these narratives, and one that makes deciding which foods to choose even more complex, is that the amount of food or the frequency of its consumption is important. In other words, the excessive or abusive consumption of any product can have a negative impact on people's health.

"- .... But if you haven't got much time, and now you're going to do the shopping, are you going to look at the label on every single product? I don't know, that would drive you ... you'd spend all day in the supermarket.

- What I do, at most, is to look later at home, though ... the first few times I've bought something ...

- I always buy the same things, that's all. But at first, I used to stop and pay good attention to the E, the stabilisers, the sweeteners, the acidulants, the E340, the E three hundred and whatever. Because I remembered really well that here in Cabra, at school, the teacher sent us all to the supermarkets to write down all the E's in the food products. So, later on, we were well aware of what we were doing ... dairy this, meat that, whatever the other, and we realised that almost everything was carcinogenic.

- If you start reading, you won't eat anything".

(Cabra focus group)

3.1. The Trust of Pregnant and Breastfeeding Women in Food

The *nonmetric multidimensional scaling (nMDS)* performed for confidence in food revealed five associative subdomains in the proximity/distance map of the categories, according to the perceptions of the women participating (Figure 2).

The clusters or associative subdomains of the *nMDS* graphical representation of trust in food were given these labels: 1. items in which trust arises from the nutritional properties of the food itself and/or its origin and manipulation; 2. cereals, legumes and nuts; 3. dairy products; 4. eggs; 5. items in which participants expressed ambivalence in terms of (mis)trust.

In the focus groups, various categories and items related to trust in food emerged from the participants' narratives (Figure 3).

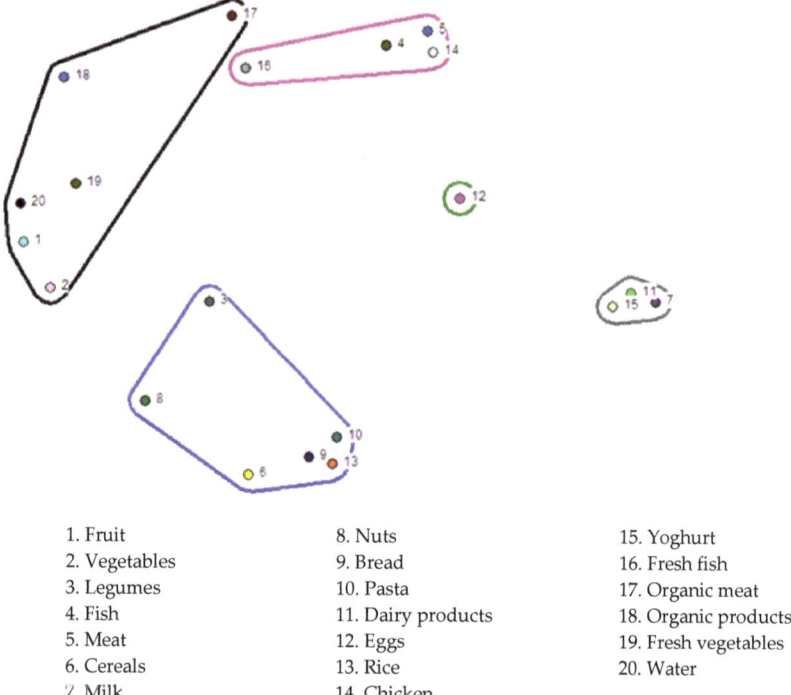

1. Fruit	8. Nuts	15. Yoghurt
2. Vegetables	9. Bread	16. Fresh fish
3. Legumes	10. Pasta	17. Organic meat
4. Fish	11. Dairy products	18. Organic products
5. Meat	12. Eggs	19. Fresh vegetables
6. Cereals	13. Rice	20. Water
7. Milk	14. Chicken	

Figure 2. Nonmetric multidimensional scaling (nMDS) of trust in food. Representation of the total number of pile sorts ($n = 62$), showing the proximity/distance of the categories in the women's perceptual universe. The nMDS model allows for various interpretations, and therefore the proposed item areas are tentative. Interpretation of the clusters or dimensions: blue: cereals, legumes and nuts; black: trusted items due to the nutritional properties of the food itself and/or its origin and manipulation; pink: items characterised by ambivalence regarding (mis)trust; green: eggs; grey: dairy products.

The first area of items in the nMDS model of trust in food revealed two related categories: on the one hand, fruits and vegetables, in which trust is based on their inherent nutritional properties; on the other, organic meats and products linked by trust based on their origin and handling.

"In relating these groupings with the narratives drawn from the focus groups, it can be seen that, in reference to trust in the nutritional properties of fruits and vegetables, the participants remarked that natural, fresh products contain the best nutritional components, vitamins and minerals. Furthermore, these nutrition-based attitudes towards the properties of foods are reinforced by biomedical care during pregnancy and childbirth, although taste also plays an important role; thus, some mothers emphasised that fresh fruit had a better flavour: 'Exactly, so they can grow them faster, because when you see a tomato that's this big, but when you eat it, it doesn't have any taste!'".

(Tíjola focus group)

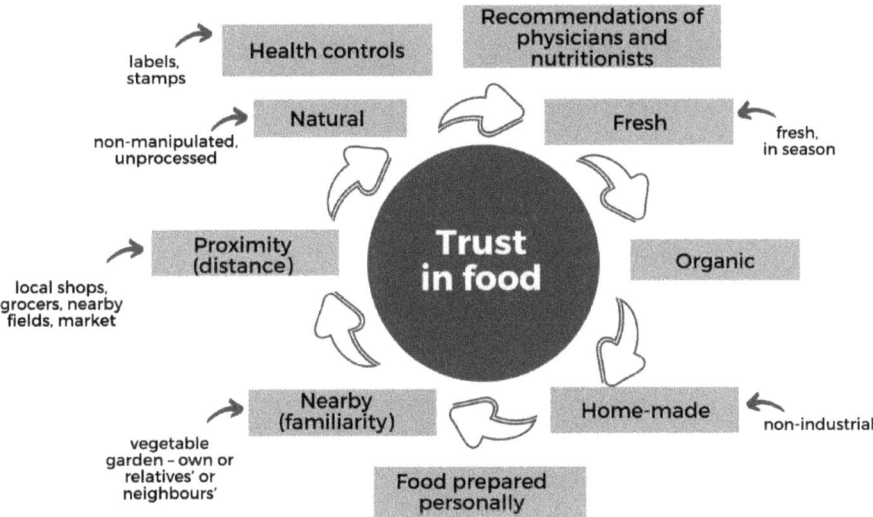

Figure 3. Categories and items arising from the focus groups in relation to trust in food.

Although fruits and vegetables are trusted and considered to be healthy and nutritious, some of the women consulted compared the use of pesticides and fertilisers in intensive agriculture (unfavourably) with the absence of these products from their own and relatives' vegetable gardens. They provided an environmental justification in relation to a growing distrust toward chemical substances derived from agricultural production [18,36], and they argued that intensive agriculture harms plant health and growth by degrading the soil and water. Some of the women commented that although they tried to avoid using pesticides in their gardens, this was not always possible:

> "Because they've made [the fruit, vegetables] bigger, oh yes, with fertilisers and the like… I know that my father-in-law has to use something to kill the bugs, because nowadays the soil isn't good, the water isn't good. So, I don't know, your plants die. If you don't use something extra, the tomatoes won't grow".
>
> *(Tíjola focus group)*

Nevertheless, these women distinguish between the products of intensive agriculture and what comes from their own or their family's gardens, which they know is much healthier:

> "My father-in-law has a vegetable garden and we used to help him out. The best thing is… there's no comparison, you pick a tomato from there… the bunch of tomatoes or the peppers in season, … we grew it ourselves, that's what I really trust".
>
> *(Cabra focus group)*

In relation to organic meat and other organic products, and people's trust based on the origin and handling of the food, the participants in our focus groups remarked that they had more trust in this type of product, which they considered less industrially manipulated and contained fewer chemical additives such as pesticides, herbicides and hormones. In their opinion, organic certification gives a sense of security backed by production controls, where the legal discourse of certification generates trust associated with healthy living and sustainability. A woman who works in a meat producing company shared her experience:

> "- Even if there are lots of controls, industrial methods will never be as natural as what you do at home. But it is true that the industrial scene has all the veterinary controls. When you slaughter at home, well yes, the vet is usually there. Except when he isn't. That's the thing. So, it's a bit complicated.

- And when you buy from the local man, you don't know if the pig has been sick, either...

- That's right.

- And, for example, the animal could have been given antibiotics, right?

- Sure. So, I know that my company has passed all the quality controls. I would trust the food completely if I did this at home, you know, but someone else who does it, well, you don't know what they're feeding the pig, you don't know if the vet has been to... to make sure that the meat is in good condition. So, really, I'd eat my company's meat, that's the truth".

(Tíjola focus group)

The *nMDS* model of consumer trust also contained a second set of items that were a little more widely separated: an associative subdomain comprised of cereals, legumes and nuts.

In their words, the members of the focus groups trusted cereals, viewing them as products that usually keep well without spoiling. In this respect, they placed special emphasis on bread, pasta and rice, which were termed "balanced" foods and a source of energy.

"What would give me the most confidence would be, as I said before, pasta and legumes, because they give me more peace of mind".

(Antequera focus group)

The levels of trust in cereals were determined by notions of their origin, price and degree of manipulation.

"For example, because I see it in my work, maybe... "Look, I'm going to buy these cereals for my child, because they're the best, because they are more expensive", and you compare them with another brand and it has a lot of added sugar ... ".

(Cabra focus group)

Many of the participants trusted legumes because this type of food has many nutritional properties with proteins and iron. For these mothers, it is important that legumes are subject to very little processing and manipulation and are easy to store.

"Well, the thing is to have a balanced diet, a little of everything. With legumes, fish, a bit of everything. In pregnancy, sometimes, I don't know, sometimes it does something to you, but well. Sure, dairy products and all that, yes".

(Tarragona focus group)

It is these very characteristics that are apparent in legumes, which are seen as trusted products, like nuts. The mothers in the focus groups also indicated that legumes are very "natural", being rich in healthy fats and providing a lot of energy.

"For I eat a few nuts, too. They give me energy, I think. I don't know if it's psychological, but I think they do me good".

(Sant Feliu focus group)

"Nuts, perhaps, is what I trust most. Because I think everything else is more adulterated, and ... With animals, it's hormones. With fish, heavy metals. Fruit and vegetables, they're full of pesticides. Unless you're going to buy organic, then you know there are more guarantees. Nuts, I would say, maybe. And seeds".

(Tarragona focus group)

Considered in a similarly positive light are two associative subdomains, dairy products and eggs.

Dairy foods, especially milk and yogurt, also generated confidence among the participants, who referred to these products as complete and nutritious with a high calcium content and which undergo strict controls in their preparation process.

Eggs were also among the foods that were generally well trusted by the mothers in the study groups, who emphasised that it provides lots of protein and is subject to little industrial manipulation. However, this trust depends on the production methods used; eggs from free-range hens are trusted because this status affects the way the hens are treated, their behaviour and, ultimately, the quality of the food. By contrast, the intensive production model is criticised, and this negative view influences consumer choice.

> "Eggs, for example, before, the chickens lived free, they were... now we eat eggs from chickens that are stressed out because they are locked up. It's true, they are psychologically stressed, they're pressured to lay eggs, come on, lay eggs that need to be sold, do this, do that ... I don't like eggs very much. I'll often buy from someone who's got a bit of land, I'll buy just a few eggs from them... I also buy in supermarkets, because you've got to do the shopping, ...".
>
> *(Tíjola focus group)*

Finally, another set of items in the *nMDS* trust model formed an associative subdomain characterised by ambivalence between trust and distrust. This ambivalence concerned two types of food in particular: fish and meat.

On the one hand, fish generated trust due to the properties of the food itself, its proteins, minerals and omega 3 content. On the other hand, distrust could occur depending on the origin, manipulation and conservation of this food. As one of the mothers pointed out:

> "For example, I eat a lot of fresh fish, my father goes out fishing, and you can't even trust that, really, because of the plastics in the water, the spills from the boats...".
>
> *(Vera focus group)*

Meat is another food that generated trust due to its natural properties, providing proteins and containing a lot of iron. However, concerns about production and manipulation reduced the level of trust in this respect as well.

> "- I prefer to go to the butcher's and have the meat minced there, rather than buy packaged minced meat from...
>
> - But you don't know what you're eating from the butcher's either. I can tell you, because I work a lot there.
>
> - Yes, of course, obviously... But at least you can see the piece of chicken and the piece that they're mincing.
>
> - They put it in the display case and say, how good it looks, how clean it is, but they also add salt water and leave it for 24 h to turn white...
>
> - Yes, of course, of course.
>
> - At present, I'd rather trust the meat, for example, from the M. supermarket than from the butcher's. In my experience, anyway".
>
> *(Antequera focus group)*

> "Well, the thing is to have a balanced diet, a little of everything. With legumes, fish, a bit of everything. In pregnancy, sometimes, I don't know, sometimes it does something to you, but well. Sure, dairy products and all that, yes".
>
> *(Tarragona focus group)*

3.2. The Distrust of Pregnant and Breastfeeding Women in Food

The illustration of *nonmetric multidimensional scaling (nMDS)* on distrust in food shows that there are five associative subdomains in the proximity/distance map of the food categories according to the pregnant and breastfeeding women participating in this study (Figure 4).

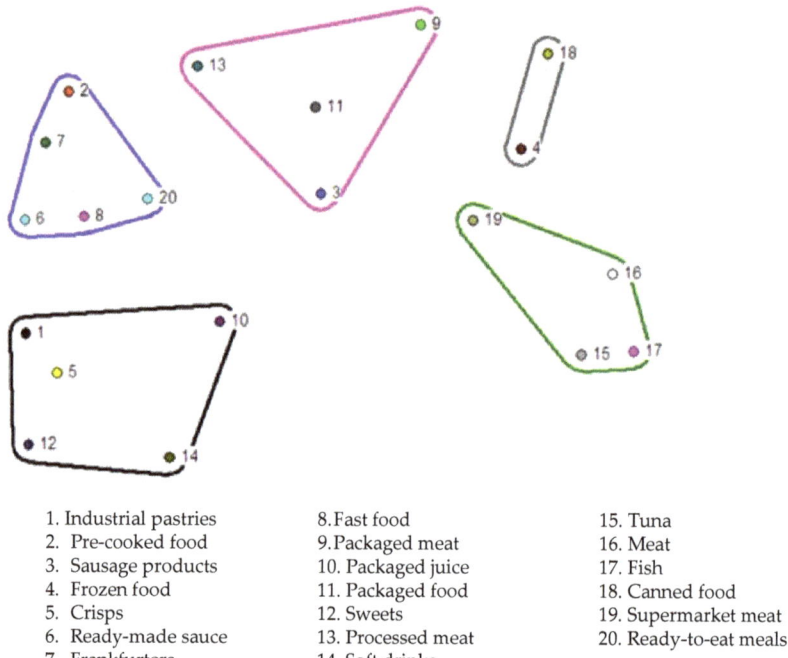

1. Industrial pastries	8. Fast food	15. Tuna
2. Pre-cooked food	9. Packaged meat	16. Meat
3. Sausage products	10. Packaged juice	17. Fish
4. Frozen food	11. Packaged food	18. Canned food
5. Crisps	12. Sweets	19. Supermarket meat
6. Ready-made sauce	13. Processed meat	20. Ready-to-eat meals
7. Frankfurters	14. Soft drinks	

Figure 4. Nonmetric multidimensional scaling (nMDS) of distrust in food. Representation of the total number of pile sorts (n = 62) showing the proximity/distance of the categories in the women's perceptual universe. The nMDS model allows for various interpretations and therefore the proposed item areas are tentative. Interpretation of the clusters or dimensions: blue: prepared or pre-cooked food; black: highly artificial processed products with many added chemical substances; pink: basic processed products; green: products that are distrusted due to their origin, manipulation and/or distribution; grey: products that are distrusted because of concerns about added preservatives.

The different clusters or associative subdomains in the nMDS graphical representation of distrust in food are labelled as: 1. prepared or precooked products; 2. basic processed products; 3. highly artificial processed products with many added chemical substances; 4. items distrusted due to their origin, manipulation and/or distribution; 5. items distrusted due to concerns about added preservatives.

The discussions held in the focus groups gave rise to the following categories and items related to trust in food (Figure 5).

Continuing with the first area of items in the nMDS model of food distrust, there were three subdomains of items that grouped a large body of foods that generated suspicion according to the way in which they were manipulated: these were prepared or precooked products, basic processed products and highly artificial products with chemical additives.

In relating these groupings with the narratives from the focus groups, it can be seen that the participants distrusted prepared or precooked products because they do not know what substances they may contain; they also had serious reservations concerning how these foods are processed, manipulated, cooked, preserved and packaged.

"- Very good. What foods do you think contain chemicals?

- Almost everything.

- It depends. If you are going to buy fresh, well . . .

- Pre-cooked ones, definitely.

- Fresh ones, too, now... there'll be something in them.

- The fresh ones will have less. Fresh products always have ... there'll be less, that's why they have a shelf life. But there'll be preservatives in canned goods, preserves, all of that".

(Vera focus group)

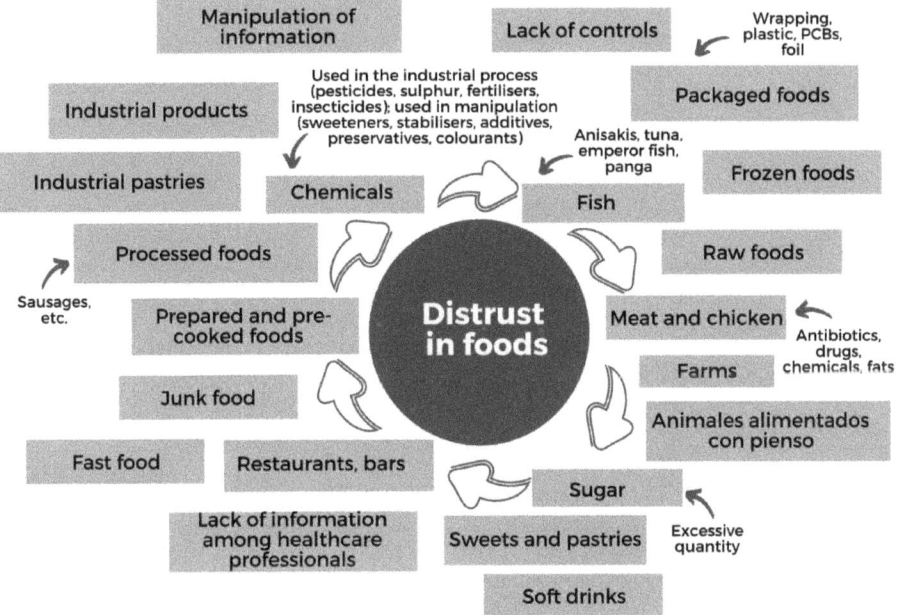

Figure 5. Categories and items arising from the focus groups in relation to distrust in food.

In relation to basic processed foods, such as meat, the participants said they distrusted those that have been "processed" or "treated", referring in particular to the addition of preservatives, stabilisers and colourants, which they perceived as "unnatural".

"- Yes, I'm not so keen on packaged food. For example, take minced meat; if you read the label on the pack you'll see it contains more things that are not meat than what is meat. But if you go to the butcher's, they'll be mincing it right there, in front of you, to give an example. Or pork loin, when you see it's full of water or, I don't know, maybe it isn't water, I don't even know what it might be. It doesn't give you much confidence.

- I think it's ... sausages and all that. Since I started reading the labels, I haven't bought them again. I haven't bought them again because it makes me uneasy. But packaged meat, well, sometimes, yes".

(Tíjola focus group)

Processed products that are considered highly artificial or which contain large amounts of chemical additives—such as industrial pastries, crisps, packaged juices and soft drinks—provoke great suspicion. This is especially the case with industrial pastries, due on the one hand to the presence of saturated fats and sugars and, on the other, to the existence of chemical additives such as sweeteners, colourants, flavourings and preservatives.

"Looking after children, I think, is much more complicated than controlling your own diet. The children who eat worse than... Well, I don't know if it's worse, but they eat what is sold as food for children, and it has such an enormous amount of sugar; I always say, go to the supermarket and get a My First Danone, and a normal Danone, and look at the amount of sugar in My First Danone. Your heart sinks. And it is very difficult to escape from those kinds of foods, no matter how much you want to. At home you can give them the healthiest, really the healthiest food, look out for them... But they are in the world ... It's really very difficult".

(Antequera focus group)

In a similar way to the above-mentioned groups, there was an ambivalent associative subdomain in the participants' (mis)trust in food depending on its origin, manipulation and distribution. Concerning meat, the mothers distrusted meat from animals that had been fed with fodder, with "chemical substances" or that had been injected with hormones or other drugs. Instead, they preferred meat that was more "natural", from animals allowed to freely graze in the open.

"The fewer the additives, the fewer the extra preservatives that aren't natural, for me that's closer to being healthy. I mean, for example, before on the label there was the word 'tuna', which is a fish that, within a balanced diet ... fish, well, you consider it... well, me at least, I consider it part of a balanced diet. But it's not a fish that gives me much confidence, because it reminds me of mercury, pollution, all that. And I'd almost rather eat canned tuna or tuna that comes from a fish farm, than the natural fish, because, perhaps because of the context of mercury that's been related with tuna and suchlike ... it depends on the food. The more natural, the less it's packaged, the fewer preservatives added, the more natural it is. For me, that's the best".

(Antequera focus group)

There was a tendency to distrust large fish and to prefer smaller ones, caught near the coast, since there is a widespread belief that big fish may have consumed more heavy metals and mercury.

Finally, one area of item grouping in the *nMDS* model of distrust was spatially separated from the rest. This associative subdomain was related to (mis)trust in relation to food preservation. For example, in the narratives obtained from the focus groups, the case of frozen fish highlights the doubts and uncertainty created by this form of food preservation. Although most of the women believed they can trust this food, because freezing the fish keeps it in a good state of preservation, they also feared that there may have been a break in the cold chain before it reached the consumer. The doubts raised by this concern, not knowing whether the frozen food maintains the same properties as fresh fish, makes them somewhat distrust it.

"But when you're pregnant, you get more cautious. You wash the vegetables much better than before. You even freeze the food. Maybe you're not pregnant and you say, "Well, look, I eat fresh fish, freshly cooked". But now, being pregnant, it's different; I prefer to freeze it. You do that, whatever, just to be on the safe side ... ".

(Antequera focus group)

4. Discussion

Pregnancy and lactation are vital stages in a woman's life, during which food becomes a central issue in relation to her health, and the changes in her body are experienced with fear and trepidation [17]. These feelings are associated with the fact that mothers, in this cycle of their lives, are marked by the discourse of risk and the precautionary principle as strategies to manage uncertainty [18] and to protect the foetus or the baby [19].

Food insecurity can affect all stages of life. However, women are at greater risk of suffering from this condition due to gender determinants as the result of inequalities arising from risk factors such as gender violence or unequal access to employment and education [47]. A balanced diet and appropriate weight gain during pregnancy are associated with better maternal and perinatal outcomes. Therefore, weight gain and nutrition are significant areas of public health concern during this stage of life [48]. Conversely, overnutrition and undernutrition both increase the risk of an adverse perinatal outcome, including excessive or inadequate foetal growth, gestational diabetes mellitus, preterm birth and pre-eclampsia. Furthermore, the absence of proper nutrition in early childhood can have life-long consequences. Therefore, it is important to explore the social representations around 'healthy eating' of these women and the factors that influence their trust or distrust in food.

The pregnant and breastfeeding mothers consulted expressed great concern about the quality of the food they consume and about its possible effects on their own health and on that of their child. Regarding which foods they can trust, these women must sometimes make highly complex decisions. The participants in our study emphasised the importance of reading food labels, of knowing the composition of the products consumed and of seeking information on any foods that might seem suspicious. However, they also recognised that worrying excessively about food quality could mean, ultimately, not eating anything.

In addition, the participants mentioned other factors that make it even more difficult to decide which foods to choose. They realise that caution is more important than the pleasure of eating. Therefore, although they like many of the foods referred to with distrust, for reasons of health they prefer to avoid them. Some women also observed that the amount of food and the frequency of its consumption are important factors, and that any excessive consumption can be harmful.

In the opinion of the pregnant and breastfeeding mothers consulted, an adequate diet is one based on the consumption of fruits and vegetables (preferably fresh) and of organic meats. However, these preferences are not always applied in practice since other factors such as price and availability (not addressed in this study) must also be taken into account. Although the medical–nutritional discourse based on sustainability has steadily gained strength among consumers as a significant criterion in their food choices [49], this environmental discourse (recommending a diet based on the production and consumption of organic meats, fruits and vegetables) does not constitute the subdomain most frequently identified in our analysis. Proximity and taste remain the preferred criteria for choosing fruits and vegetables, while "fresh" is considered synonymous with "natural" and with not having undergone cold storage for preservation.

Legumes and cereals are easier to store and hence are more generally trusted than other foods. In no case did the study participants question the production process for cereals (with the exception of transgenics) or legumes. On the contrary, although eggs and dairy products are trusted foods, they are often viewed with some suspicion due to industry involvement in the manufacturing process.

Fish and meat generate serious concern as their properties are considered ambivalent depending on the food's origin and mode of production. According to the UN Food and Agriculture Organisation [50], Spain is the fourth country in the world in fish consumption, with an annual per capita consumption of 45.6 kg. The origin and type of fish products—from various countries, fresh or frozen, large and small—creates some disquiet. Medical discourses favour the consumption of small fish in order to enhance the nutritional properties of this type of food [51] and advise against the consumption of large fish, which are subject to the risk of mercury contamination.

Ambivalence among the participants regarding the consumption of meat is due to the high consumption of sausage products in Spain. Many types are specifically warned against during pregnancy. Ambivalence is also due to the influence of discourses in the media concerning how the animals are fed [52] and because of medical warnings about effects on cardiovascular health [53].

In summary, the women consulted in this study expressed ambivalence between trust and distrust in meat, fish, dairy products and eggs, mainly regarding the ways in which these foods are produced. The participants, however, were in close agreement in classifying prepared or precooked products, basic processed products and highly artificial products with added chemical substances as foods to be distrusted due to suspicions about the manufacturing process.

5. Conclusions

The pregnant and breastfeeding women in our study groups classified various foods and assigned certain attributes to them according to the level of trust and mistrust inspired in each case, thus providing a social representation of food risks. These criteria are perceived by women as relevant to their food decisions and, therefore, emic knowledge should be taken into account when developing food safety programmes and planning actions aimed at pregnant and breastfeeding women.

We believe that achieving a better understanding of what women consider 'healthy eating' and determining the factors that influence their trust or distrust in the food consumed is critical. This is one of the main contributions of this article. These findings could be very useful for health professionals, revealing which criteria determine trust/mistrust among this population group and highlighting similarities and differences with regard to medical–nutritional recommendations.

Author Contributions: Conceptualization and design, A.M. and C.L.-K.; methodology and software, A.M., A.F.-N. and M.C.-M.; formal analysis and data curation, A.M., C.L.-K. and M.C.-M.; investigation, A.M., C.L.-K., A.F.-N. and M.C.-M.; writing—original draft preparation, A.M. and C.L.-K.; writing—review and editing, A.M., C.L.-K., A.F.-N. and M.C.-M.; supervision and project administration, M.C.-M. All authors have read and agreed to the published version of the manuscript.

Funding: The first phase of this research was financed by the Ministry of Economy and Competitiveness, the State Programme for the Promotion of Scientific and Technical Research of Excellence, the State Subprogramme for the Generation of Knowledge, Spain (reference: CSO2014-58144-P). The second phase of the study was funded by Fundación Pública Andaluza Progreso y Salud de la Junta de Andalucía, Spain (reference: AP-0139-2017). Dr. M. Company-Morales obtained a scholarship for this part of the research from the Ministry of Health of the Junta de Andalucía, Spain (A-0043-2018).

Institutional Review Board Statement: This study was conducted according to the guidelines of the Declaration of Helsinki and was approved by the following ethics committees: "Parc de Salut Mar" Clinical Research Ethics Committee (Ref: 2015/6459/I), IDIAP Jordi Gol Ethics Committee for Clinical Research (Ref. P15/135) and the Research Ethics Committee of the Andalusian Health Service in Almería (Ref: 66/2017).

Informed Consent Statement: Informed consent was obtained from all subjects involved in the study.

Data Availability Statement: The data presented in this study are not publicly available due to privacy and confidentiality reasons.

Acknowledgments: The authors would like to thank all the pregnant and breastfeeding women who took part in this study for their attentiveness, effort and participation in the focus groups and in making the pile sorts.

Conflicts of Interest: The authors declare no conflict of interest.

References

1. Fox, E.; Davis, C.; Downs, S.M.; McLaren, R.; Fanzo, J. A focused ethnographic study on the role of health and sustainability in food choice decisions. *Appetite* **2021**, *165*, 105319. [CrossRef]
2. Gaspar, M.C.; Juzwiack, C.; Muñoz, A.; Larrea-Killinger, C. Las relaciones entre salud y alimentación: Una lectura antropológica. In *Polisemias de la Alimentación*; Gascón, J., Ed.; Promocions UB: Barcelona, Spain, 2018; p. 3248.
3. Lupton, D. Risk as moral danger: The social and political functions of risk discourse in public health. *Int. J. Health Serv.* **1993**, *23*, 425–435. [CrossRef]
4. Contreras, J. A modernidade alimentar: Entre a superabundância e a insegurança. *História Questões Debates Curitiba* **2011**, *54*, 19–45. [CrossRef]
5. Fischler, C. La maladie de la 'vache folle'. In *Risques et Peurs Alimentaires*; Apfelbaum, M., Ed.; Odile Jacob: Paris, France, 1998; pp. 45–56.
6. Yates, J.; Gillespie, S.; Savona, N.; Deeney, M.; Kadiyala, S. Trust and responsibility in food systems transformation. Engaging with Big Food: Marriage or mirage? *BMJ Glob. Health* **2021**, *6*, e007350. [CrossRef]

7. Rupprecht, D.D.; Fujiyoshi, L.; McGreevy, S.R.; Tayasu, I. Trust me? Consumer trust in expert information on food product labels. *Food Chem. Toxicol.* **2020**, *137*, 111170. [CrossRef]
8. Fischler, C. *El (h)omnívoro. El gusto, la Cocina y el Cuerpo*; Anagrama: Barcelona, Spain, 1995.
9. Ramakrishnan, U.; Grant, F.; Goldenberg, T.; Zongrone, A.; Martorell, R. Effect of women's nutrition before and during early pregnancy on maternal and infant outcomes: A systematic review. *Paediatr. Perinat. Epidemiol.* **2012**, *26*, 285–301. [CrossRef] [PubMed]
10. Company-Morales, M.; Casadó, L.; Zafra Aparici, E.; Rubio Jiménez, M.F.; Fontalba-Navas, A. The sound of silence: Unspoken meaning in the discourse of pregnant and breastfeeding women on environmental risks and food safety in Spain. *Nutrients* **2022**, *14*, 593. [CrossRef] [PubMed]
11. Fontalba-Navas, A.; Zafra Aparici, E.; Prata-Gaspar, M.C.d.M.; Herrera-Espejo, E.; Company-Morales, M.; Larrea-Killinger, C. Motivating pregnant and breastfeeding women in Spain to avoid persistent toxic substances in their diet. *Int. J. Environ. Res. Public Health* **2020**, *17*, 8719. [CrossRef] [PubMed]
12. Blázquez, M.I. Aproximación a la antropología de la reproducción. *AIBR Rev. Antropol. Iberoam.* **2005**, *42*, 1–25.
13. Montes, M.J. Culturas del Nacimiento. Representaciones y Prácticas de las Mujeres Gestantes, Comadronas y Médicos . Doctoral Thesis, Universitat Rovira i Virgili, Tarragona, Spain, 2007. Available online: http://hdl.handle.net/10803/8421 (accessed on 20 April 2022).
14. Gracia-Arnaiz, M. Comer bien, comer mal: La medicalización del comportamiento alimentario. *Salud Pública Mex.* **2007**, *49*, 236–242. [CrossRef]
15. Imaz, E. Mujeres gestantes, madres en gestación. Metáforas de un cuerpo fronterizo. *Política Soc.* **2001**, *36*, 97–111.
16. Lupton, D. 'Precious cargo': Foetal subjects, risk and reproductive citizenship. *Crit. Public Health* **2012**, *22*, 329–340. [CrossRef]
17. Montes, M.J.; Bodoqué, Y. *Cuerpo y Nacimiento: Análisis Antropológico del Poder en la Reproducción de los Cuerpos*; Actas del IX Congreso de Antropología de la Federación de Asociaciones de Antropología del Estado Español (FAAEE): Barcelona, Spain, 2002.
18. Larrea-Killinger, C.; Muñoz, A.; Begueria, A.; Mascaró, J. "Como un sedimento que se va quedando en el cuerpo": Percepción social del riesgo sobre compuestos tóxicos persistentes y otras sustancias químicas sintéticas en la alimentación entre mujeres embarazadas y lactantes en España. *Rev. Antropol. Iberoam.* **2019**, *14*, 121–144. [CrossRef]
19. Leppo, A.; Hecksher, D.; Tryggvesson, K. 'Why take chances?' Advice on alcohol intake to pregnant and non-pregnant women in four Nordic countries. *Health Risk Soc.* **2014**, *16*, 512–529. [CrossRef]
20. Tesha, A.P.; Mwanri, A.W.; Nyaruhucha, C.N. Knowledge, practices and intention to consume omega 3 and omega 6 fatty acids among pregnant and breastfeeding women in Morogoro Municipality, Tanzania. *Afr. J. Food Sci.* **2022**, *16*, 125–136. [CrossRef]
21. Zimmerman, E.; Gachigi, K.K.; Rodgers, R.F.; Watkins, D.J.; Woodbury, M.; Cordero, J.F.; Alshawabkeh, A.; Meeker, J.D.; Huerta-Montañez, G.; Pabon, Z.R.; et al. Association between Quality of Maternal Prenatal Food Source and Preparation and Breastfeeding Duration in the Environmental Influences on Child Health Outcome (ECHO) Program. *Nutrients* **2022**, *14*, 4922. [CrossRef]
22. Larrea-Killinger, C.; Muñoz, A.; Begueria, A.; Mascaro-Pons, J. Body representations of internal pollution: The risk perception of the circulation of environmental contaminants in pregnant and breastfeeding women in Spain. *Int. J. Environ. Res. Public Health* **2020**, *17*, 6544. [CrossRef] [PubMed]
23. Spradley, J. *The Ethnographic Interview*; Holt, Rinehart & Winston: New York, NY, USA, 1979.
24. Ryan, G.W.; Bernard, H.R. Data management and analysis methods. In *Handbook of Qualitative Research*; Denzin, N.K., Linconl, Y.S., Eds.; Sage Publications: Thousand Oaks, CA, USA, 2000.
25. De Munck, V. *Research Design and Methods for Studying Cultures*; AltaMira Press: Lanham, MD, USA, 2009.
26. Kanter, R.; León Villagra, M. Participatory methods to identify perceived healthy and sustainable traditional culinary preparations across three generations of adults: Results from Chile's metropolitan region and region of La Araucanía. *Nutrients* **2020**, *12*, 489. [CrossRef]
27. Kodish, S.; Grey, K.; Matean, M.; Palaniappan, U.; Gomez, C.; Timeon, E.; Northrup-Lyons, M.; Mclean, J. Improving knowledge is not enough: Multi-level determinants of maternal, infant, and young child nutrition identified through formative research in the Republic of Kiribati (P10-037-19). *Curr. Dev. Nutr.* **2019**, *3* (Suppl. 1), 3013371. [CrossRef]
28. Kodish, S.; Grey, K.; Matean, M.; Palaniappan, U.; Gwavuya, S.; Gomez, C.; Iuta, T.; Timeon, E.; Northrup-Lyons, M.; McLean, J.; et al. Socio-ecological factors that influence infant and young child nutrition in Kiribati: A biocultural perspective. *Nutrients* **2019**, *11*, 1330. [CrossRef]
29. de M. Sato, P.; Lourenço, B.H.; Silva, J.G.S.T.D.; Scagliusi, F.B. Food categorizations among low-income women living in three different urban contexts: The pile sorting method. *Appetite* **2019**, *136*, 173–183. [CrossRef]
30. Schwendler, T.; Senarath, U.; Jayawickrama, H.; Abdulloeva, S.; Rowel, D.; De Silva, C.; Mastrorilli, J.; Kodish, S. Using cultural domain analysis to understand community perceptions of infant and young child foods in Sri Lanka. *Curr. Dev. Nutr.* **2021**, *5* (Suppl. 2), 684. [CrossRef]
31. Schwendler, T.; Senarath, U.; De Silva, C.; Abdulloeva, S.; Jayawickrama, H.; Rowel, D.; White, C.; Kodish, S. An ethnomedical perspective: Understanding young child illness in Sri Lanka using cultural domain analysis. *Curr. Dev. Nutr.* **2021**, *5* (Suppl. 2), 991. [CrossRef]
32. Trotter, R.T.; Potter, J.M. Pile sorts, a cognitive anthropological model of drug and AIDS risks for Navajo teenagers: Assessment of a new evaluation tool. *Drugs Soc.* **1993**, *7*, 23–39. [CrossRef]

33. Zobrist, S.; Kalra, N.; Pelto, G.; Wittenbrink, B.; Milani, P.; Diallo, A.M.; Ndoye, T.; Wone, I.; Parker, M. Results of applying cultural domain analysis techniques and implications for the design of complementary feeding interventions in Northern Senegal. *Food Nutr. Bull.* **2017**, *38*, 512–527. [CrossRef] [PubMed]
34. Zycherman, A. An introduction to cultural domain analysis in food research: Free lists and pile sorts. In *Food Culture: Anthropology, Linguistics and Food Studies*, 1st ed.; Chrzan, J., Brett, J., Eds.; Berghahn Books: New York, NY, USA, 2019; Volume 2, pp. 159–169. [CrossRef]
35. Company-Morales, M.; Zafra Aparici, E.; Casadó, L.; Alarcón Montenegro, C.; Arrebola, J.P. Perception and demands of pregnant and breastfeeding women regarding their role as participants in environmental research studies. *Int. J. Environ. Res. Public Health* **2021**, *18*, 4149. [CrossRef] [PubMed]
36. Muñoz, A.; Fontalba-Navas, A.; Arrebola, J.P.; Larrea-Killinger, C. Trust and distrust in relation to food risks in Spain: An approach to the socio-cultural representations of pregnant and breastfeeding women through the technique of free listing. *Appetite* **2019**, *142*, 104365. [CrossRef]
37. Zafra-Aparici, E.; Company, M.; Casado, L. Escenarios urbanos y subjetividades en la construcción de discursos y prácticas sobre cuerpo, género y alimentación: Una etnografía alimentaria sobre mujeres embarazadas y lactantes en España. In *Consumos Alimentares em Cenarios Urbanos: Multiplos Olhares*; Barcellos, D.M.N., Amaro, F., Freitas, R.F., Prado, S.D., Eds.; ED UERJ/Gramma: Rio de Janeiro, Brazil, 2020; pp. 299–328.
38. Bernard, H.R.; Wutich, A.; Ryan, G.W. *Analyzing Qualitative Data: Systemic Approaches*, 2nd ed.; SAGE: Thousand Oaks, CA, USA, 2017.
39. Borgatti, S.P. Elicitation techniques for cultural domain analysis. In *The Ethnographic Toolkit*; Schensul, J., Weeks, M., Eds.; Altamira Press: Walnut Creek, CA, USA, 1998.
40. Weller, S.C.; Romney, A.K. *Systematic Data Collection*; Sage: Newbury Park, CA, USA, 1988.
41. Borgatti, S.P. *ANTHROPAC 4.0 Methods Guide and Reference Manual*; Analytic Technologies: Natick, MA, USA, 1996.
42. Walliman, N. *Social Research Methods*; Sage Publications: London, UK, 2006.
43. Bernard, H.R. *Research Methods in Anthropology: Qualitative and Quantitative Approaches*, 4th ed.; AltaMira Press: Lanham, MD, USA, 2006.
44. Callejo, J. *El grupo de Discusión: Introducción a Una práctica de Investigación*; Editorial Ariel: Barcelona, Spain, 2001.
45. Glaser, B.G.; Strauss, A.L. *The Discovery of Grounded Theory: Strategies for Qualitative Research*; Aldine Publishing Company: Chicago, IL, USA, 1967.
46. Strauss, A.L.; Corbin, J. *Basics of Qualitative Research: Grounded Theory Procedures and Techniques*; Sage: Newbury Park, CA, USA, 1990.
47. Bastian, A.; Parks, C.; Yaroch, A.; McKay, F.H.; Stern, K.; van der Pligt, P.; McNaughton, S.A.; Lindberg, R. Factors associated with food insecurity among pregnant women and caregivers of children aged 0–6 years: A scoping review. *Nutrients* **2022**, *14*, 2407. [CrossRef] [PubMed]
48. De Vito, M.; Alameddine, S.; Capannolo, G.; Mappa, I.; Gualtieri, P.; Di Renzo, L.; De Lorenzo, A.; D'Antonio, F.; Rizzo, G. Systematic review and critical evaluation of quality of clinical practice guidelines on nutrition in pregnancy. *Healthcare* **2022**, *10*, 2490. [CrossRef] [PubMed]
49. Iqbal, S.; Ali, I. Maternal food insecurity in low-income countries: Revisiting its causes and consequences for maternal and neonatal health. *J. Agric. Food Res.* **2021**, *3*, 100091. [CrossRef]
50. FAO. *World Food and Agriculture—Statistical Yearbook 2021*; Food and Agriculture Organization of the United Nations: Rome, Italy, 2021. [CrossRef]
51. Taylor, C.M.; Emmett, P.M.; Emond, A.M.; Golding, J. A review of guidance on fish consumption in pregnancy: Is it fit for purpose? *Public Health Nutr.* **2018**, *21*, 2149–2159. [CrossRef] [PubMed]
52. Jardí, C.; Aparicio, E.; Bedmar, C.; Aranda, N.; Abajo, S.; March, G.; Basora, J.; Arija, V. Food consumption during pregnancy and post-partum. ECLIPSES Study. *Nutrients* **2019**, *11*, 2447. [CrossRef] [PubMed]
53. Perak, A.M.; Lancki, N.; Kuang, A.; Labarthe, D.R.; Allen, N.B.; Shah, S.H.; Lowe, L.P.; Grobman, W.A.; Lawrence, J.M.; Lloyd-Jones, D.M.; et al. Associations of maternal cardiovascular health in pregnancy with offspring cardiovascular health in early adolescence. *JAMA* **2021**, *325*, 658–668. [CrossRef] [PubMed]

Disclaimer/Publisher's Note: The statements, opinions and data contained in all publications are solely those of the individual author(s) and contributor(s) and not of MDPI and/or the editor(s). MDPI and/or the editor(s) disclaim responsibility for any injury to people or property resulting from any ideas, methods, instructions or products referred to in the content.

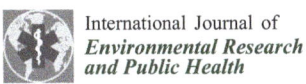

Article

Protein Supplementation in a Prehabilitation Program in Patients Undergoing Surgery for Endometrial Cancer

Josep M. Sole-Sedeno [1,2,*], Ester Miralpeix [1,2], Maria-Dolors Muns [3], Cristina Rodriguez-Cosmen [4], Berta Fabrego [1], Nadwa Kanjou [1], Francesc-Xavier Medina [5] and Gemma Mancebo [1,2]

1. Department of Obstetrics and Gynecology, Hospital del Mar, E-08003 Barcelona, Spain; gmancebo@psmar.cat (G.M.)
2. Campus del Mar, Universitat Pompeu Fabra, E-08003 Barcelona, Spain
3. Department of Endocrinology, Hospital del Mar, E-08003 Barcelona, Spain
4. Department of Anesthesia, Hospital del Mar, E-08003 Barcelona, Spain
5. FoodLab & UNESCO Chair on Food, Culture, and Development, Faculty of Health Sciences, Open University of Catalonia, E-08018 Barcelona, Spain
* Correspondence: jsole@psmar.cat

Abstract: Enhanced recovery after surgery (ERAS) and prehabilitation programs are multidisciplinary care pathways to reduce stress response and improve perioperative outcomes, which also include nutritional interventions. The aim of this study is to assess the impact of protein supplementation with 20 mg per day before surgery in a prehabilitation program in postoperative serum albumin, prealbumin, and total proteins in endometrial cancer patients undergoing laparoscopic surgery. Methods: A prospective study including patients who underwent laparoscopy for endometrial cancer was conducted. Three groups were identified according to ERAS and prehabilitation implementation (preERAS, ERAS, and Prehab). The primary outcome was levels of serum albumin, prealbumin, and total protein 24–48 h after surgery. Results: A total of 185 patients were included: 57 in the preERAS group, 60 in the ERAS group, and 68 in the Prehab group. There were no basal differences in serum albumin, prealbumin, or total protein between the three groups. After surgery, regardless of the nutritional intervention, the decrease in the values was also similar. Moreover, values in the Prehab group just before surgery were lower than the initial ones, despite the protein supplementation. Conclusions: Supplementation with 20 mg of protein per day does not impact serum protein levels in a prehabilitation program. Supplementations with higher quantities should be studied.

Keywords: prehabilitation; ERAS; endometrial cancer; surgery; protein supplementation

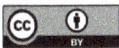

1. Introduction

Endometrial cancer is today the most common gynecological cancer in the European Union and in the United States [1]. Risk factors include medical and public health conditions such as obesity, diabetes, and polycystic ovary syndrome [2]. Diagnosis is usually carried out in the early stages, given the appearance of metrorrhagia. The primary treatment is surgery, such as hysterectomy and bilateral adnexectomy. These interventions are generally carried out through a minimally invasive approach [3]. In any case, it should be noted here that even minimally invasive surgery entails aggression for the patient's physiology [4].

In this context, the ERAS (Enhanced Recovery After Surgery) protocol emerges to reduce surgical aggression, and to obtain an earlier recovery of the patient, reducing complications. This protocol includes recommendations for perioperative and postoperative management that have been widely described in the existing literature [5,6].

The concept of prehabilitation was also created to improve the results. The objective of the prehabilitation is to prepare the patient for surgical treatment and to improve functional capacity and metabolic reserves, including medical, physical, nutritional, and psychological interventions [7,8]. Prehabilitation programs include recommendations to increase protein intake, as it has been proved that the increase in protein consumption reduces the number and severity of postoperative complications [9]. Nonetheless, we must also highlight here that there is no clear guidance or conclusive information about the quantity of protein to intake in prehabilitation programs.

The WHO (World Health Organization, Geneva, Switzerland) recommendations for protein intake in healthy adults are 0.66 g/kg per day (OMS recommendations in 2007) [10]. This UN organization shows different recommendations for special groups, such as children and pregnant women, but not for situations such as preparing for surgery or having cancer or other special health conditions.

Following this premises and the present lack of existing information, the aim of our study was to analyze whether supplementation with 20 g of daily protein would be sufficient to maintain serum albumin, prealbumin, and total protein levels during the prehabilitation period.

2. Materials and Methods

2.1. Design and Subjects of This Study

A prospective pilot observational study of patients undergoing laparoscopic surgery for endometrial cancer was conducted for more than two years, between January 2018 and March 2020, at the Department of Obstetrics and Gynecology of the Hospital del Mar in Barcelona (Spain).

Eligible patients for the study were, uniquely, women diagnosed with endometrial cancer and suitable for laparoscopic surgical treatment. As exclusion criteria, we included patients who declined surgery, an inability or incapacity to give an informed consent, the fact of having a non-resectable disease, having a degree of cognitive deterioration limiting or impeding their adherence to the program, or having surgery via laparotomy. The nutritional intervention was a feature of the prehabilitation program implemented in our hospital department in January 2018, and is extensively described in a previous paper [11]. Patients treated previously (before January 2018) were used as a control group and were classified according to the preoperative program followed: ERAS program (Enhanced Recovery After Surgery Program, without prehabilitation nor nutritional intervention), and PreERAS program (conventional preoperative program, which included only preoperative studies and anesthesiologist evaluation, and used before the establishment of the ERAS protocol).

The prehabilitation program was explained to the patients during the first oncologic gynecological visit and began on that day. The program involved preoperative and postoperative periods, and was maintained until 8 weeks after surgery. The preoperative part, the one analyzed in this paper, ranges between 2 and 6 weeks.

2.2. Nutritional Prehabilitation Intervention

Patients in the prehabilitation program were screened for malnutrition with the Malnutrition Universal Screening Tool (MUST) test, where a score of 2 or more indicates high risk, a score of 1 indicates intermediate risk, and 0 indicates low risk for malnutrition [12]. In addition to the MUST score, serum total protein, albumin, and prealbumin were assessed at baseline. All patients with a MUST score of 2 or more, or with albumin levels below 3 g/dl, were also previously treated by a nutritionist, trying to revert the eventual malnutrition status.

All patients in the prehabilitation group received a nutritional education program involving food selection and meal planning patterns, including an easy and feasible list of recipes for the homemade creation of protein supplements (mainly shakes and smoothies, always created with natural and non-processed ingredients such as fruits, vegetables, dried fruits, etc.) and adapted to diabetic patients, if necessary. These recipes included around 20 g of protein per day. All patients involved were previously instructed to take those oral protein supplements daily, always 30 min after exercise training, to enhance muscle hypertrophy. Those protein supplements prescribed did not alter the normal protein intake during meals. The food selection was made according to the WHO recommendations for healthy adults.

Patients in the PreERAS or ERAS program did not receive nutritional advice about increasing the protein intake, nor the recipes or strategies to achieve this. They were only assessed with the MUST test and serum albumin levels at baseline regarding nutritional aspects.

2.3. Variables and Outcomes

We used medical registries to retrospectively collect demographic and clinical baseline information. The nutritional status of women involved in this study was evaluated with the following indicators: total serum protein, prealbumin levels, and albumin in the prehabilitation patients' group. Measurements were recorded baseline at the time of the first visit, immediately before the surgery, and 24–72 h post surgery. Patients in the preERAS or the ERAS group were only evaluated at baseline and 24–72 h after surgery with serum protein and albumin, adding the prealbumin level in the ERAS group.

2.4. Statistical Methods

The statistical analysis applied in this study was performed using SPSS 25.0 (Chicago, IL, USA), accepting a statistically significant level of 5% ($p < 0.05$). Both the demographic and clinical characteristics of our patients were summarized using descriptive statistics. Continuous variables were reported as mean (range) or mean ± standard deviation (SD) when indicated. Categorical variables were reported as frequency and percentage (%). We used, when appropriate, the Pearson's chi-square test or the Fisher's exact test to compare efficiently categorical variables. We used the Student's t-test or the non-parametric Mann–Whitney test to compare continuous variables.

3. Results

A total of sixty-eight consecutive patients undergoing laparoscopy surgery for endometrial cancer were included in the prospective prehabilitation cohort of the study. In the historical cohorts, 60 patients were included in the ERAS group and 57 in the preERAS group.

The mean patient age in the prehabilitation group was 66.4 years (range, 35–86 years), with no differences with the two other groups. The median time of patients who followed the prehabilitation program before surgery, which includes the protein supplementation, was 25 days (Interquartile 18–35) days. The baseline demographic and clinical characteristics of the study population according to the perioperative program are shown in Table 1. The groups were comparable in baseline characteristics in terms of age, BMI, comorbidities, ASA, and cancer stage.

Table 1. Baseline patients' characteristics according to the followed perioperative program.

	PreERAS (n = 57)	ERAS (n = 60)	Prehab (n = 68)	p Value
Age (years), mean [range]	64.1 [39–88]	67.4 [44–92]	66.4 [35–86]	0.310
BMI kg/m², mean (SD)	32.0 ± 7.1	29.1 ± 6.5	31.0 ± 7.1	0.062
Smoking, n (%)	14 (24.6)	9 (15.0)	9 (13.2)	0.211
Hypertension, n (%)	31 (54.4)	37 (61.7)	40 (58.8)	0.724
Dyslipidemia, n (%)	18 (31.6)	21 (35.0)	23 (33.8)	0.924
Diabetes, n (%)	13 (22.8)	11 (18.3)	15 (22.1)	0.813
ASA, n (%)				0.578
I	7 (12.3)	4 (6.7)	5 (7.4)	
II	36 (63.2)	39 (65.0)	51 (75.0)	
III	14 (24.6)	16 (26.7)	11 (16.2)	
IV	0	1 (1.7)	1 (1.5)	
Disease Stage (FIGO), n (%)				0.496
IA-IB	41 (71.9)	43 (71.7)	56 (82.4)	
II	7 (12.3)	7 (11.7)	7 (10.3)	

Table 1. Cont.

	PreERAS (n = 57)	ERAS (n = 60)	Prehab (n = 68)	p Value
IIIA-IIIC	9 (15.8)	10 (16.7)	5 (7.4)	
IV	0	0	0	

ASA: American Society of Anesthesiologists, BMI: body mass index, SD: standard deviation.

According to the MUST score, only six patients (9.8%) were at high risk of malnutrition (five patients scored 2, one scored 1). All other patients had a MUST score of 0 (90.2%).

The values of serum total protein, albumin, and prealbumin at baseline were similar in the three groups (Table 2), although there was a trend toward better values in the prehabilitation group. It should be noted that these values are previous to any intervention.

Table 2. Nutritional parameter value evolution according to the followed perioperative program (preERAS vs. ERAS vs. Prehab).

		PreERAS (n = 57)	ERAS (n = 60)	Prehab (n = 68)	p Value
Baseline	Total proteins (g/dL)	7.01 ± 0.42	7.04 ± 0.40	7.17 ± 0.45	0.076
	Albumin (g/dL)	4.41 ± 0.29	4.38 ± 0.25	4.48 ± 0.33	0.138
	Prealbumin (mg/dL)	NA	21.02 ± 4.16	24.12 ± 6.95	0.288
Preoperative	Total proteins (g/dL)	NA	NA	6.33 ± 0.70	NA
	Albumin (g/dL)	NA	NA	3.92 ± 0.46	NA
	Prealbumin (mg/dL)	NA	NA	20.51 ± 5.29	NA
Postoperative	Total proteins (g/dL)	5.58 ± 0.57	5.73 ± 0.57	5.93 ± 0.66	0.085
	Albumin (g/dL)	3.47 ± 0.31	3.49 ± 0.36	3.63 ± 0.43	0.128
	Prealbumin (mg/dL)	NA	15.66 ± 4.17	18.14 ± 4.74	0.194
Decrease	Total proteins (g/dL)	1.49	1.30	1.23	0.376
	Albumin (g/dL)	0.93	0.89	0.85	0.758
	Prealbumin (mg/dL)	NA	5.73	5.82	0.970

NA: non applicable.

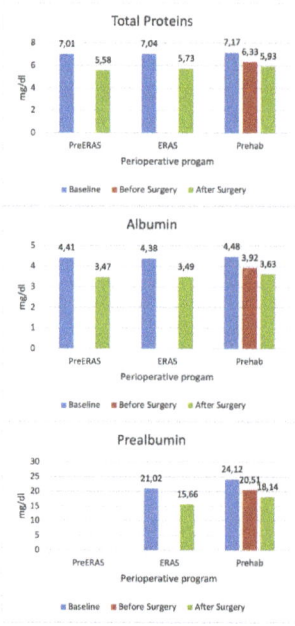

Figure 1. Variation of serum levels according to intervention groups.

Results comparing the impact of the nutritional intervention program on blood analysis just before surgery and 24–72 h after we recorded it are in Table 2 and Figure 1. Values after surgery decreased in all three groups. The prehabilitation group was the only one which had blood tests before surgery. The values showed a decrease in serum albumin, prealbumin, and total proteins, even with the nutritional intervention. Differences in basal and after surgery data were not statistically significant between the three groups.

Table 2 also shows the variation between the values after surgery and baseline. Although the decrease was lower for all parameters in the prehabilitation group compared to the preERAS and ERAS groups, the difference was not statistically significant.

4. Discussion

This research reported our experience with implementing protein supplementation intervention in a prehabilitation program for endometrial cancer patients undergoing laparoscopic surgery. We would like to assess the impact of this nutritional intervention on serum total protein, albumin, and prealbumin. The main results failed, nevertheless, to confirm a real nutritional improvement among women included in the prehabilitation group.

Our prehabilitation programs consist of the earlier preparation of patients between diagnosis and surgery. This preparation allows the patients to improve functional capacity and metabolic reserves before surgical intervention. It includes physical, emotional, and nutritional interventions. Previous published papers confirmed that multimodal prehabilitation programs used in cases of major cancer surgeries show a positive impact on the patients' outcomes [11,13]. Nutritional support comprises pre-operative carbohydrate loading just before surgery, and nutritional interventions aim to increase the protein intake [5].

The main objective of improving the nutritional status of the patients is its potential role in reducing perioperative and postoperative complications. In our study, serum levels of albumin and prealbumin were proposed for preoperative risk stratification [14]. In their review article, Loftus et al. show that low albumin and prealbumin levels are associated with an increase in surgical complications. In this regard, the authors address the inability to differentiate between malnutrition and acute inflammation, since those parameters are also altered because of inflammation. Nevertheless, and even having in mind those significant limitations, there are data that protein supplementation could decrease complication rates, as shown in the classical study from the Veterans Affairs' where it was demonstrated that severely malnourished patients supplemented with parenteral nutrition in the perioperative period had better surgery outcomes (veterans). There are conflicting data about this topic. Van Venrooij [13] studied the complication rate in patients well-nourished undergoing cardiac surgery, showing no improvement in preoperative protein and energy intake.

Salvetti et al. showed that in patients undergoing elective spine surgery, a threshold of <20 mg/dl for prealbumin was correlated with an increase in surgical site infection (17.8% versus 4.8%) [15]. A meta-analysis and a systematic review performed by Liu showed that decreased preoperative albumin in patients undergoing surgery for urothelial carcinoma predicted poor overall survival, cancer-specific survival, recurrence-free survival, 30-day complications after surgery, and 90-day mortality after surgery [16]. Kabata also published a randomized control trial of preoperative nutritional support in cancer patients with no clinical signs of malnutrition and undergoing abdominal cancer surgery. Patients receiving nutritional supplementation for 14 days before surgery had a lower rate of postoperative complications. Serum total protein and albumin were stable compared to the control group, where the levels decreased [17].

Previously, we analyzed the role of nutritional prehabilitation in women with ovarian cancer [18]. We selected patients undergoing a prehabilitation program during neoadjuvant chemotherapy and interval cytoreductive surgery. The data showed an increased postoperative recovery and decreased intraoperative complications (40% vs. 14.3%) in the prehabilitation group.

Hamaker et al. published a systematic review of nutritional status in patients with cancer, showing values as high as 49% of patients malnourished [19]. There are no data about this in endometrial cancer specifically, but our data show low levels of malnourished patients. This is the reason why we supplemented diets with only 20 mg of protein a day and kept patients on their normal daily eating habits (which is the easiest way to obtain useful comparative results). Nevertheless, we must remark that our study failed to improve nutritional status, even with the mentioned protein supplementation. This was not, however, the only unexpected result; in addition, the serum nutritional status even decreased during the prehabilitation program before surgery, which was a very unexpected finding in the framework of this study.

Other studies have shown interesting results improving nutritional status with higher levels of supplementation. In this regard, ERAS protocols recommend protein intakes of 1.2–2.0 g/kg/day from high-quality protein sources [20,21], including normal diet and supplementation. In a randomized trial carried out by Kabata, the prescribed dose was 40 mg of protein per day. In this study, modest increases in albumin and total protein were found, while, however, in the control group, the levels decreased [17]. Following these premises, our recommendation was to half this intake quantity. Additionally, this is probably the main reason we have found no improvement in the intervention group.

One of the most unexpected results was that even with the protein supplementation, our patients had a decrease in the serum levels of total protein, albumin, and prealbumin. This variation occurred in only 25 days, in patients non-malnourished and with neoplasia with little systemic affectation. ESPEN guidelines (European guideline on obesity care in patients with gastrointestinal and liver diseases) recommend perioperative support only in patients with malnutrition or at nutritional risk, and do not provide any information about how they should be supplemented [9]. In our case, we found that even patients not at risk for malnutrition could also benefit from protein supplementation.

We have also to remark that one of the reasons why we have not observed any benefit in our study could be the period time during which the patients take the protein supplements. The mean time of protein supplementation in our series was 25 days, which could explain why no benefit was observed. However, in Kabata et al.'s study [17], with only 14 days of supplementation, they observed beneficial effects in terms of morbidity and stability in nutritional parameters. The protein supplementation was also 20 g of protein per day, although from a commercial preparation. We might think that the homemade natural shakes or smoothies are not as effective, perhaps due to bioavailability issues, as the commercial ones.

Strengths and Weaknesses

This research also presents different strengths that we would like to remark on. As far as we know (and as far as we have been able to verify from the published literature), this is the first piece of research studying the evolution of nutritional parameters in patients with endometrial cancer during the prehabilitation and after-surgery periods. Additional strengths include this being a homogeneous study (both in demographics and clinical characteristics) regarding a population with endometrial cancer undergoing laparoscopic surgery.

Potential weaknesses of our research also include, on the other hand, the non-randomized control trial design, and the limitations usually associated with comparing results with retrospective cohorts. Another weakness is that we have not recorded the adherence of the patients to the recommended supplements, and the results could be a result of low adherence to them. Finally, we must note also that we could not address aspects that should affect results such as the bioavailability of the nutrients.

5. Conclusions

As we have highlighted throughout this article, the aim of this study was to assess the impact of protein supplementation (with 20 mg per day) before surgery in a prehabilitation program. This impact was supposed to affect postoperative serum albumin, prealbumin, and total proteins in endometrial cancer patients undergoing laparoscopic surgery.

A prospective study including patients who underwent laparoscopy for endometrial cancer was conducted, with a total of 185 patients divided into three groups (68 in the prehabilitation group). Surprisingly, there were no basal differences in serum albumin, prealbumin, or total proteins between the three groups. After surgery, and regardless of the type of nutritional intervention, the decrease in values was also similar. The values in the Prehab group before surgery were even lower than the initial ones, despite protein supplementation.

In view of all the above, we can conclude that supplementation with 20 mg of protein a day, in patients undergoing laparoscopic surgery for endometrial cancer, is not sufficient to maintain the levels of serum total protein, albumin, and prealbumin. Higher supplementation is necessary, considering that, even with this extra protein intake, the observed levels decreased.

Author Contributions: Conceptualization, E.M. and M.-D.M.; Data curation, E.M.; Investigation, J.M.S.-S.; Methodology, J.M.S.-S. and E.M.; Writing—original draft, J.M.S.-S.; Writing—review and editing, J.M.S.-S., F.-X.M., E.M., C.R.-C., M.-D.M., B.F., N.K. and G.M. All authors have read and agreed to the published version of the manuscript.

Funding: This research received no external funding.

Institutional Review Board Statement: The study was conducted in accordance with the Declaration of Helsinki and approved by the Ethics Committee of the Hospital del Mar (protocol code No. 2017/7770/I, 14 June 2018) for studies involving humans. A waiver of informed consent for the control groups was obtained from the Institutional Ethical Review Board from the home institution.

Informed Consent Statement: Informed consent was obtained from all subjects involved in the study, except for the historical control cohorts where a waiver of informed consent was obtained from the Ethics Committee of the Hospital del Mar.

Data Availability Statement: The data presented in this study are available on request from the corresponding author. The data are not publicly available due to privacy reasons.

Conflicts of Interest: The authors declare no conflict of interest.

References

1. Siegel, R.L.; Miller, K.D.; Fuchs, H.E.; Jemal, A. Cancer Statistics. *CA Cancer J. Clin.* **2021**, *71*, 7–33. [CrossRef] [PubMed]
2. Crosbie, E.J.; Kitson, S.J.; McAlpine, J.N.; Mukhopadhyay, A.; Powell, M.E.; Singh, N. Endometrial cancer. *Lancet* **2022**, *399*, 1412–1428. [CrossRef] [PubMed]
3. Concin, N.; Matias-Guiu, X.; Vergote, I.; Cibula, D.; Mirza, M.R.; Marnitz, S.; Ledermann, J.; Bosse, T.; Chargari, C.; Fagotti, A.; et al. ESGO/ESTRO/ESP guidelines for the management of patients with endometrial carcinoma. *Int. J. Gynecol. Cancer* **2021**, *31*, 12–39. [CrossRef] [PubMed]
4. Gillis, C.; Carli, F. Promoting Perioperative Metabolic and Nutritional Care. *Anesthesiology* **2015**, *123*, 1455–1472. [CrossRef] [PubMed]
5. Nelson, G.; Bakkum-Gamez, J.; Kalogera, E.; Glaser, G.; Altman, A.; Meyer, L.A.; Taylor, J.S.; Iniesta, M.; LaSala, J.; Mena, G.; et al. Guidelines for perioperative care in gynecologic/oncology: Enhanced Recovery After Surgery (ERAS) Society recommendations-2019 update. *Int. J. Gynecol. Cancer* **2019**, *29*, 651–668. [CrossRef] [PubMed]
6. Miralpeix, E.; Nick, A.M.; Meyer, L.A.; Cata, J.; Lasala, J.; Mena, G.E.; Gottumukkala, V.; Iniesta-Donate, M.; Salvo, G.; Ramirez, P.T. A call for new standard of care in perioperative gynecologic oncology practice: Impact of enhanced recovery after surgery (ERAS) programs. *Gynecol. Oncol.* **2016**, *141*, 371–378. [CrossRef] [PubMed]
7. Li, C.; Carli, F.; Lee, L.; Charlebois, P.; Stein, B.; Liberman, A.S.; Kaneva, P.; Augustin, B.; Wongyingsinn, M.; Gamsa, A.; et al. Impact of a trimodal prehabilitation program on functional recovery after colorectal cancer surgery: A pilot study. *Surg. Endosc.* **2013**, *27*, 1072–1082. [CrossRef] [PubMed]
8. Minnella, E.M.; Carli, F. Prehabilitation and functional recovery for colorectal cancer patients. *Eur. J. Surg. Oncol.* **2018**, *44*, 919–926. [CrossRef] [PubMed]
9. Weimann, A.; Braga, M.; Carli, F.; Higashiguchi, T.; Hübner, M.; Klek, S.; Laviano, A.; Ljungqvist, O.; Lobo, D.N.; Martindale, R.G.; et al. ESPEN practical guideline: Clinical nutrition in surgery. *Clin. Nutr.* **2021**, *40*, 4745–4761. [CrossRef] [PubMed]
10. *Protein and Amino Acid Requirements in Human Nutrition: Report of a Joint WHO/FAO/UNU Expert Consultation*; Weltgesundheitsorganisation; FAO; Vereinte Nationen (Eds.) (WHO technical report series); WHO: Geneva, Switzerland, 2007; 265p.

11. Miralpeix, E.; Mancebo, G.; Gayete, S.; Corcoy, M.; Solé-Sedeño, J.M. Role and impact of multimodal prehabilitation for gynecologic oncology patients in an Enhanced Recovery After Surgery (ERAS) program. *Int. J. Gynecol. Cancer* **2019**, *29*, 1235–1243. [CrossRef] [PubMed]
12. Elia, M. *The "MUST" Report. Nutritional Screening of Adults: A Multidisciplinary Responsibility. Development and Use of the "Malnutrition Universal Screening Tool" ('MUST') for Adults*; BAPPEN: Redditch, UK, 2003; (Chairman of MAG and Editor Advancing Clinical Nutrition, a Standing Committee of BAPEN); Available online: https://www.bapen.org.uk/pdfs/must/must-report.pdf (accessed on 15 December 2022).
13. de Klerk, M.; van Dalen, D.H.; Nahar-van Venrooij, L.M.W.; Meijerink, W.J.H.J.; Verdaasdonk, E.G.G. A multimodal prehabilitation program in high-risk patients undergoing elective resection for colorectal cancer: A retrospective cohort study. *Eur. J. Surg. Oncol.* **2021**, *47*, 2849–2856. [CrossRef] [PubMed]
14. Loftus, T.J.; Brown, M.P.; Slish, J.H.; Rosenthal, M.D. Serum Levels of Prealbumin and Albumin for Preoperative Risk Stratification. *Nutr. Clin. Pract.* **2019**, *34*, 340–348. [CrossRef] [PubMed]
15. Salvetti, D.J.; Tempel, Z.J.; Goldschmidt, E.; Colwell, N.A.; Angriman, F.; Panczykowski, D.M.; Agarwal, N.; Kanter, A.S.; Okonkwo, D.O. Low preoperative serum prealbumin levels and the postoperative surgical site infection risk in elective spine surgery: A consecutive series. *J. Neurosurg. Spine* **2018**, *29*, 549–552. [CrossRef] [PubMed]
16. Liu, J.; Wang, F.; Li, S.; Huang, W.; Jia, Y.; Wei, C. The prognostic significance of preoperative serum albumin in urothelial carcinoma: A systematic review and meta-analysis. *Biosci. Rep.* **2018**, *38*, BSR20180214. [CrossRef] [PubMed]
17. Kabata, P.; Jastrzębski, T.; Kąkol, M.; Król, K.; Bobowicz, M.; Kosowska, A.; Jaśkiewicz, J. Preoperative nutritional support in cancer patients with no clinical signs of malnutrition—Prospective randomized controlled trial. *Support. Care Cancer* **2015**, *23*, 365–370. [CrossRef] [PubMed]
18. Miralpeix, E.; Sole-Sedeno, J.-M.; Rodriguez-Cosmen, C.; Taus, A.; Muns, M.-D.; Fabregó, B.; Mancebo, G. Impact of prehabilitation during neoadjuvant chemotherapy and interval cytoreductive surgery on ovarian cancer patients: A pilot study. *World J. Surg. Oncol.* **2022**, *20*, 46. [CrossRef] [PubMed]
19. Hamaker, M.E.; Oosterlaan, F.; van Huis, L.H.; Thielen, N.; Vondeling, A.; van den Bos, F. Nutritional status and interventions for patients with cancer—A systematic review. *J. Geriatr. Oncol.* **2021**, *12*, 6–21. [CrossRef] [PubMed]
20. Smith-Ryan, A.E.; Hirsch, K.R.; Saylor, H.E.; Gould, L.M.; Blue, M.N.M. Nutritional Considerations and Strategies to Facilitate Injury Recovery and Rehabilitation. *J. Athl. Train.* **2020**, *55*, 918–930. [CrossRef] [PubMed]
21. Gillis, C.; Wischmeyer, P.E. Pre-operative nutrition and the elective surgical patient: Why, how and what? *Anaesthesia* **2019**, *74* (Suppl. S1), 27–35. [CrossRef] [PubMed]

Disclaimer/Publisher's Note: The statements, opinions and data contained in all publications are solely those of the individual author(s) and contributor(s) and not of MDPI and/or the editor(s). MDPI and/or the editor(s) disclaim responsibility for any injury to people or property resulting from any ideas, methods, instructions or products referred to in the content.

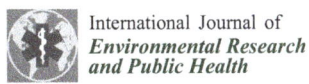

Article

Preference-Based Determinants of Consumer Choice on the Polish Organic Food Market

Agnieszka Dudziak [1] and Anna Kocira [2,*]

1. Department of Power Engineering and Transportation, Faculty of Production Engineering, University of Life Sciences in Lublin, 20-612 Lublin, Poland
2. Institute of Human Nutrition and Agriculture, The University College of Applied Sciences in Chełm, 22-100 Chełm, Poland
* Correspondence: akocira@panschelm.edu.pl

Abstract: **Background:** The development of the organic food market in Poland is currently at a fairly high level. There is a growing demand for organic food, but the share of total sales remains low. There are still many barriers related to the availability of organic food and information about it. In addition, consumers are skeptical of the inspection system in organic farming and admit that these foods do not meet their expectations regarding sensory qualities. **Methods:** The article conducted its own research, using an author's survey questionnaire, which was distributed in Lublin Province. The research sample consisted of 342 respondents and was diverse in terms of gender, age and place of residence. The purpose of the analysis was to ascertain the determinants affecting the choice of organic food. For the study, the method of correspondence analysis was used, the purpose of which was to isolate characteristic groups of consumers who exhibit certain behaviors towards organic products. **Results:** Respondents admitted that they buy organic food several times a month, most often spending an amount of EUR 10–20 (per month). They also paid attention to product labeling, with labels read mostly by residents of small towns (up to 30,000 residents). Respondents were also asked about the reasons why they do not buy organic food. The results of the analysis show that respondents believe it is too expensive, but they also cannot point out differences with other products. **Conclusions:** The main purpose of this article was to study the preferences of organic food buyers and to identify factors that determine their choice but that may also be barriers to purchasing this category of food. These issues need to be further explored so as to create recommendations in this regard for various participants in the organic food market.

Keywords: sustainability; consumer attitudes; organic food; consumer behavior; sustainable food

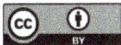

1. Introduction

Growing interest in various products offered on the organic food market is now observed, related not only to concerns about food safety [1] and sustainable agricultural production [2,3]. It is also motivated by the health impact of the diet [4]. This, in turn, encourages the introduction of healthy organic food into the food market, in line with the natural cycle [5,6]. In addition, the introduction of the Farm to Fork Strategy, a key component of the European Green Deal, whose overarching goal is to build a food chain that works for consumers, producers, the climate and the environment, is expected to enable the transition to a sustainable food system in EU countries while ensuring food security for people, as well as access to healthy food. This will ensure that Europeans have access to affordable and sustainable food with the support of measures to combat climate change, promote environmental protection, preserve biodiversity and support organic farming. One of the goals of the strategy is to allocate 25% of the EU's arable land to organic farming, which, in addition to promoting sustainable food consumption and facilitating the transition to healthy, sustainable diets, can have a positive impact on the consumption of organic products [7].

Eyinade et al. [7] showed that consumer preferences for organic food are based on the general belief that it has more desirable characteristics than "traditional" produce [8].

However, the development of the market for organic products depends on the structure of sales channels, the level of prices, long-term trends in increasing standard of living and environmental awareness [9]. Furthermore, the diversified assortment caused by market development causes consumers to follow different opportunities related to purchasing or obtaining organic products, inducing competition in the organic market. In Poland, the organic food market is growing at 20% year to year and is one of the fastest growing sectors of the economy, and the growing competition balances its prices. Poland is perceived as an EU country with great potential for organic farming and the organic food market [10]. However, the products offered on the organic market should be approached with caution because, as the price of a product decreases, so does the quality. The growing demand is encouraging more and more specialized healthy food providers to emerge, and more and more Polish farmers are inclined toward ecology. This, in turn, causes new certified farms to emerge.

Consumer preferences for organic food are based on the general belief that it has more desirable characteristics than "traditional" produce. Consumer product choices are influenced by several factors, including status and lifestyle, as well as financial situation. Those who are not concerned with the origin of the produce can actually hinder the development of the organic market. On the other hand, consumers who are the most willing buyers of organic products treat the origin of products as part of a healthy lifestyle philosophy or a means to rational nutrition [11].

Furthermore, consumers are driven more by desires than by needs when purchasing food products. This forces them to search for additional features that add value to the product. For the organic food market, this means that meeting emotional needs is as important as ensuring the functional potential of the product. This requires creating an emotional bond with the consumer, who is more likely to purchase a product if they perceive it as a psychological and emotional benefit in addition to its expected functional properties. Therefore, the study of consumer preferences regarding organic food products should focus not only on the products' attributes but also on the benefits they represent to the consumer [12].

This article aims to analyze the determinants that affect the choice of organic food by Poles to show the emerging trends in the Polish market related to the purchase of organic food.

2. Factors Determining Consumers' Choice of Organic Market Products

A dynamic model of food quality, which assumes that a food product has functions determined by its properties, can help in understanding consumer perceptions of organic food. Properties are objective characteristics, independent of the user and determined by the composition of raw materials and conditions of the production process. Functions are subjective characteristics that relate to the product and exist in the interaction between the consumer and the product. They are also the main concern of the consumer, and, from the point of view of the manufacturer, it is important to control the properties and determine the relationship between functions and product properties. Appropriate shaping of product properties makes it possible to obtain the functional characteristics desired by consumers [13]. Product quality is multidimensional, and a product can be described by a universal set of attributes. In defining food product quality, four dimensions can be identified: hedonic, health, process and convenience. Hedonic quality refers to the pleasure of consumption based on sensory qualities, primarily taste, smell and appearance of the product. Health quality refers to the impact of the product on the consumer's health. The quality dimension related to convenience consists of issues related to the processes of purchasing, storing, preparing and consuming the product. The process dimension is related to the characteristics of the production process and relates directly to the other quality dimensions [14].

There are many variations in the grouping of consumers with respect to food choice. One such example of consumer segmentation research was conducted by Roper Starch Worldwide, which approached the problem from the point of view of different consumer priorities. Their characteristics are shown in Table 1.

Table 1. Division of consumers by views on organic food.

Consumer Group	Group Characteristics
True Blues	They are politically active, want to have a say in current affairs and prefer not to use environmentally unfriendly products.
Greenback Greens	They have a strong value system but are not interested in political issues and also prefer to avoid environmentally unfriendly products.
Sprouts	For them, nature conservation is important but does not go hand in hand with their food choices.
Grousers	They are unwilling to change and know little about environmental protection. They consider organic products too expensive, yet they are not really different from conventional products.
Apathetics	They are completely uninterested in the natural environment, sustainability and "green" products.

[15–22].

The second division was created by the Natural Marketing Institute (NMI), who have also distinguished five different consumer groups. These characteristics are presented in Table 2.

Table 2. Division of consumers according to the NMI.

Consumer Group	Group Characteristics
LOHAS (Lifestyles of Health and Sustainability)	They care about sustainability and healthy living. This group adopts an ecological lifestyle as its philosophy of life and wants to influence the environment with their actions.
Naturalites	They consider an active lifestyle and a healthy diet important to them, but this is not fully reflected in their purchasing decisions.
Conventionals	They are involved in environmental initiatives, but this is not their main concern. They choose food products that are attractively priced and will save them money.
Drifters	For them, environmental issues are a temporary fad. They want to be identified as environmentally conscious but do not apply the necessary principles in everyday life.
Unconcerneds	Similar to Apathetics, this group is not concerned with the environment and is not interested in organic foods, least in purchasing them.

[15–22].

Upon analyzing these two divisions, it can be observed that the results are very similar and the groups highlighted had similar priorities. The groups can be observed in all societies [16].

In the food market, many consumers are buying organic products, but there is also a large segment of the population that is not interested in buying them and does not identify with them for a number of reasons. One reason is the lack of clear differentiation between conventional and organic products and the higher price of the latter. According to a 2006 survey of Polish consumers, more than half of respondents who shopped for organic food were willing to pay only 10% more for organic food. Almost a fourth (23.5%) were willing to pay 11–25% more for healthy food and the rest of the respondents even more. It follows that price is a factor that is largely responsible for the level of sales of organic food as most consumers are not willing to spend more on it than on conventional food [23–25]. However, consumers often consider organic food to be a valuable alternative to popular conventionally produced food brands [26].

Organic food buyers are often advocates of regional food as a result of their views. They are in good shape and willing to take their time searching for the right food. They spend a large portion of their money on organic foods and are most likely to source them from specialized stores. In addition, they pay attention to the origin of the products and the ecological packaging [24]. According to some researchers, consumers pay attention to the origin of the product, and this information influences their purchasing decisions [27]. They divided the origin of food into "local" and "imported", with the former perceived more positively. In contrast, Fehse et al. (2017) confirm that branding has a significant impact on the purchase decision of these products. Generally, branding is identified as environmental consciousness; in the eyes of customers, organic food is of higher quality [9,24]. Consumers relate the high quality of these products, also perceived as healthy foods, to their lifestyle habits, which has great potential as a foundation for marketing strategies [12].

Culture, or, more precisely, the principles learned in a family home, are of great importance among the factors that motivate and influence purchasing decisions. Poland is dominated by a traditional cuisine based on simple, unprocessed, all-available ingredients. However, the eating behaviors of Poles are shaped by economic and environmental factors that influence Polish culture and are related to consumption.

In Poland, the market for organic food is developing dynamically. Poland is also seen as a European Union country with a huge potential for organic farming, if only in terms of the area under organic farming and the number of organic farms. In addition, there is a growing number of conscious consumers in Poland convinced of its health benefits. Nowadays, more people are interested in product labeling, description and composition of product contents. Nevertheless, there is also a large group of consumers who, for many reasons, do not buy organic food, discouraged by, among other things, the high price or lack of confidence in products described as organic. Research conducted by Jarczok-Guzy indicates that the scope of promotion of organic food is narrow and prices are too high; moreover, organic food is difficult to access. Most consumers have heard of the food, but they mainly seek information on the Internet or by reading product labels, and there is still a large group of people who cannot correctly identify the labels for organic food [10].

Economic status has a huge impact on consumer choices and is related to education and social status. A relationship between income and food consumption was also observed. Often, people with a lower food budget pay attention to the price rather than the origin of food, while those with a higher budget pay attention to quality and origin, but also, although to a lesser extent, to price. Consumers with lower incomes often have to compromise on the quality and nutritional value of food, which contributes to a reduction in the pleasure derived from food shopping and consumption, linked to the awareness of one's inability to choose from the 'better' quality brands and products [28]. Marketing related to promoting healthy lifestyles is an important factor that influences consumer behavior. Consumers often look up information they have found on television, radio or online and thus become informed consumers. This situation changed significantly during the COVID-19 pandemic, when many food establishments were temporarily closed. Then, consumer spending on groceries increased and shifted largely to the Internet [29].

According to Shepherd et al. [30], in addition to the factors that influence the type of food purchased and its consumption, there are a variety of food-related considerations: aroma, texture, palatability and food buyer reasons. Equally important are the nutritional value of the product, its price, the broad range of available products and brand and product awareness among consumers [31].

Based on the observations of the organic food market, it can be concluded that Poles are motivated to buy organic products due to their beneficial health effects, taste and presentation of the product. Above all, they want to protect the environment that way [32]. However, it is not always environmental concerns that influence the purchase of these types of foods, as confirmed by Le-Anh and Nguyen-To [33]. On the other hand, Barrena et al. [12] found that the two main elements that determine the final choice to purchase organic foods are health and self-image. This is due to the health benefit effect, nutritional value and health safety guarantee of organic food, which are related to its perception as healthy food, ensuring healthy eating habits and quality of life, as well as security or peace of mind, dignity and self-respect. However, the reason why consumers choose conventional food over organic worldwide is because its price is too high, its availability is poor and it offers little variety [32].

Despite the abundance of information on consumer habits, it should be noted that it is difficult to clearly define the segment of the Polish consumer. Nevertheless, the profile is constantly changing. More and more people are aware of their food consumption needs. An interesting proposal for segmenting consumers in terms of the shopping habits and habits of Polish households was presented by Bilska et al. [34]. Nevertheless, the authors focused mainly on the problem of food waste. In the research conducted by Smiglak-Krajewska and Wojciechowska-Solis [35], the following groups of consumers were distinguished: eco-activists, eco-dietitians, eco-traditionalists and eco-innovators. An analysis of the motives for choosing organic products by selected types of consumers by Śmiglak-Krajewska and Wojciechowska-Solis shows that eco-activists pay more attention to marketing and practical features than to sensory attributes. Eco-dietitians, when deciding to buy organic products, take into account practical features first while paying slightly less attention to sensory features. A similar distribution of importance of the features of organic products can be noticed in the case of eco-traditionalists; however, the obtained values are lower. Sensory characteristics are of the least importance to the eco-innovator consumer type. A comparison of the groups of consumers showed that the most informed customers of organic products are eco-activists and eco-dietitians, who are able to notice all the benefits of organic products, which is reflected in the obtained values. Eco-activists and eco-innovators pay the most attention to marketing features and the least to sensory features, whereas eco-dietitians and eco-traditionalists pay the most attention to practical features and the least to marketing features [35].

3. Forecasted Directions of Changes in the Polish Organic Food Market

Since health-conscious communities are now emerging, organic producers are constantly looking for innovative solutions in agricultural production that could totally replace conventional ones. The growth of the organic food market is likely to involve the elimination of meat or the introduction of dairy substitutes. This is because consumers who prefer organic products also tend to have healthy eating habits that include many fruits and vegetables but less meat [36]. The Internet, especially social media, e.g., Instagram, Facebook, which educate the public, have a major impact on these changes, becoming the main source of information, entertainment and informal education and the chief communication space that shapes people's tastes, knowledge and lifestyles [37]. Social media have been shown to play a major role in society, creating the meaning of diet and influencing food choices [38].

According to Adewuyi and Adefemi, together with the emergence of a green lifestyle, social media nowadays also become a crucial part of people's daily life as they play an important role in spreading awareness of important information [39]. In their research, Nguyen and Zhang showed that social media influencers can moderate the intention–behavior gap within ecological lifestyle adoption by directly affecting consumers' green behaviors. The influence includes the quality and quantity of contents, the authenticity and credibility from influencers and information and their personal background and characteristics [40]. The lack of trust and fear of conventional foods will increase the interest in the organic market, especially reliable and certified products.

Increasingly important in the organic market is the share of "free from food", i.e., products in which specific ingredients were eliminated due to adverse effects on the human body (e.g., lactose-free, gluten-free or sugar-free). This is due to the increasing rate of diagnosed food intolerances and allergies. This trend is becoming more and more popular and is related to the wellness trend, which involves self-care. By 2021, its popularity was projected to grow at an average annual rate. However, consumers who do not have food allergies but care about the quality of the products they eat are also interested in "free from foods" [41].

Emerging technologies will allow every consumer to track a product "Farm to Fork" using a new generation of barcodes and blockchain. All it takes to find out the path a product has taken before it got into the consumer's hands is a smartphone. According to public preference studies, consumers will prefer foods with a clear label and transparent packaging (if transparent packaging is used for the product). This is important for raw products (fruits and vegetables) for direct consumption because the freshness and quality of the product can be visually assessed, and this may influence the decision to purchase these foods by consumers who prefer healthy foods [2]. In 2018, an increased interest in a variety of supplements that have a positive impact on the health of the digestive system and mind can be observed [42,43]. The value of the market related to consumption and the proper functioning of the human body is bound to increase. Therefore, the willingness to purchase products that are beneficial to health will follow [28,29]. The popularity of various diets is also generating interest in edible insects, which contain high amounts of protein. Less surprising but increasingly popular are legumes. Vegans and vegetarians seek plant-based snack alternatives that resemble the taste of meat. Interest in such products has been growing since early 2019 [44,45]. This is why meat-based treat producers constantly expand the range and quantity of their offer [30,31].

The organic market is expected to grow steadily by 20% per year until 2030, which makes it a worthwhile investment. It can be expected that sales and availability of organic food will increase in the coming years [46–50].

In Central and Eastern Europe, a number of large-scale specialized organic food stores with a large selection of products and attractive prices are likely to appear. Moreover, small organic stores, offering only a selected category of products, e.g., only bread or vegetables, will become more and more popular. Moreover, online stores of large retail chains, such as Auchan or E. Leclerc, as well as Foodini.pl, have opened specialized "Eco" or "Bio" departments, offering organic food, and more and more brick-and-mortar organic stores are offering their products online. By innovating and creating online platforms, retailers communicate more effectively with consumers [51,52]. According to the study "Food Trade in Poland in 2010–2020" by Roland Berger, the food market will have to adapt to many factors related to the modern consumer. Food sales should combine traditional and online channels, taking into account products of the highest possible quality, grown in harmony with nature. This sales model fits best into the lifestyle of modern consumers who use technology to shop for groceries [53].

According to specialists, the organic market in Poland has positive prospects, and, in a few years, it should be on par with that in the EU. Consumers who want organic foods will not have a problem sourcing such products in Poland in the coming years.

4. Materials and Methods

A consumer study was conducted using a proprietary survey questionnaire (The Research questionnaire—Supplementary Materials). The research involved 342 respondents who were residents of Lublin Province in the south-eastern part of Poland. Grouping variables such as place of residence, age and gender were used to differentiate the respondents in a more detailed and additional way and were aimed at pointing to differences in the perception of the problem in the purchasing of organic products by consumers. The survey was conducted via the Internet, and the selection of respondents was random selection using the so-called the "snowball" method due to the fact that mainly young people use Internet resources; hence, their number turned out to be the largest.

The aim of the study was to analyze the determinants influencing the choice of organic food by the inhabitants of Lubelskie Voivodeship. However, since many respondents admitted that they buy food sporadically, in the further part of the analysis, the respondents were asked what the reasons for this situation were. Therefore, the analysis also includes the reasons for these negative attitudes towards organic food; the aim was to investigate the barriers that prevent consumers from buying organic food products.

The dominant group of respondents in this study were consumers aged 18–25, of which 68% were women (Table 3). Since consumers of organic products living in rural areas are less frequently analyzed in this type of research, this group of people constituted a large proportion of the respondents in the study (39%). The varied characteristics of the respondents allowed the demonstration of the differences in attitude toward the study subject and to show the relationship between the characteristics and their choices.

Table 3. Socio-demographic profile of the respondents.

In Total	Number of Respondents 342	Percentage 100.0
Gender:		
female	232	68.0
male	110	32.0
Age:		
up to 18 years	12	4.0
18–25 years old	236	69.0
26–40 years old	24	7.0
41–60 years old	46	13.0
60 years and more	24	7.0
Place of residence:		
rural area	132	39.0
city to 30,000 residents	48	14.0
30–300,000 residents	86	25.0
city with more than 300,000 residents	76	22.0

The survey was anonymous. The questions were related to the purchase of organic food products, the level of interest in them, reading the labels and knowledge of the packaging designation, the budget allocated for organic products and factors that encourage and discourage the purchase of this type of product and the attitude towards organic products. The responses allowed analyzing and evaluating the behavior of consumers in the organic food market and to interpret their attitude towards organic food products.

Data analyses were carried out on the basis of the statistical processing software Statistica 13.3 (Set Plus, version 5.0.96, license for University of Life Sciences in Lublin, Lublin, Poland) and Excel 2013 (Microsoft Office Professional Plus 2013, license for University of Life Sciences in Lublin, Lublin, Poland).

5. Results and Discussion

Among the various issues raised in the research, the key issue was knowledge of organic products and the respondents' declarations regarding their purchase. Most of the respondents declared that they knew and bought organic food. Figure 1 shows slight differences between individual groups of respondents depending on age and gender. However, among the largest group of respondents, i.e., aged 18–25, the majority of women declared that they buy organic food, while the opposite correlation was noted in men. Furthermore, there was greater interest in this type of product among women in two age groups, 26–40 years and 41–60 years old, who purchased only organic products. In the case of men, the age groups 18–25 and 41–60 purchased organic food more frequently. Please note that, in this study, women were twice as large a group of respondents as they are more often responsible for grocery shopping than men.

Table 4 provides more detailed information on the survey's respondents by participation in each category of gender and place of living.

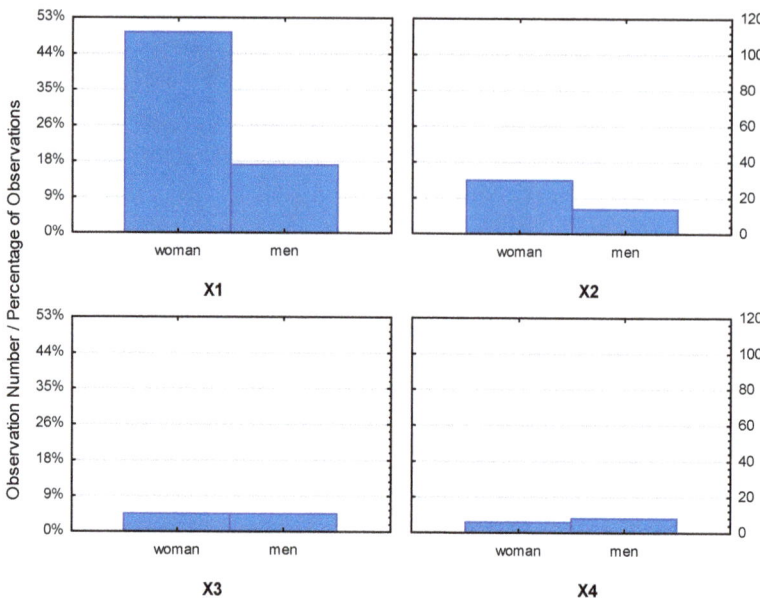

Figure 1. Graph of interaction of consumers declaring the purchase of organic food in relation to the sex of the respondents. (Abbreviations: X1—several times a month; X2—several times a year; X3—every day; X4—never).

Table 4. Respondents' attitudes toward organic food by gender and place of living.

		Gender		Place of Living			
		F n (%)	M n (%)	RA n (%)	C30 n (%)	C30–300 n (%)	C300 n (%)
Buying Organic Food	yes	150 (61.2)	58 (27.8)	76 (36.5)	44 (21.2)	50 (24.0)	38 (18.3)
	no	82 (61.2)	52 (38.8)	56 (41.7)	4 (3.0)	36 (26.9)	38 (28.4)
Frequency of Organic Food Purchases	every day	10 (50.0)	10 (50.0)	10 (50.0)	4 (20.0)	2 (10.0)	4 (20.0)
	several times a month	112 (74.7)	38 (25.3)	50 (33.3)	34 (22.7)	38 (25.3)	28 (18.7)
	several times a year	30 (68.2)	14 (31.8)	18 (40.9)	6 (13.7)	10 (22.7)	10 (22.7)
	never	6 (42.9)	8 (57.1)	2 (14.2)	2 (14.3)	4 (28.6)	6 (42.9)
Amount of Money Spent on Organic Food Purchases (Per Month)	<EUR 2.5	6 (100.0)	0 (0.0)	0 (0.0)	2 (3.3)	4 (66.7)	0 (0.0)
	EUR 2.5-10	50 (67.6)	24 (32.4)	26 (35.2)	16 (21.6)	10 (13.5)	22 (29.7)
	EUR 10-20	56 (70.0)	24 (30.0)	26 (32.5)	20 (25.0)	24 (30.0)	10 (12.5)
	>EUR 20	12 (50.0)	12 (50.0)	14 (58.4)	0 (0.0)	2 (8.3)	8 (33.3)
	I do not care about this	30 (78.9)	8 (21.1)	14 (36.8)	6 (15.8)	12 (31.6)	6 (15.8)
Reasons to Stop Buying Organic Food	too expensive	134 (72.0)	52 (28.0)	62 (33.3)	34 (18.3)	50 (26.9)	40 (21.5)
	are no different from any other food	22 (61.0)	14 (39.0)	16 (44.4)	10 (27.8)	6 (16.7)	4 (11.1)
	widespread availability of products from supermarkets	0 (0.0)	2 (100.0)	2 (100.0)	0 (0.0)	0 (0.0)	0 (0.0)
	no interest in organic food	0 (0.0)	4 (100.0)	0 (0.0)	0 (0.0)	2 (50.0)	2 (50.0)
Reading Labels of Organic Products	yes	66 (66.0)	34 (34.0)	44 (44.0)	22 (22.0)	16 (16.0)	18 (18.0)
	sometimes	80 (74.1)	28 (25.9)	36 (33.3)	22 (20.4)	32 (29.6)	18 (16.7)
	I don't pay attention at all	8 (57.1)	6 (42.9)	2 (14.3)	0 (0.0)	4 (28.6)	8 (57.1)

Abbreviations: F—female; M—male; RA—rural area; C30—city up to 30,000 residents; C30–300—city 30–300,000 residents; C300—city of more than 300,000 residents.

The literature confirms that women buy organic food more often than men [54–56]. However, men have a higher level of awareness of organic food [57,58] and are more confident in their knowledge of organic products [59]. The results of our own research in relation to gender are shown in Figure 1. Taking into account the factor of age, it has been shown that younger consumers are more aware of organic food, prompting them to buy it more often [58,60]. For young people, a lifestyle based on organic food provides a sense of mental stability in life, a life lived in harmony with nature, history and their perception of health. Such a lifestyle ensures vitality as it relates its existence to the natural world [61]. Therefore, it is gaining more and more followers among young people. The results of our own research in relation to age and gender are shown in Figure 2.

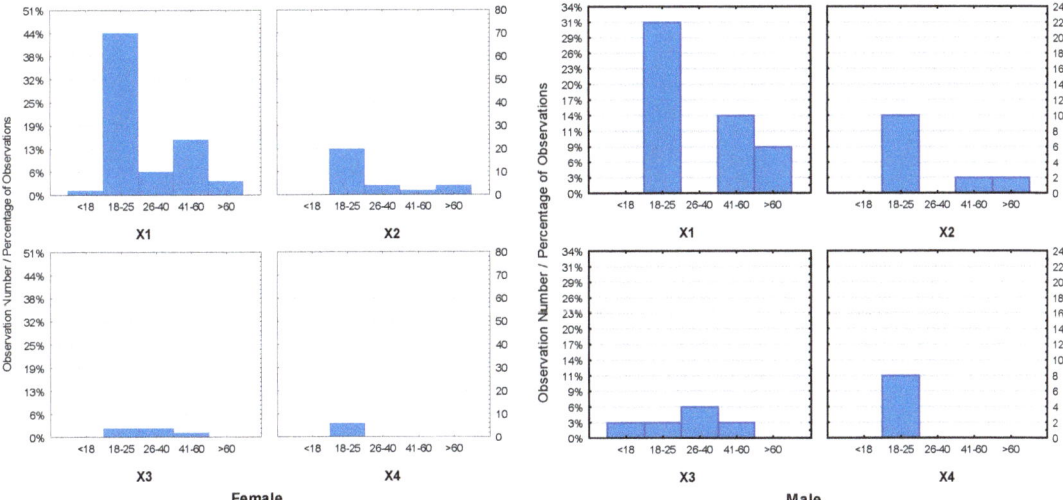

Figure 2. Graph of interaction of consumers declaring the purchase of organic food in relation to the sex and age of the respondents. (Abbreviations: X1—several times a month; X2—several times a year; X3—every day; X4—never).

The label on organic food packaging confirms that organic products are produced and processed according to the requirements related to the use of additives and artificial ingredients, pesticides, soil quality or the husbandry and processing of animal products. In addition, all ingredients and processing aids must be certified organic [62]. Given these stringent labeling requirements for organic products, it has been shown that most consumers have a broad and general understanding of what the name "organic product" on the packaging label means, including an understanding of how this food was produced and processed [62]. In terms of place of residence, it was found that consumers in cities with more than 30,000 residents prefer organic food, while consumers living in rural areas or cities with a population below 30,000 buy local rather than organic food [63–65].

The amount of funds allocated to the purchase of organic food is also an important issue. A clear differentiation can be observed in the group of respondents divided by gender (Figure 3), but, in division by age, these differences are small (Figure 4). Men declared specific amounts allocated to the purchase of organic food. On the other hand, some women declared that they were not interested in this issue.

Most often, the respondents spend EUR 10–20 (approximately PLN 45–90) of their monthly expenditure on organic food. Less than EUR 2.5 (approximately PLN 10) is spent mainly by people aged 18–25; this age group also often responded that they were not interested in spending money on organic products.

In the case of the declared expenditure of EUR 2.5–10 on organic products, three age groups, 18–25, 26–40 and 41–60, declared it. On the other hand, in the case of the amount exceeding EUR 20, it was declared in the age group of 18–60 years. Therefore, it is clearly visible that the budgets allocated to the purchase of organic food are not high.

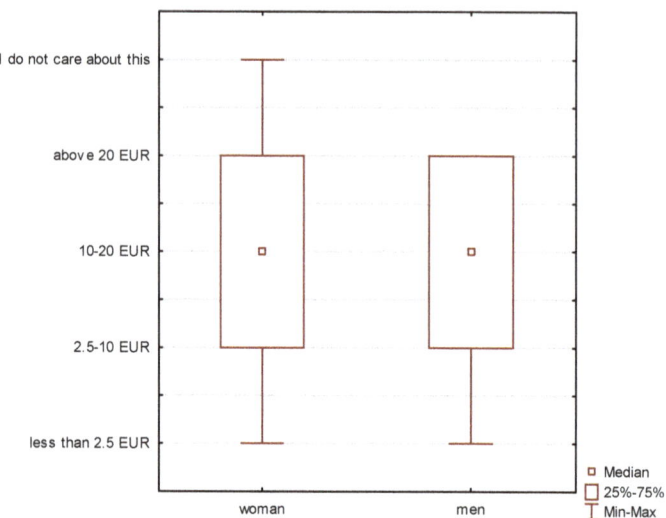

Figure 3. Declaration of the amount of money earmarked for the purchase of organic food depending on the gender of the respondents.

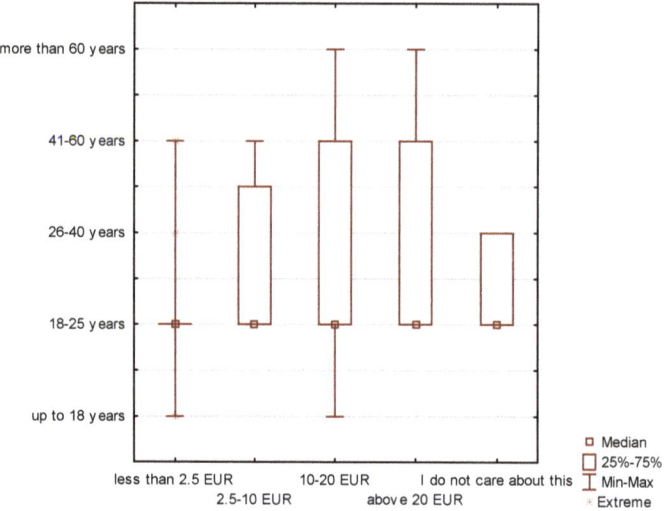

Figure 4. Declaration of the amount of money earmarked for the purchase of organic food depending on the age of the respondents.

Statistical Analysis—Correspondence Analysis

Correspondence analysis (CA) is a multivariate statistical method for analyzing tables of categorial data or any data on a common ratio scale. Correspondence analysis is a descriptive and exploratory technique for analyzing two-way and multi-way tables containing certain measures that characterize the relationship between columns and rows. The obtained results provide information and allow for the analysis of the structure of qualitative variables making up the table. Therefore, as a result of the analyses, a two-dimensional contingency table was obtained, where the frequencies in the contingency table were first standardized in such a way that the relative frequencies were calculated, which, when summed up in all fields (cells) of the table, provide 1.0. One way to show the goals of a typical analysis is to express the relative frequencies by the distance between individual rows or columns in a space with a small number of dimensions. In correspondence analysis, inertia is defined as the quotient of the Pearson chi-squared statistic calculated from the two-way table by the total count (in the example presented, the total count is 342) [66].

Therefore, to analyze the market of organic products in Lubelskie Province, the correspondence between three groups of characteristics was analyzed: knowledge of the labels of organic products (three groups), place of residence (four groups) and gender (two groups). To present the configuration of the points representing the input data, a two-dimensional factor space was selected.

The first factor allows reproducing 80.04% of the input data variation (i.e., total inertia), and the second one 19.96% (Table 5).

Table 5. Information resources factors.

Number of Dimensions	Eigenvalues and inertia, Total inertia = 0.23810 χ^2 = 52.859 df = 14 p = 0.0000				
	Singular Value	Eigenvalues	Percentage of Inertia	Cumulative Percentage	χ^2
1	0.436548	0.190574	80.03881	80.0388	42.30747
2	0.218009	0.047528	19.96119	100.0000	10.55123

The greatest share in a two-dimensional factor space was related to the knowledge of ecological product labels, namely the answers that respondents "sometimes" read labels and that they "did not" pay attention to it—coordinate I. On the other hand, in the case of coordinate II, the answers related to reading labels were: "always" and "sometimes".

On the other hand, men living in a city of 30–300,000 and men living in a village had the largest share in the creation of a two-dimensional factor space, taking into consideration the place of residence and gender. Coordinate I was male residents of cities and coordinate II was male residents of rural areas (Figure 5).

The study distinguished three groups of consumers whose indicator structure depends on their interest in the label of the product they intend to buy (Figure 5). The first group (G1) is made up of people who "sometimes" read product labels and make a purchase. The second group (G2) includes customers who "do not" pay attention to the labels, and the third group (G3) is made up of people who "always" read the product labels. The fourth group consists of women living in rural areas and women living in large cities with more than 300,000 residents. This group's structure is the closest to the average.

The strongest relationship was observed between people who "sometimes" read product labels: these are women living in cities of 30,000 to 300,000 residents and men living in cities with more than 300,000 residents. The group in question stands out from the others due to the index value of this factor. On the other hand, the respondents' declaration that they "always" read labels is quite strongly related to men living in rural areas, as well as women and men living in small towns (up to 30,000 residents). In turn, consumers who "do not" pay attention to product labels are mainly men living in cities of 30–300,000 residents.

As the research conducted earlier shows, purchases of organic products are still not a common phenomenon among Polish consumers. The main reasons for the lack of confidence of consumers in the rationality of purchasing organic food include, first of all, their high price. Other reasons include a lack of conviction about their nutritional value, or, as the respondents claim, "no difference" between organic and conventional products (Figure 6).

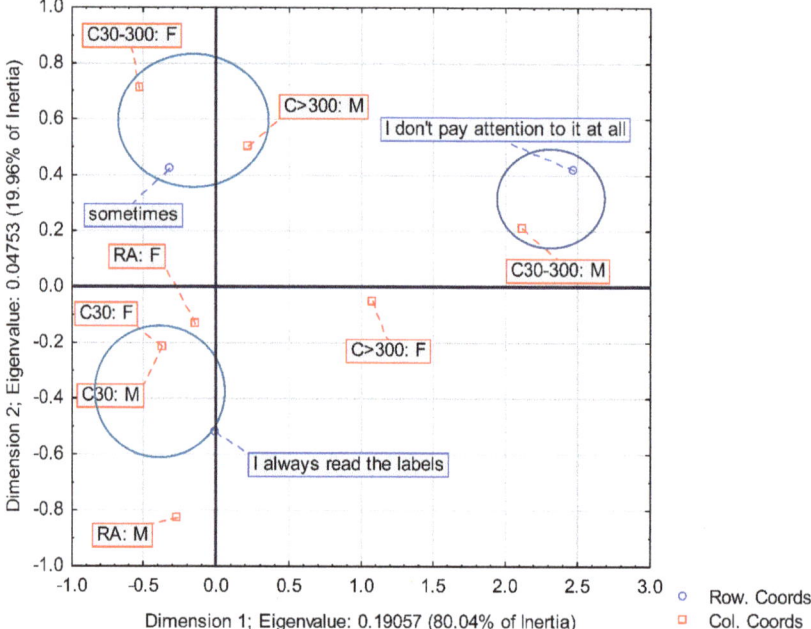

Figure 5. Correspondence analysis results between three groups of characteristics: knowledge of the labels on the packaging of organic products, place of residence of respondents and gender, canonical standardization. (Abbreviations: RA—rural area; C30—city to 30,000 residents; C30–300—city 30–300,000 residents; C > 300—city with more than 300,000 residents; Row. Coords—row coordinates; Col. Coords—column coordinates; F—female; M—male).

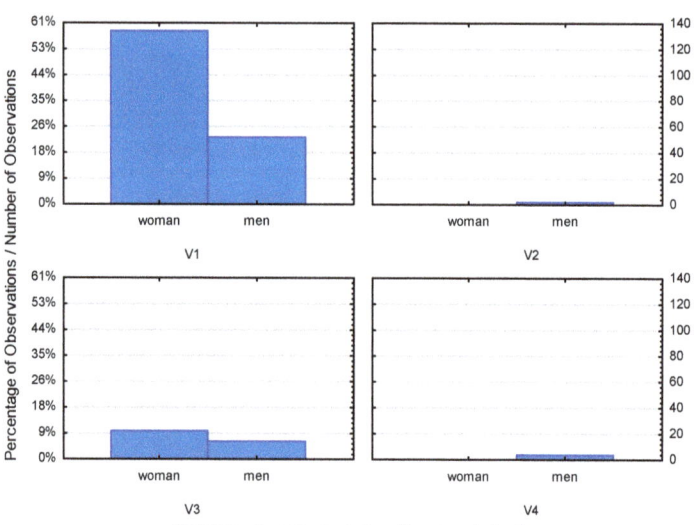

Figure 6. Categorized histogram describing the reasons that prevent consumers from buying organic food in relation to the gender of the respondents. (Abbreviations: V1—high price of eco food; V2—widespread availability of products from supermarkets; V3—no difference between products; V4—no interest in eco products).

As shown in Figures 6 and 7, the variables differentiating gender and place of residence clearly indicate that there is no differentiation in these two groups. Price remains the most significant factor regardless of the gender and place of residence of the respondents. Decisions to purchase organic products often depend on the budget allocated on such a purchase. Therefore, the lack of differences between an organic and a traditional product may not be a sufficient argument to buy the former.

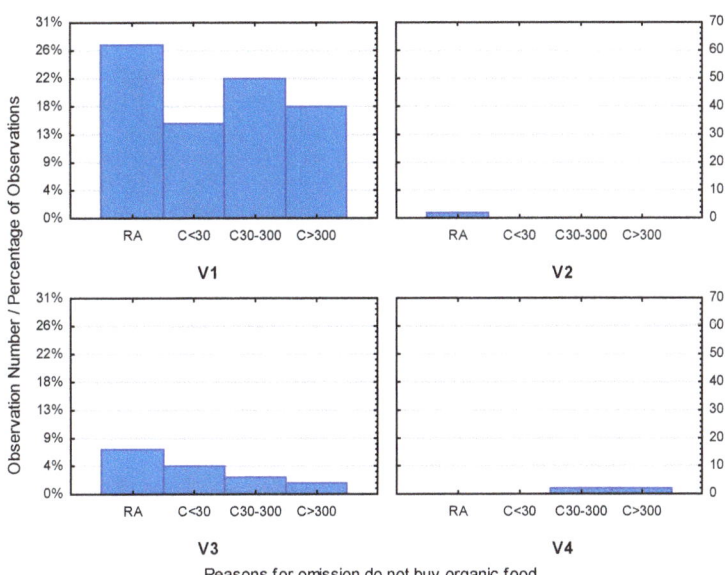

Figure 7. Categorized histogram describing reasons that prevent consumers from purchasing organic food in relation to where they live. (Abbreviations: V1—high price of eco food; V2—widespread availability of products from supermarkets; V3—no difference between products; V4—no interest in eco products; RA—rural area; C30—city to 30,000 residents; C30–300—city 30–300,000 residents; C > 300—city with more than 300,000 residents).

Davies et al. [67] confirmed that the main factors that influence the purchase of organic products are their price and availability. In turn, Kyriakopoulos and Oude-Ophuis [68] argued that the quality of organic food determines its purchase to a greater extent than the price. Therefore, consumers' knowledge and awareness of the benefits of organic food is important in the decision-making process. The inability to clearly distinguish between the two alternatives, as well as the price premium on organic produce, can complicate or influence the purchasing decision of the consumer in favor of cheap products [8,69].

However, the main factor influencing the choice of organic food is the consumer's concern for their own health and that of their loved ones. Buyers have greater certainty as to the origin and the natural method of production of the produce when organic food is certified. Baer-Nawrocka and Szalaty (2017) concluded that the main motives behind consumers' decision to purchase organic products are health considerations and the high quality of the products offered. This is demonstrated by numerous studies conducted among different groups of respondents indicating that health benefits are the most important rationale for purchasing organic food, which confirms that consumers are convinced of the health-promoting qualities of organic products [70–73]. On the other hand, concern for the environment as a reason for purchasing organic food was rated by consumers as an unimportant factor [74]. The implication is that motivation in choosing organic food is dominated by the perspective of individually perceived concern for health rather than concern for the natural environment [75].

The public is aware of the benefits of organic food, but this is often not reflected in the demand reported due to the higher price and lower availability of ecological products [59]. Organic food in specialized stores is purchased mainly by people with a higher monthly income, while people with secondary education buy organic food mainly at the bazaar due to the lower prices or the lack of specialized stores nearby. It follows that an additional barrier is hindered distribution, which is related to the fact that organic products usually have a short shelf life and, often, quick delivery to the consumer is a condition for their sale [74]. One of the barriers to the development of this market is the dispersion of supply [76]. Hence, the physical movement of products along the transportation and logistics chain plays a major role. In the market for organic products, short distribution channels that promote the sale of local products are often more advantageous from the point of view of producers because of the association with lower costs and margins, making it possible to sell products at competitive prices. At the same time, the risk of various types of damage or out-of-date food is reduced. As a result, direct sales, especially in the early stages of market development, based on sales in one's own store, on an organic farm, at a market or agricultural retail trade are advantageous. It has been shown that the profitability of selling these products depends on the location of the organic farm near the main markets, which include large and very large urban areas. The strengths of direct sales are the control of the price level by the organic food producer, the adjustment of the offer to the structure and size of demand and the possibility of obtaining information on consumer expectations and preferences. However, this type of sale requires greater involvement on the part of the consumer and creates a greater sales risk burden for the producer [74,77].

6. Conclusions

The development of the organic food market can bring significant benefits not only to organic farmers, processors and intermediaries but also to customers and, ultimately, to society. The revival of organic farming and the organic food market should come from the actions of the governments of individual countries and the EU as a whole. In Poland, the organic food market is not yet as developed as in other EU countries, but, by learning from their practice and leveraging the profile and possibilities of organic farming, these differences can be minimized in the near future.

The most important conclusions resulting from the conducted research include:
- The majority of respondents declared that they know and buy organic food;
- Many respondents, however, admitted that they buy organic food occasionally;
- Among the largest group of respondents, i.e., those aged 18–25, most women declared that they buy organic food, while the opposite relationship was noted among men;
- There was greater interest in food among women in the two age groups of 26–40 and 41–60 who bought only organic products;
- For men, organic food was more frequently purchased by those aged 18–25 and 41–60 (women made up twice as large a group of respondents as they are more likely to be responsible for grocery shopping than men);
- With regard to place of residence, it was found that consumers in cities with more than 30,000 residents prefer organic food, while consumers living in rural areas or cities with less than 30,000 residents tend to buy local food rather than organic food;
- Most often, respondents spend EUR 10–20 of their monthly expenses on organic food. Less than EUR 2.5 is spent mainly by those aged 18–25 (this age group also often responded that they were not interested in spending money on organic products);
- For declared spending of EUR 2.5–10 on organic products, it was declared by the three age groups 18–25, 26–40 and 41–60, while, for the amount above EUR 20, it was declared by those aged 18–60. Thus, budgets for buying organic food are not high.

The practical implications of this study indicate that, as much as possible, action should be taken to convince consumers of the palatability, nutritional and health values of organic food so that the higher price comes second for the potential consumer. Highlighting the quality features of organic products will undoubtedly increase their demand and thus improve the health and general well-being of the population.

Please note that the tastes and preferences of consumers are changing, especially when it comes to the food market. Therefore, it is worth taking steps to produce food that meets the expectations of various consumer groups. Such recommendations should be particularly taken into account by producers and distributors. As the market is constantly developing, it must be researched both in terms of the health benefits of organic produce on the human body and the changing preferences of consumers. This is especially important in the age of comprehensive, all-available information as, these days, healthy eating has become a kind of fad. In light of the above, the growing awareness about organic products could contribute to the growth of the organic food market in Poland. Future research should focus on the level of consumer satisfaction, which affects the demand for organic products. Research into consumer personality types is also important, allowing the design and targeting of marketing strategies. The area of consumer expectations towards innovation in organic food is also worth investigating in the future.

Supplementary Materials: The following supporting information can be downloaded at: https://www.mdpi.com/article/10.3390/ijerph191710895/s1, Research Questionnaire.

Author Contributions: Conceptualization, A.D. and A.K.; methodology, A.D. and A.K.; software, A.D. and A.K.; validation, A.D. and A.K.; formal analysis, A.D. and A.K.; investigation, A.D. and A.K.; resources, A.D. and A.K.; data curation, A.D. and A.K.; writing—original draft preparation, A.D. and A.K.; writing—review and editing, A.D. and A.K.; visualization, A.D.; supervision, A.K.; project administration, A.D. and A.K.; funding acquisition, A.D. and A.K.; All authors have read and agreed to the published version of the manuscript.

Funding: This research received no external funding.

Institutional Review Board Statement: Not applicable.

Informed Consent Statement: Not applicable.

Data Availability Statement: Not applicable.

Conflicts of Interest: The authors declare no conflict of interest.

References

1. Liang, B.; Scammon, D.L. Food Contamination Incidents: What Do Consumers Seek Online? Who Cares? *Int. J. Nonprofit Volunt. Sect. Mark.* **2016**, *21*, 227–241. [CrossRef]
2. Asioli, D.; Aschemann-Witzel, J.; Caputo, V.; Vecchio, R.; Annunziata, A.; Næs, T.; Varela, P. Making Sense of the "Clean Label" Trends: A Review of Consumer Food Choice Behavior and Discussion of Industry Implications. *Food Res. Int.* **2017**, *99*, 58–71. [CrossRef] [PubMed]
3. Aschemann-Witzel, J.; Ares, G.; Thøgersen, J.; Monteleone, E. A Sense of Sustainability?–How Sensory Consumer Science Can Contribute to Sustainable Development of the Food Sector. *Trends Food Sci. Technol.* **2019**, *90*, 180–186. [CrossRef]
4. Janssen, M.; Heerkens, Y.; Kuijer, W.; Van Der Heijden, B.; Engels, J. Effects of Mindfulness-Based Stress Reduction on Employees' Mental Health: A Systematic Review. *PLoS ONE* **2018**, *13*, e0191332. [CrossRef] [PubMed]
5. Shahabi Ahangarkolaee, S.; Gorton, M. The Effects of Perceived Regulatory Efficacy, Ethnocentrism and Food Safety Concern on the Demand for Organic Food. *Int. J. Consum. Stud.* **2021**, *45*, 273–286. [CrossRef]
6. Rana, J.; Paul, J. Health Motive and the Purchase of Organic Food: A Meta-analytic Review. *Int. J. Consum. Stud.* **2020**, *44*, 162–171. [CrossRef]
7. Schebesta, H.; Candel, J.J. Game-Changing Potential of the EU's Farm to Fork Strategy. *Nat. Food* **2020**, *1*, 586–588. [CrossRef]
8. Eyinade, G.A.; Mushunje, A.; Yusuf, S.F.G. The Willingness to Consume Organic Food: A Review. *Food Agric. Immunol.* **2021**, *32*, 78–104. [CrossRef]
9. Bryła, P. *Marketing Regionalnych i Ekologicznych Produktów Żywnościowych. Perspektywa Sprzedawcy i Konsumenta*; Wydawnictwo Uniwersytetu Łódzkiego: Łódź, Poland, 2015; ISBN 83-7969-435-X.
10. Jarczok-Guzy, M. Obstacles to the Development of the Organic Food Market in Poland and the Possible Directions of Growth. *Food Sci. Nutr.* **2018**, *6*, 1462–1472. [CrossRef]
11. Hermaniuk, T. Postawy i Zachowania Konsumentów Na Rynku Ekologicznych Produktów Żywnościowych. *Handel Wewnętrzny* **2018**, 189–199.

12. Barrena, R.; Sánchez, M. Frequency of Consumption and Changing Determinants of Purchase Decision: From Attributes to Values in the Organic Food Market. *Span. J. Agric. Res.* **2010**, *8*, 251–272. [CrossRef]
13. Peri, C. The Universe of Food Quality. *Food Qual. Prefer.* **2006**, *17*, 3–8. [CrossRef]
14. Grunert, K.G.; Bech-Larsen, T.; Bredahl, L. Three Issues in Consumer Quality Perception and Acceptance of Dairy Products. *Int. Dairy J.* **2000**, *10*, 575–584. [CrossRef]
15. Lorek, A. Światowy Kryzys Żywnościowy, Przyczyny i Wpływ Na Kraje Rozwijające Się. *Prace Nauk. Uniw. Ekon. Wrocławiu* **2011**, *231*, 38–50.
16. Lorek, E. *Biznes Ekologiczny*; Wydawnictwo Uniwersytetu Ekonomicznego: Katowice, Poland, 2015.
17. Szakály, Z.; Popp, J.; Kontor, E.; Kovács, S.; Pető, K.; Jasák, H. Attitudes of the Lifestyle of Health and Sustainability Segment in Hungary. *Sustainability* **2017**, *9*, 1763. [CrossRef]
18. Mosier, S.L.; Rimal, A.; Ruxton, M.M. A Song of Policy Incongruence: The Missing Choir of Consumer Preferences in GMO-Labeling Policy Outcomes. *Rev. Policy Res.* **2020**, *37*, 511–534. [CrossRef]
19. Sung, J.; Woo, H. Investigating Male Consumers' Lifestyle of Health and Sustainability (LOHAS) and Perception toward Slow Fashion. *J. Retail. Consum. Serv.* **2019**, *49*, 120–128. [CrossRef]
20. Choi, S.; Feinberg, R.A. The LOHAS Lifestyle and Marketplace Behavior. In *Handbook of Engaged Sustainability*; Springer: Berlin/Heidelberg, Germany, 2018; pp. 1069–1086.
21. Choi, S.; Feinberg, R.A. The LOHAS (Lifestyle of Health and Sustainability) Scale Development and Validation. *Sustainability* **2021**, *13*, 1598. [CrossRef]
22. Takada, S.; Yamamoto, Y.; Shimizu, S.; Kimachi, M.; Ikenoue, T.; Fukuma, S.; Onishi, Y.; Takegami, M.; Yamazaki, S.; Ono, R. Association between Subjective Sleep Quality and Future Risk of Falls in Older People: Results from LOHAS. *J. Gerontol. Ser. A* **2018**, *73*, 1205–1211. [CrossRef]
23. Aschemann-Witzel, J.; Zielke, S. Can't Buy Me Green? A Review of Consumer Perceptions of and Behavior toward the Price of Organic Food. *J. Consum. Aff.* **2017**, *51*, 211–251. [CrossRef]
24. Frýdlová, M.; Vostrá, H. Determinants Influencing Consumer Behaviour in Organic Food Market. *Acta Univ. Agric. Silvic. Mendel. Brun.* **2011**, *59*, 111–120. [CrossRef]
25. Reisch, L.; Eberle, U.; Lorek, S. Sustainable Food Consumption: An Overview of Contemporary Issues and Policies. *Sustain. Sci. Pract. Policy* **2013**, *9*, 7–25. [CrossRef]
26. Fehse, K.; Simmank, F.; Gutyrchik, E.; Sztrókay-Gaul, A. Organic or Popular Brands—Food Perception Engages Distinct Functional Pathways. An FMRI Study. *Cogent Psychol.* **2017**, *4*, 1284392. [CrossRef]
27. Simmons, A.L.; Schlezinger, J.J.; Corkey, B.E. What Are We Putting in Our Food That Is Making Us Fat? Food Additives, Contaminants, and Other Putative Contributors to Obesity. *Curr. Obes. Rep.* **2014**, *3*, 273–285. [CrossRef] [PubMed]
28. Kneafsey, M.; Dowler, E.; Lambie-Mumford, H.; Inman, A.; Collier, R. Consumers and Food Security: Uncertain or Empowered? *J. Rural Stud.* **2013**, *29*, 101–112. [CrossRef]
29. Grashuis, J.; Skevas, T.; Segovia, M.S. Grocery Shopping Preferences during the COVID-19 Pandemic. *Sustainability* **2020**, *12*, 5369. [CrossRef]
30. Paluck, E.L.; Shepherd, H. The Salience of Social Referents: A Field Experiment on Collective Norms and Harassment Behavior in a School Social Network. *J. Pers. Soc. Psychol.* **2012**, *103*, 899. [CrossRef]
31. Żakowska-Biemans, S.; Gutkowska, K. *Rynek Żywności Ekologicznej w Polsce Iw Krajach Unii Europejskiej*; Wydawnictwo SGGW: Warszawa, Poland, 2003; ISBN 83-7244-390-4.
32. Pilarczyk, B.; Nestorowicz, R. *Marketing Ekologicznych Produktów Żywnościowych*; Oficyna a Wolters Kluwer Business: Warszawa, Poland, 2010; ISBN 83-7526-736-8.
33. Le-Anh, T.; Nguyen-To, T. Consumer Purchasing Behaviour of Organic Food in an Emerging Market. *Int. J. Consum. Stud.* **2020**, *44*, 563–573. [CrossRef]
34. Bilska, B.; Tomaszewska, M.; Kołożyn-Krajewska, D.; Piecek, M. Segmentation of Polish Households Taking into Account Food Waste. *Foods* **2020**, *9*, 379. [CrossRef]
35. Śmiglak-Krajewska, M.; Wojciechowska-Solis, J. Consumer versus Organic Products in the COVID-19 Pandemic: Opportunities and Barriers to Market Development. *Energies* **2021**, *14*, 5566. [CrossRef]
36. Christensen, T.; Denver, S.; Bøye Olsen, S. Consumer Preferences for Organic Food and for the Shares of Meat and Vegetables in an Everyday Meal. *J. Int. Food Agribus. Mark.* **2020**, *32*, 234–246. [CrossRef]
37. Łaska-Formejster, A.; Messyasz, K. Youtuberzy Kreujący Styl Życia i Zdrowia Młodzieży. Nowe Media Jako Narzędzie Indywidualizacji Odpowiedzialności Za Zdrowie. 2020. Available online: https://depot.ceon.pl/handle/123456789/19249 (accessed on 15 June 2021).
38. Niewczas-Dobrowolska, M. Preferowane Źródła Informacji Dotyczącej Żywności w Opinii Konsumentów. *Nauka Technol. Jakość* **2021**, *28*, 132–143. [CrossRef]
39. Adewuyi, E.O.; Adefemi, K. Behavior Change Communication Using Social Media: A Review. *Int. J. Commun. Health* **2016**, *9*, 109–116.
40. Nguyen, T.H.; Zhang, H. Green Lifestyle, Where to Go?: How Social Media Influencers Moderate the Intention–Behavior Gap within the Ecological Lifestyle Context. 2020. Available online: https://www.diva-portal.org/smash/get/diva2:1430761/FULLTEXT01.pdf (accessed on 15 June 2021).

41. Joshi, V.; Kumar, S. Meat Analogues: Plant Based Alternatives to Meat Products-A Review. *Int. J. Food Ferment. Technol.* **2015**, *5*, 107–119. [CrossRef]
42. Góralczyk, K. Czy Żywność Ekologiczna Rzeczywiście Jest Najlepsza? *Stud. Ecol. Bioethicae* **2018**, *16*, 51–56. [CrossRef]
43. Kwiatkowski, C.; Harasim, E. *Produkcja Rolnicza a Bezpieczna Żywność: Wybr ane Aspekty*; Wydano Nakładem Instytutu Naukowo-Wydawniczego" Spatium": Radom, Poland, 2019; ISBN 83-66017-62-1.
44. Burlea-Schiopoiu, A.; Ogarca, R.F.; Barbu, C.M.; Craciun, L.; Baloi, I.C.; Mihai, L.S. The Impact of COVID-19 Pandemic on Food Waste Behaviour of Young People. *J. Clean. Prod.* **2021**, *294*, 126333. [CrossRef]
45. Wang, P.; McCarthy, B.; Kapetanaki, A.B. To Be Ethical or to Be Good? The Impact of 'Good Provider'and Moral Norms on Food Waste Decisions in Two Countries. *Glob. Environ. Change* **2021**, *69*, 102300. [CrossRef]
46. Bazaluk, O.; Yatsenko, O.; Zakharchuk, O.; Ovcharenko, A.; Khrystenko, O.; Nitsenko, V. Dynamic Development of the Global Organic Food Market and Opportunities for Ukraine. *Sustainability* **2020**, *12*, 6963. [CrossRef]
47. Costa, M.P.; Schoeneboom, J.C.; Oliveira, S.A.; Vinas, R.S.; de Medeiros, G.A. A Socio-Eco-Efficiency Analysis of Integrated and Non-Integrated Crop-Livestock-Forestry Systems in the Brazilian Cerrado Based on LCA. *J. Clean. Prod.* **2018**, *171*, 1460–1471. [CrossRef]
48. Keeler, B.L.; Hamel, P.; McPhearson, T.; Hamann, M.H.; Donahue, M.L.; Meza Prado, K.A.; Arkema, K.K.; Bratman, G.N.; Brauman, K.A.; Finlay, J.C. Social-Ecological and Technological Factors Moderate the Value of Urban Nature. *Nat. Sustain.* **2019**, *2*, 29–38. [CrossRef]
49. Nezamova, O.; Olentsova, J. *Adaptation Problems of the Food Market to Modern Conditions*; IOP Publishing: Bristol, UK, 2020; Volume 548, p. 082023.
50. Solopov, V.A.; Minakov, I.A. Food Safety in the Sphere of Production and Consumption of Vegetable Products. *Int. J. Eng. Technol. UAE* **2018**, *7*, 523–527. [CrossRef]
51. Jacobsen, L.F.; Stancu, V.; Wang, Q.J.; Aschemann-Witzel, J.; Lähteenmäki, L. Connecting Food Consumers to Organisations, Peers, and Technical Devices: The Potential of Interactive Communication Technology to Support Consumers' Value Creation. *Trends Food Sci. Technol.* **2021**, *109*, 622–631. [CrossRef]
52. Tyburski, J.; Zakowska-Biemans, S. Możliwości Wykorzystania Surowców z Rolnictwa Ekologicznego Do Produkcji Żywności Tradycyjnej. *Biul. Nauk. Uniw. Warm.-Mazur. Olszt.* **2009**, *30*, 79–82.
53. Mir, S.A.; Dar, B.; Shah, M.A.; Sofi, S.A.; Hamdani, A.M.; Oliveira, C.A.; Moosavi, M.H.; Khaneghah, A.M.; Sant'Ana, A.S. Application of New Technologies in Decontamination of Mycotoxins in Cereal Grains: Challenges, and Perspectives. *Food Chem. Toxicol.* **2021**, *148*, 111976. [CrossRef]
54. Lockie, S.; Lyons, K.; Lawrence, G.; Mummery, K. Eating 'Green': Motivations behind Organic Food Consumption in Australia. *Sociol. Rural.* **2002**, *42*, 23–40. [CrossRef]
55. Radman, M. Consumer Consumption and Perception of Organic Products in Croatia. *Br. Food J.* **2005**, *107*, 263–273. [CrossRef]
56. Fatha, L.; Ayoubi, R. A Revisit to the Role of Gender, Age, Subjective and Objective Knowledge in Consumers' Attitudes towards Organic Food. *J. Strateg. Mark.* **2021**. [CrossRef]
57. Briz, T.; Ward, R.W. Consumer Awareness of Organic Products in Spain: An Application of Multinominal Logit Models. *Food Policy* **2009**, *34*, 295–304. [CrossRef]
58. Kumar, S.; Ali, J. Analyzing the Factors Affecting Consumer Awareness on Organic Foods in India. In Proceedings of the 21st Annual IFAMA World Forum and Symposium on the Road, Frankfurt, Germany, 20–23 June 2011; Volume 2050, pp. 20–23.
59. Aertsens, J.; Mondelaers, K.; Verbeke, W.; Buysse, J.; Van Huylenbroeck, G. The Influence of Subjective and Objective Knowledge on Attitude, Motivations and Consumption of Organic Food. *Br. Food J.* **2011**, *113*, 1353–1378. [CrossRef]
60. Gumber, G.; Rana, J. Who Buys Organic Food? Understanding Different Types of Consumers. *Cogent Bus. Manag.* **2021**, *8*, 1935084. [CrossRef]
61. Von Essen, E.; Englander, M. Organic Food as a Healthy Lifestyle: A Phenomenological Psychological Analysis. *Int. J. Qual. Stud. Health Well-Being* **2013**, *8*, 20559. [CrossRef] [PubMed]
62. Berry, C.; Burton, S.; Howlett, E. It's Only Natural: The Mediating Impact of Consumers' Attribute Inferences on the Relationships between Product Claims, Perceived Product Healthfulness, and Purchase Intentions. *J. Acad. Mark. Sci.* **2017**, *45*, 698–719. [CrossRef]
63. Hempel, C.; Hamm, U. Local and/or Organic: A Study on Consumer Preferences for Organic Food and Food from Different Origins. *Int. J. Consum. Stud.* **2016**, *40*, 732–741. [CrossRef]
64. Cholette, S.; Özlük, Ö.; Özşen, L.; Ungson, G.R. Exploring Purchasing Preferences: Local and Ecologically Labelled Foods. *J. Consum. Mark.* **2013**, *30*, 563–572. [CrossRef]
65. Pugliese, P.; Zanasi, C.; Atallah, O.; Cosimo, R. Investigating the Interaction between Organic and Local Foods in the Mediterranean: The Lebanese Organic Consumer's Perspective. *Food Policy* **2013**, *39*, 1–12. [CrossRef]
66. Clausen, S.E. *Applied Correspondence Analysis: An Introduction*; Sage: Thousand Oaks, CA, USA, 1998; Volume 121, ISBN 0-7619-1115-4.
67. Davies, A.; Titterington, A.J.; Cochrane, C. Who Buys Organic Food? A Profile of the Purchasers of Organic Food in Northern Ireland. *Br. Food J.* **1995**, *97*, 17–23. [CrossRef]
68. Kyriakopoulos, K.; Ophuis, P.A.O. A Pre-Purchase Model of Consumer Choice for Biological Foodstuff. *J. Int. Food Agribus. Mark.* **1997**, *8*, 37–53. [CrossRef]

69. Yiridoe, E.K.; Bonti-Ankomah, S.; Martin, R.C. Comparison of Consumer Perceptions and Preference toward Organic versus Conventionally Produced Foods: A Review and Update of the Literature. *Renew. Agric. Food Syst.* **2005**, *20*, 193–205. [CrossRef]
70. Ozguven, N. Organic Foods Motivations Factors for Consumers. *Procedia-Soc. Behav. Sci.* **2012**, *62*, 661–665. [CrossRef]
71. Shafie, F.A.; Rennie, D. Consumer Perceptions towards Organic Food. *Procedia-Soc. Behav. Sci.* **2012**, *49*, 360–367. [CrossRef]
72. Bryła, P. Selected Aspects of the Marketing Strategy of a Healthy Food Retailer–a Case Study of the Słoneczko Shop in Łódź. *Mark. Zarządzanie* **2016**, *44*, 209–221. [CrossRef]
73. Nestorowicz, R.; Pilarczyk, B.; Jerzyk, E.; Rogala, A.; Disterheft, D. *Raport z Badań Przeprowadzonych w Ramach Projektu "Postawy Etnocentryczne Konsumentów (w Ujęciu Lokalnym) a Szanse i Bariery Rozwoju Rynku Żywności Ekologicznej"*; Uniwersytet Ekonomiczny w Poznaniu: Poznań, Poland, 2016.
74. Baer-Nawrocka, A.; Szalaty, N. Organic Products in the Producers' and Consumers' Opinion—Case Study. *Zagadnienia Ekon. Rolnej* **2017**, *353*, 138–153. [CrossRef]
75. Łuczka-Bakuła, W. Decyzje Zakupu Na Rynku Żywności a Świadomość i Zachowania Proekologiczne Konsumentów. *Handel Wewn.* **2011**, *3*, 52–59.
76. Blaik, P.; Matwiejczuk, R.; Pokusa, T. *Integracja Marketingu i Logistyki-Wybrane Problemy*; Politechnika Opolska: Opole, Poland, 2005; ISBN 83-88492-14-4.
77. Czubała, A. *Dystrybucja Produktów*; Polskie Wydawnictwo Ekonomiczne: Warszawa, Poland, 2001; ISBN 83-208-1324-7.

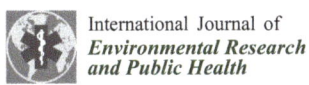 International Journal of
Environmental Research and Public Health

Article

Prospects for the Development of the Demand for Carp in Poland among Young Consumers

Magdalena Raftowicz

Department of Applied Economics, Faculty of Life Sciences and Technology, Wrocław University of Environmental and Life Sciences, 50-375 Wrocław, Poland; magdalena.raftowicz@upwr.edu.pl

Abstract: Carp fishing economy in Poland has a centuries-old tradition. However, in the last decade, as a result of changes in global market trends, this industry has experienced stagnation. Still, the elimination of this niche industry may have painful consequences for the entire ecosystem and biodiversity. Hence, every effort should be made to protect and maintain the status quo. The aim of the article is an attempt to show that the development prospects for the carp market in Poland are limited, especially in the face of little interest in carp consumption by young adult consumers, who will create the demand for carp in the near future. The remedy may be to change the image of the carp together with a territorial marketing strategy that would be consistent with the preferences of the young generation. The research was conducted on the basis of a critical analysis of the literature of the subject, focus studies, questionnaires and a case study.

Keywords: aquaculture; food heritage; carp; consumer preferences of Young Adult Populations; marketing place

Citation: Raftowicz, M. Prospects for the Development of the Demand for Carp in Poland among Young Consumers. *Int. J. Environ. Res. Public Health* **2022**, *19*, 3831. https://doi.org/10.3390/ijerph19073831

Academic Editors: F. Xavier Medina, Francesc Fusté-Forné and Nela Filimon

Received: 19 February 2022
Accepted: 22 March 2022
Published: 23 March 2022

Publisher's Note: MDPI stays neutral with regard to jurisdictional claims in published maps and institutional affiliations.

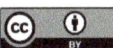

Copyright: © 2022 by the author. Licensee MDPI, Basel, Switzerland. This article is an open access article distributed under the terms and conditions of the Creative Commons Attribution (CC BY) license (https://creativecommons.org/licenses/by/4.0/).

1. Introduction

The carp economy in Poland has a tradition that goes back over eight centuries. It is assumed that knowledge about carp breeding was transferred to Poland by religious orders, and later by the secular clergy (bishoprics). The oldest order that was the first to raise fish were the Cistercians, brought to Poland in the 12th century from Belgium and France. As the Christian religion strengthened, there was a need to respect numerous church fasts, the number of which exceeded 200 days a year [1], thus increasing the national demand for fish. The turn of the 16th and 17th centuries is often considered the 'golden age of Polish pond carp fishing'. This thesis is exemplified by the fact that at that time, ponds with a unit area of 100 to over 1000 ha were built. After the Second World War, as a result of the state border change, the area of ponds in Poland decreased by over 22 thousand ha and amounted to a total of 66,525 ha, of which, until 1989 (i.e., until the political transformation in Poland), about 75% of the pond area was used by the State Fisheries Farms. The beginning of the 1990s, which initiated the functioning of the free market economy in Poland, was characterized by the appearance of completely new, private carp breeders (currently, there are about 300 carp farms in Poland) [2], who, however, still cultivated breeding traditions and the traditional form of selling carp in the form of live fish. The implementation of such sales strategies a decade ago strengthened the eating habits of Poles even more. Currently, 80–90% of carp consumption in Poland takes place around Christmas, which is closely related to Polish tradition and Christian culture, where carp is a traditional dish on the Christmas Eve table.

The aim of the article is an attempt to show that the development prospects for the carp market in Poland are limited due to the decline in domestic demand and the reluctance of the young generation to consume carp all year round. However, the elimination of this niche industry may have painful consequences for the entire ecosystem and its biodiversity. Hence, every effort should be made to protect and maintain the status quo.

Such research assumption established also the purpose of the study, which consisted in identifying consumer trends from the perspective of young consumers and changes taking place on the carp market in Poland from the carp producers' point of view.

The research was conducted on the basis of a critical analysis of the literature of the subject, focus studies, questionnaires and a case study.

The practical aspect of the issues discussed in the article will be the possibility of using the research results by the aquaculture advisory services, NGOs, local governments and carp farms themselves interested in developing and selling their products in the future.

The structure of the article is divided into seven parts. The first part is the introduction to the carp economy in Poland. The second part introduces the importance of carp in the food economy, with particular emphasis on its non-production aspects, especially those social and environmental. The third part presents new consumer trends in the agri-food sector. The fourth part illustrates the adopted research methodology. The fifth part presents the results of the focus studies and questionnaire research conducted in the chosen target selection. Parts 6 and 7 close the considerations, presenting the discussion and conclusions in turn.

2. The Importance of Carp in the Food Economy

Fish and seafood account for approx. 7% of the global food market [3]. Even at the end of the 20th century, the quantity of fish supplied for consumption was determined by catches in the seas and oceans. However, over the past two decades, there has been a significant decline in the catch dynamics of sea fish due to severe overfishing. Only thanks to the intensive aquaculture development, despite the decline in the state of sea resources, world fish production continues to show an upward trend, as illustrated in Figure 1.

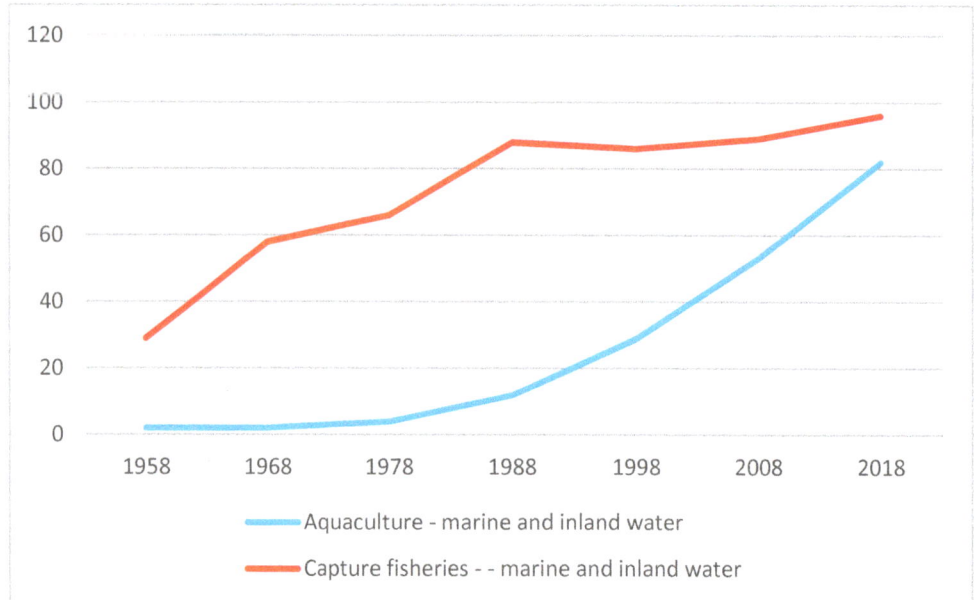

Figure 1. Capture fisheries and aquaculture production (in million tonnes). Source: own study based on [4].

Aquaculture means the breeding or farming of aquatic organisms by means of specifically developed techniques with the aim of increasing production beyond the natural environmental capacity, while the organisms remain the property of a natural or legal person throughout the breeding and farming period, up to and including the catch [5]. It covers both fish and seafood (crustaceans, mollusca and seaweed). Production takes place in ponds, pools and fairways, partitions and wells, cages, recirculation systems and other devices not mentioned above. Currently, aquaculture covers about 580 species of aquatic animals and plants [6]. World aquaculture production is dominated by China, as shown in Table 1.

Table 1. Total aquaculture production by major producers in 2017.

Country	Value [in Thousands of EUR]	% Value	Volume [in Tonnes]	% Volume
China	131,860,769	59.56	64,358,481	57.48
Indonesia	11,424,415	5.16	15,896,100	14.20
India	10,882,498	4.92	6,182,000	5.52
Chile	9,216,766	4.16	1,219,747	1.09
Vietnam	8,599,847	3.88	3,831,241	3.42
Norway	6,954,930	3.14	1,308,634	1.17
Bangladesh	5,227,379	2.36	2,333,352	2.08
UE-28	5,059,021	2.29	1,372,012	1.23
Japan	4,147,649	1.87	1,021,580	0.91
South Korea	3,037,683	1.37	2,306,280	2.06
Thailand	2,393,042	1.08	889,891	0.79
OTHERS	22,591,846	10.2	11,246,153	10.05
In total	221,395,844	100.00%	111,965,471	100.00%

Source: own elaboration based on [7].

According to FAO estimates, by 2030, the global share of aquaculture in relation to traditional fish catches will increase from 46% to 57% [8]. Aquaculture allows for the supply of natural animal protein and thus contributes to strengthening global food security. Statistics of using feed and water in breeding aquaculture products are also favorable in comparison to the to beef, pork or poultry, as shown in Table 2.

Table 2. Amount of feed and water necessary to produce 1 kg of meat.

	Feed [in kg]	Water [in Litres]
Beef	8	14,500
Pork	3	5990
Poultry	2	4330
Salmon	1.1–1.2	1500

Source: own elaboration based on [9,10].

Table 2 shows that the production of 1 kg of beef requires 8 kg of feed and 14.5 thousand liters of water. For 1 kg of pork, 3 kg of feed is needed and nearly 6 thousand liters of water, while salmon farming seems to be the most effective and ecological because it requires only 1.1–1.2 kg of feed and 1500 L of water.

The importance of the aquaculture development is evidenced by the fact that the catch of cod (Poles' favorite fish [11]) in the Baltic Sea has fallen from 50 thousand tones in 2015 to 21.6 thousand in 2018 [12]. Thus, the monthly consumption of fish and seafood in Poland decreased from 0.45 kg per person in 2010 to 0.27 kg per person in 2020 (i.e., by as much as 40% over a decade) [13].

In the world, the most popular farmed species of aquaculture are those belonging to the carp family: grass carp, silver carp and common carp, as shown in Table 3.

Table 3. Top 10 aquaculture species in the world.

	Aquaculture Species	Production in Tonnes	%	Value in 10^3 USD	%
1.	Grass carp	5,822,869	7.60	7,462,316	4.73
2.	Silver carp	5,125,461	6.69	6,776,963	4.29
3.	Common carp	4,328,083	5.65	5,905,279	3.74
4.	Japanese carpet shell	4,049,541	5.29	3,708,929	2.35
5.	Nile tilapia	3,930,579	5.13	6,017,377	3.81
6.	Whiteleg shrimp	3,879,786	5.07	18,899,320	11.97
7.	Bighead carp	3,402,870	4.42	4,373,102	2.77
8.	Catla	2,764,944	3.61	4,813,647	3.05
9.	Atlantic salmon	2,381,576	3.11	11,945,146	7.56
10.	Rohu	1,785,900	2.33	3,034,446	1.92

Source: [6].

Common carp is the third most frequently produced fish species in the world, with 97.3% of its production taking place in aquaculture [14]. Global common carp production is dominated by China. In the EU, the leader in the production of carp is Poland with an annual production of approx. 20 tons, almost entirely allocated to the domestic market (approx. 96–97%), as shown in Table 4.

Table 4. Production of common carp in the UE in 2018.

Country	Production in 2018 (in Tons)	% of Change 2018/2008
Poland	20,751	+21%
Czech Republic	18,430	+5.2%
Hungary	11,462	+9.3%
Germany	4746	−43.7%
France	Estimated: 3000–4000	Estimated: −20%

Source: [15].

For comparison, nearly 67 thousand tons of carp [16] are produced in the whole European Union. However, the consumption of carp in Poland is gradually decreasing; currently, it amounts to 0.56 kg per year/person [17]. The research has shown that it is not price that is the main obstacle to consumption, as the demand for carp is rigid. This means that lowering the price will not reflect in an increase in carp demand [18].

The non-production aspect of the carp economy in Poland also plays an important role. Social and environmental values are of particular importance here.

When it comes to the social sphere, there is a long list of benefits that local residents derive from the conducted fishing activity. In addition to traditional values such as food supply and employment guarantee, the development of fishing, processing and recreation (e.g., hotel industry, gastronomy or agritourism) may be observed, which is related to the possibility of the multifunctional development of rural areas.

When it comes to nature, research has shown that carp is a very environmentally friendly system of fish farming [19]. Moreover, carp management is one of the aquaculture systems most preferably accepted by consumers, together with their expectations for sustainable fish farming [20]. Especially the management of water resources is of great importance here. The ponds act as retention reservoirs and thus maintain a higher groundwater level. Water flow is used only in emergency situations, when the welfare of the stock is threatened as a result of e.g., high temperatures. During the season, the water is replenished only in situations of its visible losses due to evaporation or leakage through dikes. Due to the water retention system used in carp farming, these ponds have a very positive effect on the water quality in the catchment area. This contributes to the retention of very large number of factors responsible for water eutrophication during the production cycle: both nitrogen and phosphorus. The pond management also positively influences the amount of water flow in the watercourse. The research results have shown that the lower the ratio of the catchment area to the area of ponds, the more favorable this effect is [1]. Carp ponds also function as areas of rich natural value. First of all, they are a refuge for wetland birds. The extensive carp ponds serve as wetlands and provide high biodiversity habitats for protected species of birds, amphibians, reptiles, mammals and insects. Moreover, carp farms have a positive effect on the microclimate of the surrounding areas and have a much higher agro-ecological value than arable lands and grasslands. An example is the area of the Barycz Valley, where the largest carp breeding center in Europe is located (the Milicz Ponds). This area covers almost one-fifth of the total usable area of breeding ponds in Poland, while the area of land under the waters of the Barycz Valley is as much as 11%. The Barycz Valley has been included in the Ramsar Convention on Wetlands of international importance, especially as a habitat for waterfowl due to the presence of numerous ponds, wetlands, meadows and forests, which affects the development of biodiversity [21]. In the Barycz Valley, there are also three areas covered by the Natura 2000 program as areas of special protection for birds (especially white-tailed eagles, cormorants, black storks, cranes and herons (white and gray)). These are Ostoja nad Baryczą (82,026.4 ha), the Barycz Valley (55,516.8 ha) and the Lower Barycz Valley (3165.8 ha) [22]. It also houses the largest ornithological reserve, the Milicz Ponds in Poland, and the largest Landscape Park in Poland, the Barycz Valley. These areas, as one of four in Poland, have also been classified as environmentally sensitive areas, which enables the implementation of EU agri-environmental programs. Due to the unique natural and landscape values of the Barycz Valley Landscape Park, this area is an example of the need to harmonise environmental, social, economic and spatial aspects [23].

3. New Consumer Trends in the Agri-Food Sector

The changes taking place in the contemporary world as a result of the globalization and internationalization processes of the world economy have a significant impact on the modern consumers attitudes, especially the young ones. The change in consumer behaviour is caused, among others, by the awareness of the sustainable development principles, circular economy or the need to shorten the food supply chains [24]. There is also growing awareness of changes in local food production markets and the importance of the consumption of healthy, high-quality products, including local [25], regional [26], traditional [27] and natural [28] products, which is in line with the development of slow food [29,30], culture and food safety [31].

These trends are also present in Poland, where, after 1989, there has been a significant change in the approach to consumption [32]. Back in the 1990s, Polish consumers focused mainly on satisfying basic nutritional needs, which was consistent with the 'food consumption model', while in the following years, along with the economic growth and income growth, the consumption structure of Poles assumed the nature of an 'industrial model'. The beginning of the 21st century can be, quoting [33], called 'consumer capitalism' characterized by a rapid increase in consumption and a significant improvement in the living standard of the societies of middle and highly developed countries, including Poland. It was then that a peculiar McDonaldization of consumption patterns took place, consisting in the massification and unification of Western values. However, in opposition to strong Western consumerism, a model of sustainable consumption has emerged, which is based on ethnocentric, environmentally friendly patterns. This model is also related to the servicisation of consumption, in which the communication process (especially in social media) and an attractive way of spending free time are of great importance (the traditional division into work and free time is disappearing).

A new consumer trend is also prosumption [34], defined as the phenomenon of intertwining consumption and production processes, which leads to blurring the boundaries between them, where consumers become producers [35] at the same time. In other words, prosumption is the expression of consumer opposition to mass, unified and standardized production. By engaging in the production process, the consumer is able to produce the final product in line with their expectations through independent design and reconfiguration. In practice, a prosumer is a consumer who meets at least two of the three conditions [36]:

1. Becomes acquainted with the opinions of other Internet users and most often personally looks for them when planning to purchase a product;
2. Describes products online or asks questions about them;
3. Participates in promotions and co-creates products, slogans or advertising campaigns.

There is also a slow change in consumer orientation on the food market from a quantitative to a qualitative approach, which is exemplified by the diminishing role of price in making decisions about food purchases [18]. In recent years, there has also been a dynamic increase in the number of Polish consumers who are looking for high-quality products with high nutritional value, produced using methods consistent with the idea of sustainable development, including organic food, produced locally and sold in short supply chains [37].

4. Materials and Methods

The research area was narrowed down to the Barycz Valley in Poland, where the largest carp breeding center in Poland and Europe is located, as shown in Table 5 and Figure 2.

Table 5. Fish farms in the Barycz Valley.

Number of Fish Fams	The Total Area of the Ponds [in ha]	Production Value Measured in Income from Fishing Activities Together with the Total Value of Production [in PLN]	Number of People Employed on a Permanent Basis in Fish Farms
26	8253.45	25,348,966.56	271

Source: own elaboration based on [38].

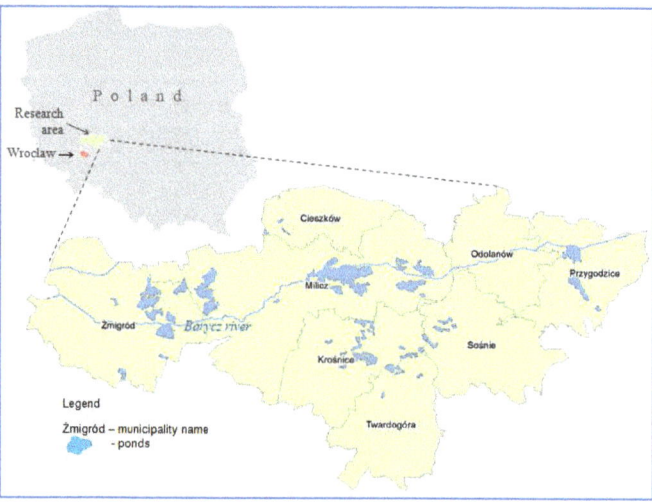

Figure 2. Barycz Valley. Source: own elaboration.

The Milicz Carp from the Barycz Valley has been entered on the List of Traditional Products of the Minister of Agriculture and Rural Development [39]. It has become a key image element of the economic, natural and cultural offer in the Barycz Valley.

The first element of the research was to conduct focus studies (10 participants) combined with in-depth expert interviews with three owners of fish farms on the specifics of the carp market and the changes that producers have observed on the market. These studies were conducted in October 2019. A focus group is a qualitative research method that brings together a small group of people to answer questions in a moderating setting. The method aims to obtain data from a purposely selected group of individuals [40].

The focus study, through direct contact with producers enables the acquisition of hard-to-reach data and information. In addition, it allows for a better understanding and grasping of changes and challenges in production. In the literature, focus studies in the carp sector in Barycz Valley were already conducted in 2016 by [41].

The second element of the research was an electronic questionnaire addressed to the target group of people aged 18 to 26, which belong to the Generation Z (people born in the period of 1997–2012). The questionnaire (see Appendix A) was disseminated among students of the University of Life Sciences in Wrocław (60 km from the Barycz Valley) by e-mail and using social networks in May 2021. The selection of the sample was deliberate, and the results presented here concern 169 people. The majority of the sample was female (79%), which is correlated with the global trend, because 80% of purchasing decisions are made by women [42].

5. Results

Focus studies have shown that carp producers are aware of the changes taking place on the market. In their opinion, contemporary retail consumers of carp (especially young people) value a healthy lifestyle combined with healthy eating and outdoor activities (bicycles, kayaks) combined with self-realization and passion (fishing, nature walks). The aesthetics of the place and the locality of production are also important for consumers. They put emphasis on ecology combined with convenience and comfort (e.g., the possibility of making cashless transactions).

Hence, focus studies have shown that the era of live carp wholesale is about to end forever in favour of shortening food supply chains and diversifying activities. Traditional fishing farms (in a three-year production cycle with the avarage cost of production about 8–10 PLN/kg), which, until now, were mainly involved in the pre-Christmas sale of live fish, are currently obliged to expand the range of activities with new elements, as shown in Table 6.

Table 6. Diversification of the fish farms activities.

Activities	
• Year-round sale of live fish	• Sale of stocking material
• Gastronomy	• Agricultural retail trade
• Processing—pre-treatment	• Agritourism
• Processing—advanced treatment	• Live fish sale before Christmas
• Growing cereals	• Cyclical sale (e.g., gastro-zone)
• Nature education	• Services for anglers

Source: own study based on the conducted research.

The results have shown that diversification for fishing farms often means investing additional funds (usually EU funds) for the construction of restaurants, processing plants, smokehouses or mobile fish sales points, which leads to an increase in the number of employees, taking up new managerial skills and implementing new organizational and technological solutions. An important element of diversification is also the use of modern communication tools with the client through social media (e.g., Facebook, Google) and care for the company's image. This raises the need to create completely new B2C relationships, in which the manufacturer must take care of partner relationships with customers and provide information about the origin of products, their history and quality. In particular, the traditional generation of Poles with carp swimming in the tub before Christmas, as a result of the natural aging process of the society, is irretrievably gone. That is why it was so important in the research to capture the perception of carp by Generation Z, who will shape the demand for carp for the next decades.

The results of research among young Polish consumers have shown that fish are present on their menu: 40% of the surveyed consumers declared that they eat fish once a week and 33% once a month, which means that the fish diet is widely accepted by young consumers, as shown in Figure 3.

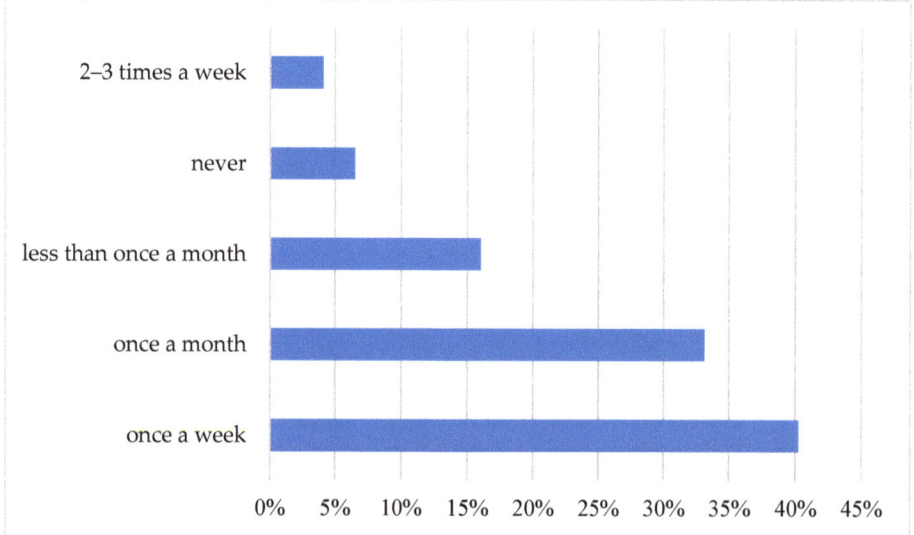

Figure 3. Frequency of fish consumption in Poland among the Young Adult Populations. Source: own elaboration based on data of [43].

It can also be concluded that young consumers are aware of the benefits of eating fish, even though some of the respondents do not consume it because of their vegetarian or vegan diet. As for the fish species most eaten by young consumers, studies have shown that the most consumed fish is salmon (at least once a week—9%; once a month—22%). The results of the research clearly show that carp is a fish that is eaten once a year (58% of responses) or never 30%, as shown in Figure 4.

Focusing strictly on the consumption of carp, the research has shown that the Christmas tradition was a key factor motivating the consumption of this fish for over 60% of consumers. The second of the most encouraging factors turned out to be taste, which accounted for 18% of all the answers provided. For comparison, the questions were also asked about the factors discouraging the consumption of this fish. Research has shown that the number of fish bones in the meat is the most frequently reported deterrent to eating carp. As many as 40% of respondents have a problem with the comfortable preparation or consumption of this fish because of bones. For 32% of consumers, the smell of silt is discouraging, and 10% of respondents indicated the lack of availability of carp in stores, as shown in Figure 5.

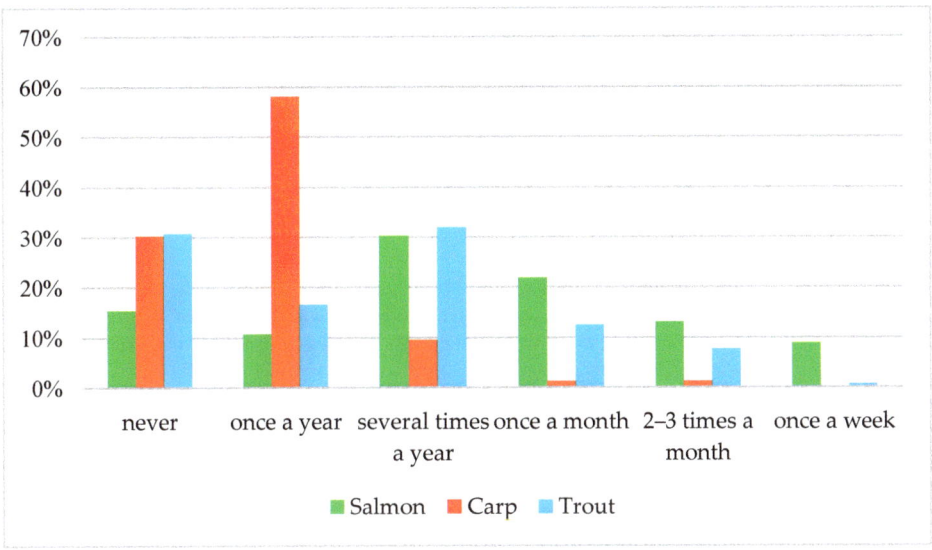

Figure 4. Frequency of salmon, carp and trout consumption in Poland among the Young Adult Populations. Source: own elaboration based on data of [43].

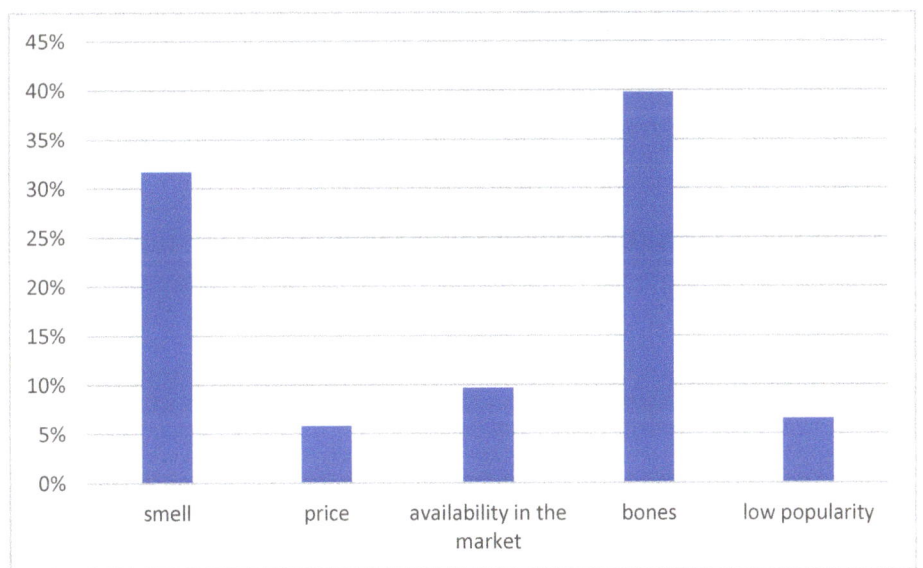

Figure 5. Factors discouraging the consumption of carp among the Young Adult Populations. Source: own elaboration based on data of [43].

In fact, during the year, apart from the Christmas season, there is no sale of carp in popular stores and discount retailers, and it is almost exclusively possible to buy it directly from the farm. As for the price, only 6% of interviewees indicated this factor as a disincentive to consumption. Due to the fact that for many years carp was a fish prepared exclusively at home, the respondents were not inclined to order carp in a restaurant (as much as 71%). Only 14% of the respondents are willing to consider the choice of a carp dish, and 13% admit that they would be willing to order it. The price was another studied factor that could affect the attitude of young adult consumers to carp. It was assumed that the affordable price could have an incentive effect on potential carp buyers and contribute to the popularization of the carp meat consumption. The research has shown that the price would not affect their attitude to the purchase or consumption of carp, which was declared by as many as 64% of the respondents. According to the preferences of consumers, the most affordable price range per kilogram of fish in the form of a fillet is from PLN 20 to PLN 25. This option was chosen by 41% of respondents; 31% of consumers would prefer to pay less than PLN 20 per kilogram of fish fillet—this option is one of the most economical and affordable.

In the case of a kilogram of fish fillet in the range from PLN 26 to PLN 30 and above PLN 30/kg, both variants gained 14% of the respondents' votes. As a result, it turns out that only 14% of the respondents could afford to buy carp in the form of a boneless fillet, considering that the price per kilogram of fish in this form falls within this price range, as shown in Figure 6. It should be added that the price for 1 kg of fillet salmon is at least twice as much.

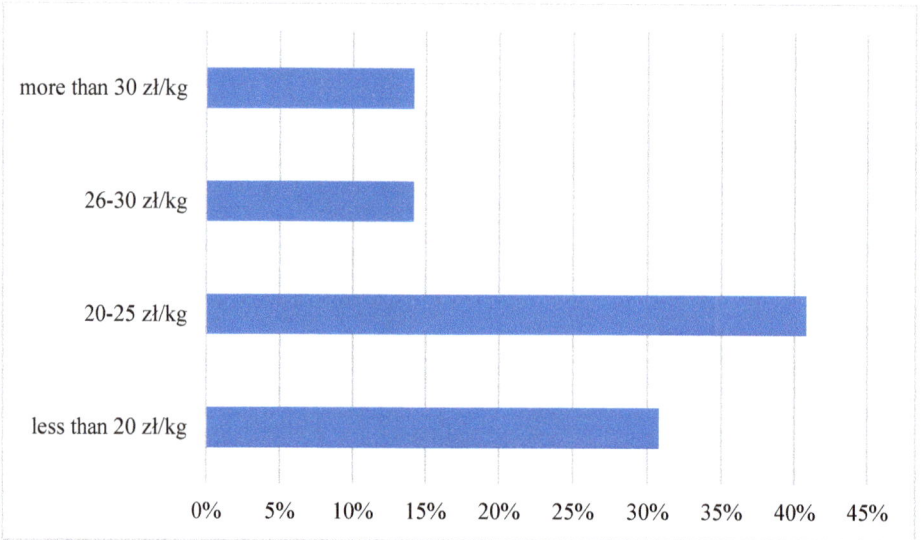

Figure 6. Price preferences for the boneless fillet of carp among the Young Adult Populations. Source: own elaboration based on data of [43].

Another question in the survey was to explain why the respondents prefer sea fish more than carp. Among the proposed marine fish, several examples of the most popular species have been mentioned, including salmon, cod, flounder, salt and turbot. The results of the research have shown that as many as 47% of answers indicate that the sea fish mentioned in the question are perceived as tastier than the carp itself and that sea fish are more available in stores (17%). According to 16% of people filling in the questionnaire, the proposed sea fish has better nutritional values than carp, while according to 12%, it is easier to prepare, as shown in Figure 7.

The next issue in the survey was the place where consumers prefer to buy carp. The answers to this question may explain their relation to both the quality and the price of the purchased fish, which may vary depending on the place of purchase. Hypermarkets, supermarkets, discount retailers (33%) and fishing farms (32%) turned out to be the places preferred by most of the surveyed consumers to buy carp. About 25% of respondents to the questionnaire buy supplies from a fish shop. Carp at the marketplace are purchased by 7% of respondents, and the remaining 3% choose the local store, as shown in Figure 8.

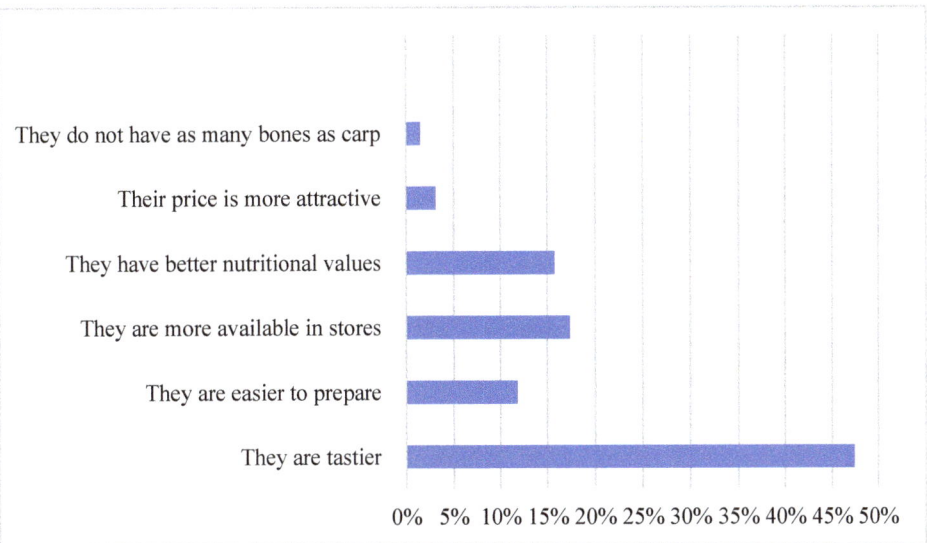

Figure 7. Preferences for sea fish among the Young Adult Populations in relation to carp. Source: own elaboration based on data of [43].

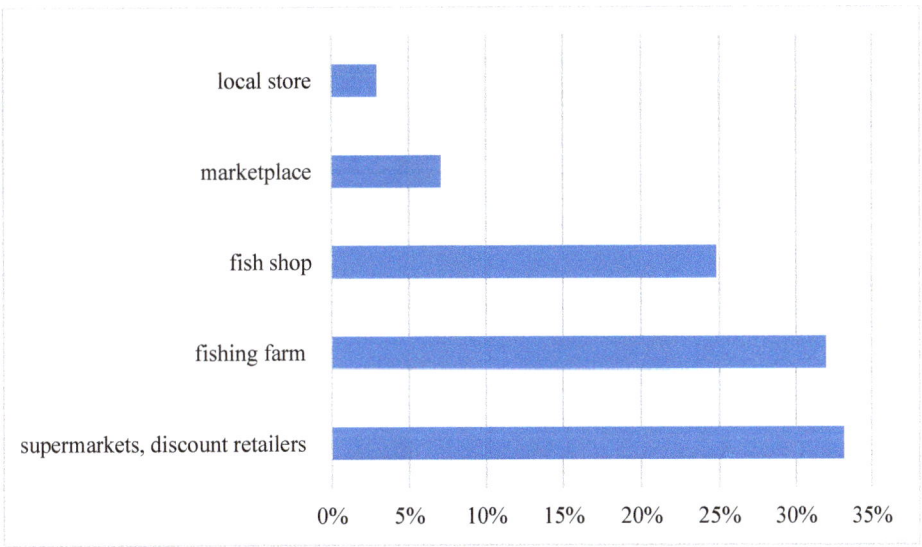

Figure 8. Shopping location preferences for carp among the Young Adult Populations in relation to carp. Source: own elaboration based on data of [43].

The questionnaire also included a question about the importance attached to the origin of the purchased carp. For the majority of respondents, the source of the carp is important: 'yes' 32%, 'rather yes' 31%. In total, as many as 63% of respondents usually pay attention to where the fish they chose to buy was previously bred, as shown in Figure 9.

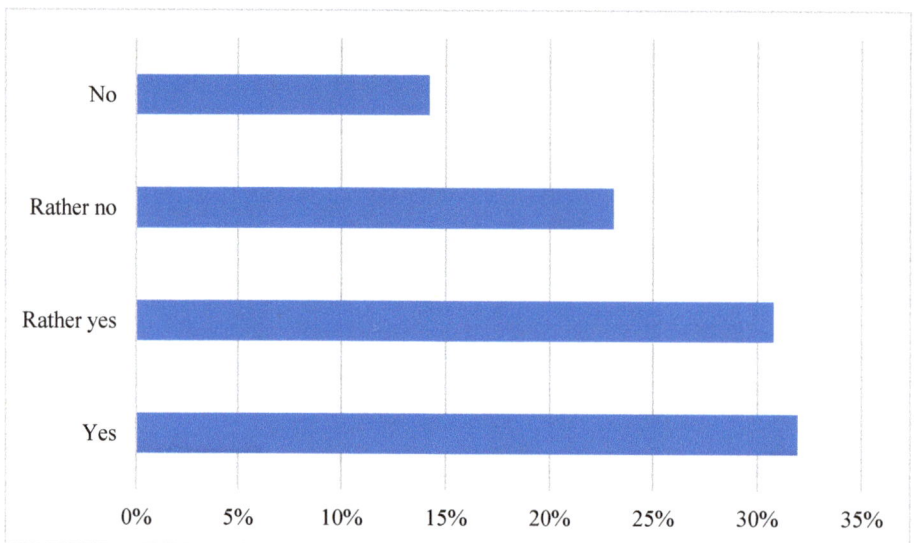

Figure 9. The importance of the origin of the purchased carp. Source: own elaboration based on data of [43].

When it comes to the form in which young consumers buy carp the most, nearly 60% declared that the most popular type of carp is fresh fish, most often found as a whole carcass with a head and scales, which must be trimmed and self-prepared. About 28% of the respondents choose a carp fillet, carcass or bells, which are much easier to prepare, but usually belong to the more expensive forms in which it is sold. The least popular are smoked carp, 4%, and carp preserves, 2%, which are, however, extremely rarely available on the market, as shown in Figure 10.

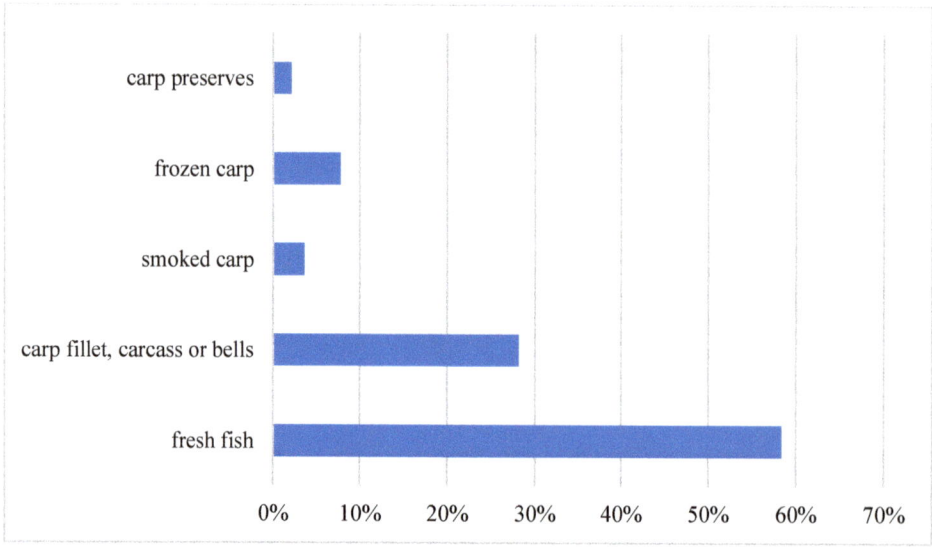

Figure 10. The preferences for the form of the purchased carp. Source: own elaboration based on data of [43].

6. Discussion

The research has proved that in order to encourage young consumers to eat fish more often, including carp, the low-intensity aquaculture sector should build a solid carp market as soon as possible that meets the expectations of young consumers and matches current nutritional trends. However, this requires a fresh look at the issue of selling fish, which will be based on the commercial, promotion and marketing offers extended with new products. Carp has enormous market potential, which, however, requires the introduction of innovative products. This thesis is confirmed by the research by [44,45], according to which consumers pay more and more attention to farming and breeding methods and expect documented transparency of catches. Poles, and especially the younger generations, are becoming more and more aware of the negative practices of selling carp. Most of all, the promotion of the elimination of live carp sales, a humane way of killing them and the origin certification of fish from domestic farms are of increasing importance. Customers demand a product that will go to the most popular discount retailers in an easy-to-prepare form and convenient packaging. This thesis is supplemented by studies conducted by [21], which focused on the approach of Polish and German consumers to carp and the demand for new, innovative products from this fish. For this purpose, the surveyed consumers were asked to express their attitude to the new carp products. Research has shown that German consumers focus not only on the taste and ease of preparation but also on the convenience that comes with the appropriate grammage of the product. Among the preferred products were boneless carp fillet, vinegar carp balls, carp chips and carp ham. Polish consumers expressed a positive opinion mainly about boneless carp fillet. They decided that it would be the tastiest, the best for health and also easy to prepare, but they would also like to try carp ham or carp balls in vinegar. Research by [46] has confirmed that carp has a chance to be recognized on the Polish market. In their opinion, 'the circle of potential carp consumers willing to buy and eat carp products more than once a year is very large and there is a possibility of increasing market demand for carp and carp preserves, provided that the product offer is adjusted to the needs and expectations of consumers'.

A positive example of activities promoting carp is conducted by the Association Partnership for the Barycz Valley, which for years has been focusing on achieving the sustainable development of tourism and expanding the market of local products and services based on specific natural and cultural conditions through [47]:

- Building the recognition of the Barycz Valley as a tourist area, especially good for active tourism surrounded by world-class nature;
- Using the promotion of tourism to endorse a sustainable fashion for local products and linking producers and service providers with the Barycz Valley;
- The use of world-class nature in building a brand that positively integrates the local community and creates a separate tourist model of the Barycz Valley.

Thanks to the Association's initiative, Carp Days have been organized from September to November since 2005. In 2021, during the 16th edition of Carp Days, over 97 events (gastronomic, fishing, educational and outdoor) were organized, in which 32 entities (economic, social and public) were involved. A statistical participant of the Carp Days in the Barycz Valley was 31–45 years old, had higher education and was a resident of villages and large cities with over 100,000 inhabitants [48]. As the research has shown, product tasting is a very effective marketing tool supporting consumers' interest in innovative products and increasing sales [49]. Highlighting local origin corresponds to consumer preferences for locally produced food [50] and can therefore support the demand for carp products, showing that carp also fits in with modern cuisine.

The findings of this study have to be seen in light of some limitations. First of all, they were conducted on a relatively small fraction of the Young Adult Populations. Secondly, they were carried out only in one area. However, due to the fact that the Barycz Valley is the biggest carp breeding center in Poland, and students from Wrocław University of Environmental and Life Study are in its proximity and have at least basic knowledge of sustainable development, it can be concluded that the research is representative for a wider population of young generation.

7. Conclusions

Based on the analysis, it can be concluded that changes on the demand side can be noticed in the agri-food products market. Increasingly noticeable is the emphasis on a healthy lifestyle combined with healthy, ecological food and outdoor activities in valuable natural areas combined with self-realization and passion. The aesthetics of the consumption area and the locality of production, as well as the convenience and comfort of transactions, are also gaining new value. However, this does not go hand in hand with the consumption of carp in Poland, which for most young consumers is associated mainly with a traditional Christmas dish and not an organic, healthy meal.

Even if the carp farming contributes to sustainable development, the consumption of the younger generation is definitely dominated by imported salmon, despite its higher price.

Young Adult Populations negatively relate to the carp fish bones and the smell, which is questionable, because of the past stereotypes that the carp ponds are slimy and muddy. They prefer sea fish because of the taste and availability of the stores, but this is due to the fact that there is simply no possibility to consume carp more frequently. Carp is available commonly in supermarkets and discout retailers only in the first half December. At other times, consumers have to go directly to the carp producer. The short supply chain in the carp market is still insufficiently developed, even if the origins of the production and the carp freshness are very important for Young Adult Populations.

On the basis of conducted analysis, it can be concluded that the situation on the carp market in Poland is not determined by the price level, but rather by factors beyond the price ones related to consumer tastes, or more broadly by sociological and psychological factors. This means that the development of the carp market in Poland requires diversification of the offer and marketing activities that influence the fashion and consumer preferences. Information activities are also necessary to highlight the health-promoting properties of carp meat.

The carp industry has great potential to create regional products, which is due to, among others, the rich national heritage, traditional carp breeding methods or the specific values of the natural environment. On the other hand, the main barrier to the development of these products is the relatively low knowledge about the possibility of selling them in other forms than before or the lack of financial resources dedicated to the development of marketing. A large number of regional products (including carp products) are not placed on the market, due to the fact that their production takes place occasionally, during local festivals and markets or is produced only for their own needs. Strengthening the marketing potential and increasing the frequency of visitors to carp regions is crucial for attracting potential customers, especially young, active consumers looking for an additional culinary and aesthetic experience. Therefore, without radical changes, it will not be possible to save the tradition of Polish carp fishing and at the same time protect valuable natural values.

Funding: The APC is financed by Wroclaw University of Environmental and Life Sciences.

Institutional Review Board Statement: Not applicable.

Informed Consent Statement: Not applicable.

Data Availability Statement: The data presented in this study are available on request from the corresponding author. Part of the research data come from the Master thesis of Aleksandra Kondela "Prospects for the development of aquaculture in Poland" under supervision of dr. Magdalena Raftowicz, Wrocław University of the Environmental and Life Sciences.

Acknowledgments: The author would like to thank Aleksandra Kondela for cooperation.

Conflicts of Interest: The authors declare no conflict of interest.

Appendix A

- How often do you eat a fish meal?
- How often do you eat any of the listed species of fish?
- How often do you eat a meal that includes carp (any form?)
- What are the factors that encourage your carp consumption?
- Identify factors that discourage carp consumption
- If you were in a restaurant, would you decide to eat a carp dish?
- Would easier and year-round access to carp encourage you to consume this fish more often
- Could a relatively low and affordable price mean that carp would appear on your table more often?
- What price are you willing/willing to pay per kilogram of fish as fillet?
- Why do you prefer sea fish such as salmon, cod, flounder, sole, turbot, rather than carp?
- Identify the place where you most often buy carp
- Do you pay attention to the origin of the carp you buy?
- What form do you purchase carp in?

References

1. Guziur, J. Z dziejów chowu ryb w Polsce i na świecie [From the history of fish farming in Poland and in the world]. In *Technologia Produkcji Rybackiej a Jakość Karpia [Fishing Production Technology and the Quality of Carp]*; Szarek, J., Skibniewska, K., Guziur, J., Eds.; Pracownia Wydawnicza ElSe: Olsztyn, Poland, 2008; p. 13.
2. FAO. National Aquaculture Sector Overview Poland. 2022. Available online: https://www.fao.org/fishery/countrysector/naso_poland/ (accessed on 18 February 2022).
3. Fish & Seafood Report 2021. Available online: https://www.statista.com/study/48828/fish-and-seafood-report/ (accessed on 18 February 2022).
4. Regulation (EU) No 1380/2013 of the European Parliament and of the Council of 11 December 2013 on the Common Fisheries Policy, Amending Council Regulations (EC) No 1954/2003 and (EC) No 1224/2009 and Repealing Council Regulations (EC) No 2371/2002 and (EC) No 639/2004 and Council Decision 2004/585/EC. Available online: https://eur-lex.europa.eu/legal-content/EN/TXT/PDF/?uri=CELEX:32013R1380&from=EN (accessed on 18 February 2022).
5. FAO. Available online: www.fao.org/aquaculture/en (accessed on 18 February 2022).
6. FAO. The State of World Fisheries and Aquaculture 2020. Available online: https://www.fao.org/state-of-fisheries-aquaculture (accessed on 18 February 2022).
7. European Commission. Oceans and Fisheries. Available online: https://ec.europa.eu/oceans-and-fisheries/facts-and-figures/facts-and-figures-common-fisheries-policy/fisheries-and-aquaculture-production_en (accessed on 18 February 2022).
8. FAO. The State of World Fisheries and Aquaculture. 2020. Available online: https://reliefweb.int/sites/reliefweb.int/files/resources/The%20State%20of%20World%20Fisheries%20and%20Aquaculture%202020.%20In%20brief.pdf (accessed on 18 February 2022).
9. Moffit, C.M. Environmental, Economic and Social Aspects of Animal Protein Production and the Opportunities of Aquaculture. *Fisheries* **2005**, *30*, 37–40.
10. Seafood from Norway. Available online: https://salmon.fromnorway.com/pl/sustainable-aquaculture/future-prospects/ (accessed on 18 February 2022).
11. Consumer and Market Insights: Fish & Seafood in Poland. Available online: https://www.marketresearch.com/Canadean-Ltd-v132/Consumer-Insights-Fish-Seafood-Poland-10014792/ (accessed on 18 February 2022).
12. OCEANA. Eastern Baltic Cod. Available online: https://europe.oceana.org/en/eastern-baltic-cod (accessed on 18 February 2022).
13. Statista, Monthly Consumption of Fish and Seafood per Capita in Poland from 2000 to 2020. Available online: https://www.statista.com/statistics/1197197/poland-monthly-consumption-of-fish-and-seafood/ (accessed on 18 February 2022).
14. Karnai, L.; Szucs, I. Outlooks and perspectives of the common carp production. *Pol. Assoc. Agric. Econ. Agribus.* **2018**, *1*, 64–72. [CrossRef]
15. OECD. Stat, 2021, Aquaculture Production, Common Carp, 2005–2018. Available online: https://stats.oecd.org/Index.aspx?DataSetCode=FISH_AQUA (accessed on 18 February 2022).
16. Production from Aquaculture. 2019. Available online: https://ec.europa.eu/eurostat/databrowser/view/FISH_AQ2A__custom_1938198/default/table?lang=en (accessed on 18 February 2022).
17. Raftowicz, M.; Kalisiak-Mędelska, M.; Kurtyka-Marcak, I.; Struś, M. *Krótkie Łańcuchy Dostaw na Przykładzie Karpia Milickiego [Short Supply Chains on the Example of the Milicz Carp]*; Raftowicz, M., Kalisiak-Mędelska, M., Eds.; CeDeWu: Warszawa, Poland, 2019.
18. Raftowicz, M.; Struś, M.; Nadolny, M.; Kalisiak-Mędelska, M. The Importance of Price in Poland's Carp Market. *Sustainability* **2020**, *12*, 10416. [CrossRef]
19. Mergili, S. Der Karpfen—prädestiniert für die Öko-Aquakultur. *Okol. Landbau* **2009**, *151*, 24.

20. Feucht, Y.; Zander, K. Of earth ponds, flow-through and closed recirculation systems—German consumers' understanding of sustainable aquaculture and its communication. *Aquaculture* **2015**, *438*, 151–158. [CrossRef]
21. Raftowicz-Filipkiewicz, M. Wpływ rybactwa śródlądowego na rozwój obszarów przyrodniczo cennych w Dolinie Baryczy [The impact of the inland fishing on the development of naturally valuable areas in the Barycz Valley]. *Pol. Assoc. Agric. Econ. Agribus.* **2013**, *15*, 175–179.
22. Natura 2000, Fundacja Ekorozwoju. Available online: obszary.natura2000.pl (accessed on 18 February 2022).
23. Warczewska, B.; Szewrański, S.; Mastalska-Cetera, B. *Zrównoważony Rozwój Gmin Leżących w Granicach Parku Krajobrazowego [Sustainable Development of Municipalities Located within the Landscape Park]*; Wydawnictwo Uniwersytetu Przyrodniczego we Wrocławiu: Wrocław, Poland, 2015; p. 7.
24. Kapała, A.M. Legal Instruments to Support Short Food Supply Chains and Local Food Systems in France. *Laws* **2022**, *11*, 21. [CrossRef]
25. Cappelli, L.; D'Ascenzo, F.; Ruggieri, R.; Gorelova, I. Is Buying Local Food a Sustainable Practice? A Scoping Review of Consumers' Preference for Local Food. *Sustainability* **2022**, *14*, 772. [CrossRef]
26. Lombart, C.; Labbé-Pinlon, B.; Filser, M.; Antéblian, B.; Louis, D. Regional product assortment and merchandising in grocery stores: Strategies and target customer segments. *J. Retail. Consum. Serv.* **2018**, *42*, 117–132. [CrossRef]
27. Skalkos, D.; Kosma, I.S.; Chasioti, E.; Bintsis, T.; Karantonis, H.C. Consumers' Perception on Traceability of Greek Traditional Foods in the Post-COVID-19 Era. *Sustainability* **2021**, *13*, 12687. [CrossRef]
28. Roman, S.; Sánchez-Siles, L.M.; Siegrist, M. The importance of food naturalness for consumers: Results of a systematic review. *Trends Food Sci. Technol.* **2017**, *67*, 44–57. [CrossRef]
29. Simonetti, L. The ideology of Slow Food. *J. Eur. Stud.* **2012**, *42*, 168–189. [CrossRef]
30. Mariani, M.; Casabianca, F.; Cerdan, C.; Peri, I. Protecting Food Cultural Biodiversity: From Theory to Practice. Challenging the Geographical Indications and the Slow Food Models. *Sustainability* **2021**, *13*, 5265. [CrossRef]
31. FAO. *The State of Food Security and Nutrition in the World*; FAO: Rome, Italy, 2021.
32. Dąbrowska, A. Trendy konsumpcji i zachowań polskich konsumentów [Consumption trends and behavior of Polish consumers] In *Konsumpcja a Rozwój Społeczno-Gospodarczy Regionów w Polsce [Consumption and the Socio-Economic Development of Regions in Poland]*; Kusińska, A., Ed.; PWE: Warszawa, Poland, 2011; pp. 173–174.
33. Bywalec, C. *Konsumpcja a Rozwój Gospodarczy i Społeczny [Consumption and Economic and Social Development]*; C.H. Beck: Warszawa, Poland, 2010; p. 7.
34. Toffler, A. *The Third Wave*; William Morrow: New York, NY, USA, 1980.
35. Jung, B. Kapitalizm Postmodernistyczny [Postmodern Capitalism]. *Ekonomista [Econ.]* **1997**, *5–6*, 715–735.
36. Collins, S. Digital fair. Prosumption and the fair use defence. *J. Consum. Cult.* **2010**, *10*, 38–39. [CrossRef]
37. Bienkiewicz, M.; Bogusiewicz, U.; Bronkowska, M.; Dmytrów, I.; Kapała, A.; Kurtyka-Marcak, I.; Kutkowska, B.; Łoźna, K.; Michniewicz, I.; Miniewska, M.; et al. *Rolnictwo Wspierane Społecznie—Zmniejszenie Barier Wejścia na Rynek dla Dolnośląskich Produktów Żywności Wysokiej Jakości [Comminity Supported Agriculture-Reducing Market Entry Barriers for High-Quality Food Products from Lower Silesia]*; Wydawnictwo Uniwersytetu Przyrodniczego we Wrocławiu: Wrocław, Poland, 2017; p. 83.
38. Strategia Rozwoju Lokalnego Kierowanego Przez Społeczność (LSR) dla Doliny Baryczy na lata 2016–2022 [Community-Led Local Development Strategy (LDS) for the Barycz Valley for 2016–2022]. Available online: http://projekty.barycz.pl/files/?id_plik=1971 (accessed on 18 February 2022).
39. The Ministry of Agriculture and Rural Development in Poland. Available online: https://www.gov.pl/web/rolnictwo/karp-milicki (accessed on 18 February 2022).
40. Silverman, D. *Doing Qualitative Research. A Practical Handbook*, 2nd ed.; Sage Publication: London, UK, 2005.
41. Lasner, T.; Mytlewski, A.; Nourry, M.; Rakowski, M.; Oberle, M. Carp land: Economics of fish farms and the impact of region-marketing in the Aischgrund (DEU) and Barycz Valley (POL). *Aquaculture* **2020**, *519*, 734731. [CrossRef]
42. Davis, K.M. 20 Facts and Figures to Know When Marketing to Women. *Forbes* **2019**, *13*. Available online: https://www.forbes.com/sites/forbescontentmarketing/2019/05/13/20-facts-and-figures-to-know-when-marketing-to-women/?sh=e8b8c021297e (accessed on 18 February 2022).
43. Kondela, A. Perspektywy Rozwoju Akwakultury w Polsce [Prospects for the Development of Aquaculture in Poland]. Master's Thesis, Department of Economics, Wrocław University of Environmental and Life Sciences, Wrocław, Poland, 2021, *unpublished*.
44. Lirski, A. Rynek i Sprzedaż ryb, Czyli co Dalej z Karpiem [The Market and the Sale of Fish, or What to Do Next with Carp]. 2019. Available online: http://www.lgropolszczyzna.pl/images/2019/jesienna_konferencja_rybacka/OPOLE_2019_Andrzej_Lirski.pdf (accessed on 18 February 2022).
45. Lirski, A. Czy grozi nam regres w sprzedaży karpia w Polsce? [Are we in danger of a regression in the sale of carp in Poland?]. *Komun. Ryb. [Fish. Messages]* **2019**, *4*, 17–21.
46. Kompleksowy System Przetwarzania Karpia na Nowoczesne Produkty Spożywcze [A Comprehensive Carp Processing System for Modern Food Products], 2014, Sprawozdanie, Koszalin. Available online: http://karp.wm.tu.koszalin.pl/dane/raport_techniczny1.pdf (accessed on 18 February 2022).
47. Golden, J.D. *Strategia Marketingowa dla Marki Lokalnej Doliny Baryczy na Lata 2008–2015 [Marketing Strategy for the Local Brand of the Barycz Valley for 2008–2015]*; 2008; p. 30. Available online: https://docplayer.pl/718486-Strategia-marketingowa-dla-marki-lokalnej-doliny-baryczy-na-lata-2008-2015.html (accessed on 18 February 2022).

48. Barycz Valley. Available online: https://dnikarpia.barycz.pl/podsumowanie-dni-karpia-16-lat-202 (accessed on 18 February 2022).
49. Heilman, C.M.; Lakishyk, K.; Radas, S. An empirical investigation of in-store sampling promotions. *Br. Food J.* **2011**, *113*, 1252–1266. [CrossRef]
50. Feldmann, C.; Hamm, U. Consumers' perceptions and preferences for local food: A review. *Food Qual. Prefer.* **2015**, *40*, 152–164. [CrossRef]

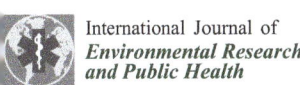

Systematic Review

Edible Insect Consumption for Human and Planetary Health: A Systematic Review

Marta Ros-Baró [1], Patricia Casas-Agustench [1,2,*], Diana Alícia Díaz-Rizzolo [1,3], Laura Batlle-Bayer [4], Ferran Adrià-Acosta [5], Alícia Aguilar-Martínez [6,7], Francesc-Xavier Medina [6,7], Montserrat Pujolà [8] and Anna Bach-Faig [6,9,*]

1 Faculty of Health Sciences, Open University of Catalonia (UOC), 08018 Barcelona, Spain
2 School of Health Professions, Faculty of Health, University of Plymouth, Plymouth PL4 8AA, UK
3 Primary Healthcare Transversal Research Group, Institut d'Investigacions Biomèdiques August Pi i Sunyer (IDIBAPS), 08018 Barcelona, Spain
4 UNESCO Chair in Life Cycle and Climate Change ESCI-UPF, Universitat Pompeu Fabra, 08003 Barcelona, Spain
5 elBullifoundation, 08004 Barcelona, Spain
6 Food Lab Research Group (2017SGR 83), Faculty of Health Sciences, Open University of Catalonia (UOC), 08018 Barcelona, Spain
7 Unesco Chair on Food, Culture and Development, Open University of Catalonia (UOC), 08018 Barcelona, Spain
8 Faculty of Agri-Food Engineering and Biotechnology, Universitat Politècnica de Catalunya BarcelonaTech, 08860 Castelldefels, Spain
9 Food and Nutrition Area, Barcelona Official College of Pharmacists, 08009 Barcelona, Spain
* Correspondence: patricia.casas@plymouth.ac.uk (P.C.-A.); abachf@uoc.edu (A.B.-F.)

Citation: Ros-Baró, M.; Casas-Agustench, P.; Díaz-Rizzolo, D.A.; Batlle-Bayer, L.; Adrià-Acosta, F.; Aguilar-Martínez, A.; Medina, F.-X.; Pujolà, M.; Bach-Faig, A. Edible Insect Consumption for Human and Planetary Health: A Systematic Review. *Int. J. Environ. Res. Public Health* **2022**, *19*, 11653. https://doi.org/10.3390/ijerph191811653

Academic Editor: Paul B. Tchounwou

Received: 27 July 2022
Accepted: 14 September 2022
Published: 15 September 2022

Publisher's Note: MDPI stays neutral with regard to jurisdictional claims in published maps and institutional affiliations.

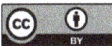

Copyright: © 2022 by the authors. Licensee MDPI, Basel, Switzerland. This article is an open access article distributed under the terms and conditions of the Creative Commons Attribution (CC BY) license (https://creativecommons.org/licenses/by/4.0/).

Abstract: This systematic review aimed to examine the health outcomes and environmental impact of edible insect consumption. Following PRISMA-P guidelines, PubMed, Medline ProQuest, and Cochrane Library databases were searched until February 2021. Twenty-five articles met inclusion criteria: twelve animal and six human studies (randomized, non-randomized, and crossover control trials), and seven studies on sustainability outcomes. In animal studies, a supplement (in powdered form) of 0.5 g/kg of glycosaminoglycans significantly reduced abdominal and epididymal fat weight (5–40% and 5–24%, respectively), blood glucose (10–22%), and total cholesterol levels (9–10%), and a supplement of 5 mg/kg chitin/chitosan reduced body weight (1–4%) and abdominal fat accumulation (4%) *versus* control diets. In other animal studies, doses up to 7–15% of edible insect inclusion level significantly improved the live weight (9–33%), reduced levels of triglycerides (44%), cholesterol (14%), and blood glucose (8%), and increased microbiota diversity (2%) *versus* control diet. In human studies, doses up to 7% of edible insect inclusion level produced a significant improvement in gut health (6%) and reduction in systemic inflammation (2%) *versus* control diets and a significant increase in blood concentrations of essential and branched-chain amino acids and slowing of digestion (40%) *versus* whey treatment. Environmental indicators (land use, water footprint, and greenhouse gas emissions) were 40–60% lower for the feed and food of edible insects than for traditional animal livestock. More research is warranted on the edible insect dose responsible for health effects and on environmental indicators of edible insects for human nutrition. This research demonstrates how edible insects can be an alternative protein source not only to improve human and animal nutrition but also to exert positive effects on planetary health.

Keywords: edible insects; health; sustainability; alternative proteins; planetary health; systematic review

1. Introduction

There is an urgent need to redesign food systems to improve human and planetary health [1]. It is likely that food systems are already operating beyond some planetary boundaries [2–4]. Therefore, more environmentally friendly but also affordable, healthy, and safe approaches need to be adopted to feed the expanding human population [5], which is projected to reach 9.7 billion by 2050 [6]. One of the major challenges is to re-align future protein supply and demand, especially animal protein [7], which is expected to rise by 70–80% between 2012 and 2050 [8]. Underutilized plants, insects, and single-cell organisms (e.g., algae, fungi, and bacteria) as well as cultured meat are being considered as novel protein sources to sustainably meet future global requirements [9,10].

Although insects have been consumed since early in human evolution, a new trend in food science began in 2013, when the Food and Agriculture Organization of the United Nations (FAO) pointed out the need to examine modern food science practices to increase the trade, consumption, and acceptance of insects [11]. In regulation 2015/2283 [12] of the European Parliament and the Council of the European Union, whole insects and their parts were included in the category of novel foods. Furthermore, in 2015, the European Food Safety Authority (EFSA) provided a scientific opinion on insect consumption and suggested a list of insect species with high potential use as food for animal feed and human food [13,14]. In 2021, the EFSA issued a positive opinion on the safety of dried yellow mealworm—*Tenebrio mellitus larvae* (TM larvae) [13], *Locusta migratoria* (LM) [15], and *Acheta domesticus* (AD) [16]—as a novel food according to European Union regulation 2015/2283 [17]. From a nutritional point of view, edible insects are being proposed as an alternative source of protein for humans and animals [18] due to their high levels of essential amino acids (EAA), unsaturated fatty acids, micronutrients (e.g., vitamin B12, iron (Fe), zinc, and calcium), and fiber [19]. Furthermore, edible insects have various bioactive compounds in their composition with potential health effects [20].

Previous systematic reviews on edible insects have focused on studying their nutritional composition [19,21,22], the presence of viruses [23], their effect on human and animal health [24–26], and allergic risks [27]. However, the global impact of edible insects on health and the environment remains to be elucidated. Previous reviews on health outcomes centered on either humans or animals and did not adopt a comprehensive approach. In the present review, data were retrieved from human studies on all relevant health outcomes (changes in growth, blood parameters, gut microbiome, changes in muscle mass composition, etc.), on the grams of edible insect, on the insect or part of insect used, and on the insect inclusion level. The aim of this systematic review was to provide an overview of human trials and animal studies to evaluate the effect of edible insect supplementation on health outcomes as well as studies on the environmental impact of edible insects as an alternative and more sustainable source of protein for humans and animals.

2. Material and Methods

2.1. Search Strategy

We conducted a systematic review in accordance with the Preferred Reporting Items for Systematic Reviews and Meta-Analyses guidelines [28] and registered it in PROSPERO (https://www.crd.york.ac.uk/prospero/ (accessed on 3 June 2021)) for humans (CRD42021243673) and animals (CRD42021243772). Following the PRISMA-P checklist, studies were identified by the electronic search of three databases (PubMed, ProQuest Medline, and Cochrane Library) for studies published between October 2010 and 28 February 2021. Combinations of the following search terms were used: "GHG", "greenhouse gas emission", "environmental impact", "environmental", "sustainability", "sustainable", "water use", "phosphor emission", "land use", "nitrogen emission", "eco-friendly", "climate-friendly", "life cycle assessment", "sustainable", "alternative animal-source", "entomophaga", "insect", "insecta", "insects", "edible", "consumption", "nutrition", "supplementation", "protein", "health", and "complementary". Boolean connectors (AND, OR) were used to search for associations between these terms.

2.2. Eligibility Criteria

Studies were eligible for inclusion if they were human investigations (experimental studies, randomized and controlled trials, and observational studies such as cohort, cross-sectional, and case-control studies) or investigated animal consumption of edible insects (placebo or reference treatment) reporting data on health and sustainability. The review also included ecological studies that evaluated greenhouse gas emission (GHG), water footprint (WFP), land use (LU), and/or energy use (EU) as environmental indicators and those that assessed the feed conversion ratio. We excluded edible insect studies on nutrition composition, acceptance, food technology, gastronomy, allergy, and toxicology. Systematic reviews, meta-analyses, and cell culture, in vitro, and ex vivo studies were all excluded.

2.3. Study Selection and Data Extraction

Search results were downloaded to EndNote (Clarivate Analytics, Philadelphia, PA) and duplicates were removed. Titles and abstracts were screened in duplicate by two of three authors (M.R.-B., P.C.-A., and A.B.-F.) for eligibility. The third author resolved disagreements. Full texts were obtained for any article that appeared to meet eligibility criteria.

Information was extracted from the animal studies on: author(s), year and country of publication, type of animal, sample size, sex, and age, length of intervention(s) (days), edible insect use, number of intervention groups with sample sizes, insect inclusion rate of complementary food product (CFP) (g/100 g expressed in %), variables/outcome, and evaluated health parameters.

Information was extracted from the human studies on: author(s), year and country of publication, sample size, sex, and age, length of intervention(s) (days), edible insect use, intervention groups with sample sizes, daily food portion of intervention with insects (g), insect inclusion rate of CFP (g/100 g expressed in %), insect inclusion level of CFP (expressed in g) per each age group, protein inclusion level of CFP per day (expressed in g), variables/outcomes, and evaluated health parameters.

Information was extracted from the sustainability articles on: GHG (Kg CO_2), which falls under the indicator global warming potential equivalent (GWP), EU (MJ) as a measure of fossil fuel depletion, LU (m^2), for the amount of arable land used in the production chain, and finally the WFP (m^3). The environmental impact was subsequently coupled with a functional unit (FU), a quantitative measure indicating the function of a product. For insects, FUs were expressed in kilograms of protein [29]. The environmental impacts of different steps within the system border were added together to express the total impact on certain environmental indicators. Finally, the total impact was divided by the number of FUs to yield the environmental impact per FU, which was used to compare environmental indicators between similar food products.

2.4. Quality Assessment

Quality and risk of bias were assessed using the Syrcle's risk of bias tool [30] for preclinical animal studies and the Cochrane risk of bias tool [31] for human studies. Both tools covered the following bias domains: selection bias (random sequence generation and allocation concealment), performance bias (blinding of participants and personnel), detection bias (blinding the outcome assessment), attrition bias (incomplete outcome data), reporting bias (selective reporting), and others. According to the score obtained, studies were classified as having a low, high, or unclear risk of bias (Table 1).

Table 1. Risk of bias in animal and human studies on the health effects of edible insects.

Animal Studies	Selection Bias	Performance Bias	Detection Bias	Attrition Bias	Reporting Bias	Others
Kim et al. [32]	-	-	-	-	-	-
Seo et al. [33]	-	-	-	-	?	?
Bergmans et al. [34]	?	-	-	-	-	-
Dabbou et al. [35]	-	-	-	-	-	?
Bovera et al. [36]	-	-	-	-	-	?
Biasato et al. [37]	-	-	-	-	-	-
Gasco et al. [38]	-	-	-	-	-	-
Agbemafle et al. [39]	-	-	-	-	-	-
Pessina et al. [40]	-	-	-	-	-	?
Ahn et al. [41]	-	-	-	-	-	?
Ahn et al. [42]	-	-	-	-	-	?
Human Studies	**Selection Bias**	**Performance Bias**	**Detection Bias**	**Attrition Bias**	**Reporting Bias**	**Others**
Skau et al. [43]	-	-	-	?	-	-
Bauserman et al. [44]	-	-	-	?	-	-
Nirmala et al. [45]	-	?	+	?	-	?
Stull et al. [46]	-	-	-	-	-	-
Vangsoe et al. [47]	-	-	-	-	-	-
Vangsoe et al. [48]	-	?	-	-	-	-

Summary of risk of bias: review of the opinions of the different authors on each element of bias risk for each study. The minus sign (-) indicates low risk of bias, plus sign (+) high risk of bias, and question mark (?) unclear risk.

Limitations of this review include gaps in the data available on the nutritional composition and quantity of edible insects administered in human studies and on the form of their administration, and some of this information could only be obtained after contacting the authors. Few studies specify the metamorphic phase of the edible insect, hampering comparisons of the % protein and composition of the complementary food product. It was also sometimes difficult to determine the stage at which values were assigned (e.g., farm gate or mill gate) and to gather information on the diet fed to the edible insects.

3. Results

3.1. Literature Search Results

The database search retrieved 4487 articles. After removing duplicates, the titles and abstracts of 3960 articles were assessed independently and in duplicate by two investigators. Eligibility criteria were finally met by 25 studies, which were included in the present systematic review (Figure 1). Tables 2–4 summarize the findings of these studies, categorized as animal [32–42,49], human [43–48], or sustainability [7,50–55] studies.

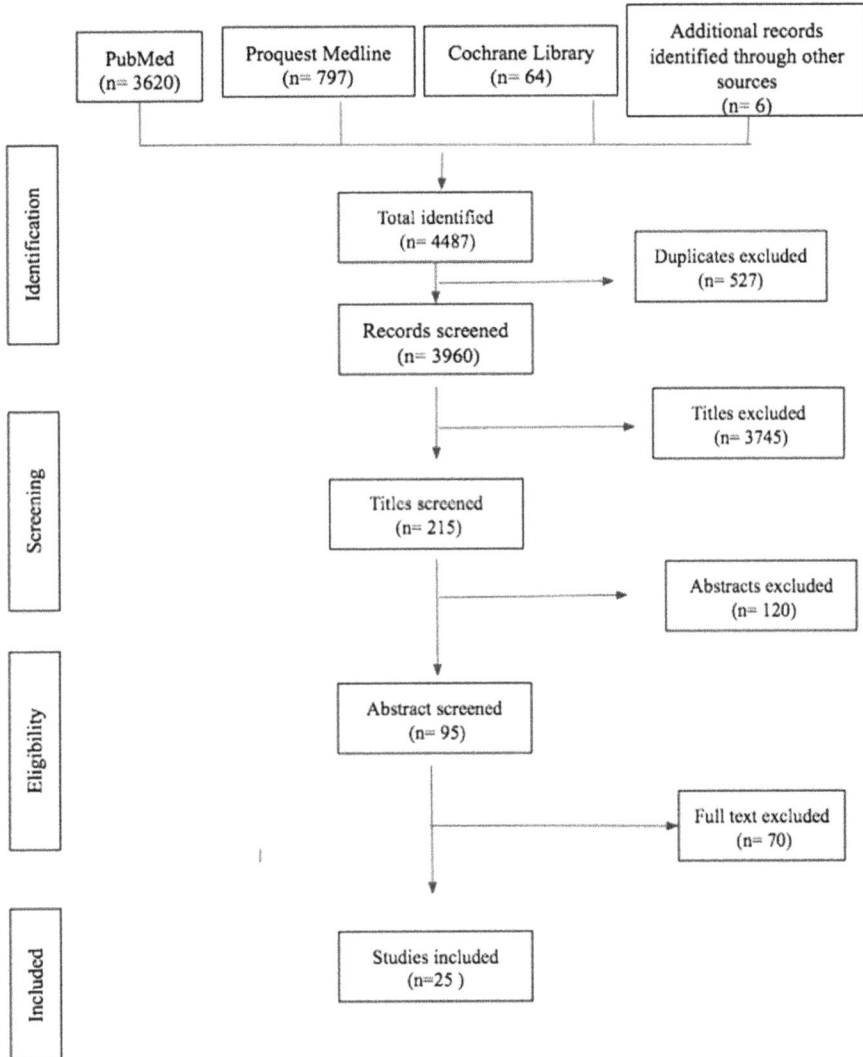

Figure 1. Flow chart of the selection of reviewed articles.

Table 2. Effect of edible insects on animal health.

Author, Year, Country	Type of Animal, Sample Size (Male/Female), Age	Duration (Days)	Insect	Intervention (n)	Insect Inclusion Level of CFP (g/100 g Expressed in %)	Variables/Outcomes	Results
Kim et al., 2016 (Korea) [32]	C57BL/6J mice 40 (40/-); 7 weeks	56	*Allomyrina dichotoma* larvae	All groups (a–e) start with: 8 weeks (diet-induced obesity): HFD, 60% fat (obese mice). (a) HFD 60% + 1 µL of 20% DMSO[1] (n = 10) (b) HFD 60% + 1 µL of ALLD[1] (10 mg/mL) (n = 10) (c) LFD 10% (n = 10) (d) LFD, 10% + 1 µL of 20% DMSO[1] (n = 10) (e) LFD, 10% + 1 µL of ALLD[1] (10 mg/mL) (n = 10)	(b) 1% [2]	***Appetite control*** (food intake and body weight) ***Metabolic traits*** (inflammatory indicators)	Food intake and body weight were reduced (b,e) compared to (a,b) respectively (S). ADE resulted in strong reduction of ER stress compared to (a) (S).
Ahn et al., 2016 (Korea) [42]	Wistar rats, 50 (50/-), 14 weeks	30	*Gryllus bimaculatus*	(a) Control + HFD (n = 10) (b) GbG5 + HFD (n = 10) (c) GbG10 + HFD (n = 10) (d) Pravastatin + HFD (n = 10) (e) Chitosan + HFD (n = 10)	(b) 0.0005 GbG (c) 0.001 GbG	***Metabolic traits*** (blood parameters and blood pressure)	Weight of abdominal and epididymal fat, AST, ALT, total cholesterol, and glucose were lower after (b,c) compared to (a) (S). Blood pressure was similar after b,c compared to (a) (NS). Anticoagulant and antithrombotic effects were seen: platelet, thrombin time, prothrombin time and factor I were increased with (b,c) treatment (S). CRP levels of (b,c) decreased compared to (a) (S).

Table 2. Cont.

Author, Year, Country	Type of Animal, Sample Size (Male/Female), Age	Duration (Days)	Insect	Intervention (n)	Insect Inclusion Level of CFP (g/100 g Expressed in %)	Variables/Outcomes	Results
Seo et al., 2017 (Korea) [33]	BALB/c mice, 35 (35/-), 5 weeks	42	*Tenebrio molitor* larvae	(a) ND (10% fat) (n = 7) (b) HFD (60% fat) (n = 7) ³ (c) HFD (60% fat) with TML (n = 7) ³ (d) HFD (60% fat) with TML (n = 7) ³ (e) HFD (60% fat) with 3000 mg/kg of yerba mate (n = 7) ³	(c) 0.01% (d) 0.30%	***Metabolic traits*** (weight gain, fat mass, hepatic steatosis, blood parameters)	Body weight gain, epididymal white adipose tissue size and volume decreased after (c,d) compared to (b) (S). Mean adipocyte volume was reduced after (d) compared to (b) (S) Hepatic lipid droplets, plasma ALT and AST levels, visceral fat were reduced after (c,d) compared to (b) (NS).
Dabbou et al., 2018 (Italy) [35]	Ross 308 CD1-IGS broiler chicken, 256 (256/-) ND	35	*Hermetia Illucens* larvae	(a) HI0 (n = 64) (b) HI5 (n = 64) (c) HI10 (n = 64) (d) HI15 (n = 64)	(a) 0% (b) 5% (c) 10% (d) 15%	***Growth performance*** (weight gain, feed intake) ***Metabolic traits*** (blood parameters, inflammatory indicators) ***Intestinal morphology***	Dietary HI inclusion (b–d) positively influenced growth performance up to 10%, in terms of improved live weight and daily feed intake during the starter period (S). At 10, 24, and 35 days of age, live weight showed a linear and quadratic response to HI meal with a maximum observed for (c) (S). HI showed a linear response ($p = 0.002$) to increases up to d) for blood or serum glutathione peroxidase (NS). Intestinal villus height was lower, crypt depth was greater, and villus height-to-crypt depth ratio was lower after (d) compared to (a–c) (S).

Table 2. Cont.

Author, Year, Country	Type of Animal, Sample Size (Male/Female), Age	Duration (Days)	Insect	Intervention (n)	Insect Inclusion Level of CFP (g/100 g Expressed in %)	Variables/Outcomes	Results
Bovera et al., 2018 (Italy) [36]	Hy-line Brown hens, 162 (−/162), 16 weeks	140	Hermetia Illucens larvae	(a) Control group: corn-soybean meal-based diet (n = 54) (b) HI25 (n = 54) (c) HI50 (n = 54)	(b) 7.3% (c) 14.6%	*Metabolic traits* (blood parameters) *Crude protein digestibility*	Serum cholesterol and triglyceride levels were reduced after (a) (S). Serum globulin levels were higher after (c) compared to (a,b) (S). Crude protein digestibility was the highest ($p < 0.05$) in (a), followed by (b,c) (NS).
Biasato et al., 2018 (Italy) [37]	Label Hubbard hybrid Chickens, 140 (−/140), 43 days	140	Tenebrio molitor larvae	(a) Control group: corn-soybean-gluten meal-based diet (n = 70) (b) TM 7.5 (n = 70)	(b) 7.5%	*Intestinal morphology*	Small intestine revealed similar villus height, crypt depth, and villus height crypt depth ratio between (a,b) (NS).
Gasco et al., 2019 (Italy) [38]	Crossbred rabbits, 200 (ND), 36 days	41	Hermetia Illucens/Tenebrio molitor larvae	(a) Control group: 1.5% soy-bean oil (n = 40) (b) H50 (n = 40) (c) H100 (n = 40) (d) T50 (n = 40) (e) T100 (n = 40)	(b) 0.75% (c) 1.5% (d) 0.75% (e) 1.50%	*Growth performance* (feed intake and body weight) *Metabolic traits* (blood parameters) *Crude protein digestibility* *Intestinal morphology*	Weight gain and feed intake was affected similarly after (a–e) (NS). Including insect lipids in rabbit diets did not influence AST, ALT, or ALP enzyme activities. Blood variables were affected similarly after (a–e) (NS). Crude protein digestibility was affected similarly after (a–e) (NS). Villi height, crypt depth, and their ratio were affected similarly after (b–e) compared to (a) (NS).

Table 2. Cont.

Author, Year, Country	Type of Animal, Sample Size (Male/Female), Age	Duration (Days)	Insect	Intervention (n)	Insect Inclusion Level of CFP (g/100 g Expressed in %)	Variables/Outcomes	Results
Agbemafle et al., 2019 (Ghana) [39]	Sprague–Dawley rats, 66 (66/-), 21 days	35	Acheta domesticus/Rhynichophorus phoenicis fabricius	(a) Normal rats + Casein + ferrous sulfate (n = 8) (b) MD⁴ (5% protein) + low protein -Fe (n = 8)-negative control (c) MD⁴ (5% protein) + S.torvum (26.7) (n = 8) (d) MD⁴ (5% protein) + AD + S. torvum (n = 8) (e) MD⁴ (5% protein) + Protein Fe sufficient (n = 8)-positive control (f) MD⁴ (5% protein) + AD (n = 8) (g) MD⁴ (5% protein) + RF (n = 8)	(d) 15.4% (f) 28.3%	*Growth performance* (body weight recovery, fat mass) *Metabolic traits* (blood parameters)	After malnourished treatment, weight gain, bone mineral content and lean and fat mass increased similarly after (d,f,g) compared to (e) (NS). Hb increased after (f,g) compared to (a) (NS).
Lokman et al., 2019 (Malaysia) [49]	Cobb500 broiler chickens, 100 (150/-), 150 days	42	Gryllodes sigillatus	(a) Control: Baseline diet (n = 30) (b) Baseline diet + 0.5 g/kg cricket chitin (n = 30) (c) Baseline diet + 0.5 g/kg cricket chitosan (n = 30) (d) Baseline diet + 0.5 g/kg shrimp chitin (n = 30) (e) Baseline diet + 0.5 g/kg shrimp chitosan (n = 30)	(b) 0.05% chitin (c) 0.05% chitosan	*Growth performance* (body weight, feed intake and fat mass)	Body weight and feed intake improved after (b) compared to (c) (S). Body weight of a) accumulated more fat compared (b–e) (S).

Table 2. Cont.

Author, Year, Country	Type of Animal, Sample Size (Male/Female), Age	Duration (Days)	Insect	Intervention (n)	Insect Inclusion Level of CFP (g/100 g Expressed in %)	Variables/Outcomes	Results
Bergmans et al., 2020 (USA) [34]	Mice, 65 (65/-), 3 weeks	66	*Gryllodes sigillatus*	(a) Control group: Standard adult diet 2018 (n = 10–12) [5] (b) HD+Cricket-based diet (n = 10–12) [5] (c) HD +Milk-based diet, (n = 10–12) [5] (d) HD+Peanut-based diet (n = 10–12) [5]		*Growth performance* (body weight recovery) *Metabolic traits* (blood parameters)	After malnourished treatment and recovery diets, there was an increment weight (34%) after (b) compared to (a) (NS). Triglycerides were reduced (47%) after (b) compared to (a) (S). After six weeks on recovery protein diets, there were no differences in the splenetic expression of select inflammatory genes among (a–c) (NS).
Pessina et al., 2020 (Brazil) [40]	Spontaneously hypertensive rats (SHR) 24 (24/-) and age-matched WKY rats (controls) 18 (18/-), 9 weeks	28	*Tenebrio molitor* larvae	(a) SHR SD (n = 8) (b) SHR SD + TM (n = 8) (c) SHR SD + captopril (n = 8) (d) WKY SD (n = 6) (e) WKY SD + TM (n = 6) (f) WKY SD + captopril (n = 6)	(b) 0.29% (e) 0.29%	*Metabolic traits* (blood parameters, blood pressure and inflammatory indicators)	Systolic BP, heart rate, and coronary perfusion pressure were reduced after (b,c) compared to (a) (S). Rat brain slices of SHR were more resistant to oxidative stress and contained lower levels of inflammatory cytokines, with no effect on vascular and liver enzyme activities (S).

Table 2. Cont.

Author, Year, Country	Type of Animal, Sample Size (Male/Female), Age	Duration (Days)	Insect	Intervention (n)	Insect Inclusion Level of CFP (g/100 g Expressed in %)	Variables/Outcomes	Results
Ahn et al., 2020 (Korea) [41]	BKS.Cg-m+/+Leprdb, heterozygous (DB-Hetero, normal) (db/+) male mice (11/-), 12 weeks and homozygous (DB-Homo, diabetes) (db/db) male db mice, 33 (33/-), 12 weeks	30	*Gryllus bimaculatus*	(a) Normal Hetero (DB-Hetero) (n = 11) (b) Control Homo (DB-Homo) (n = 11)-negative control (c) DBHomo + 5 mg/kg treatment of CaG (CaG5) (n = 11) (d) DB Homo + 5 mg/kg treatment of *GbG* (*GbG5*) (n = 11) (e) DBHomo + 10 mg/kg treatment of metformin (n = 11)-positive control	(d) 0.0005% *GbG*	**Metabolic traits** (blood parameters, and antioxidant activity)	Capacity to reduce glucose, ALT, AST, ALP, LDL-cholesterol and BUN levels increased after (d) compared to (b) (S). Antioxidant activities (catalase, SOD and GPX) increased after (d) compared to (b) (S).

[1] Injection at week 17 and week 18; [2] g/100 mL; [3] induced obesity; [4] malnourished diet; [5] Start with initial weaning diet 2020 for 10 days; S: significant; NS: non-significant; CFP: complementary food product; HFD: high fat diet; HD: Hypoprotein diet; DMSO: dimethyl sulfoxide; ALLD: *Allomyrina dichotoma* larvae; AD: *Acheta domesticus*; LFD: low-fat diet; ER: endoplasmic reticulum; ND: normal diet; TM:*Tenebrio molitor*; ALT: alanine transaminase; AST: aspartame transaminase; GS: *Gryllodes sigillatus*; HI: *Hermetia illucens*; AD: Acheta domesticus; RF: *Rhynchophorus phoenicis fabricius*; MD: malnourished; Fe: Iron; SD: standard diet; BP: blood pressure; DB: diabetes; CaG: Dung beetle (*C. molossus*) glycosaminoglycan; GbG: *Grillodes bimaculatus* glycosaminoglycan; LDL: low density lipoprotein; ALP: alanine transam:nase; SHR: spontaneously hypertension rats; WKY: Wistar Kyoto Rats; CRP:C-reactive protein; BUN: Blood urea nitrogen; SOD: Superoxide dismutase; GPX: Glutathione peroxidase.

Table 3. Effect of edible insects on human health.

Author, Year, Country	Type of Study	Subjects, Sample Size (Male/Female), Age	Duration (Days)	Insect	Intervention	Daily Food Portion of Intervention with Insects	Insect Inclusion Level of CFP (g/100 g Expressed in %)	Insect Inclusion of CFP (Expressed in g) for Each Age Group	Protein Inclusion Level of CFP: g/100 g (Expressed in %)	Protein of CFP Per Day (Expressed in g).	Variables/Outcomes	Results
Skau et al., 2015 (Cambodia) [43]	Randomized, single-blinded trial	Infants, 419 (220/119), 6 months	270	*Haplopelma species*	(a) WF: Rice-based [1] CFP with small fish and edible spiders (n = 106) (b) WF-L [1]: Rice-based CFP with small fish (n = 104) (c) CSB++ [1]: Fortified corn-soy blend product (n = 103) (d) CSB+ [1]: Fortified whole-soy (n = 106)	1. Infants 6–8 months: 50 g. 2. Infants 9–11 months: 75 g. 3. Infants 12–15 months: 125 g.	a1,a2,a3 = 1.8%	(a.1) 0.9 g (a.2) 1.35 g (a.3) 2.25 g	(a) 15.4% (b) 12.6% (c) 16.8% (d) 14.6%		*Growth performance* (food intake, body weight) *Metabolic traits* (blood parameters)	Total weight increases in a), b) compared to vs c) (NS). Similar growth observing no differences between (a–d) groups (NS) FFM no differences were observed between (a,b) (NS). Plasma ferritin, sTfR, and hemoglobin concentration no differences were observed between (a–d) (NS). Total weight increase in (a,b) compared to (c) (NS).
Bauserman et al., 2015 (Democratic Republic of Congo) [44]	Cluster-randomized controlled trial	Infants, 222 (113/109), 6 months	540	Caterpillar	(a) Usual diet [2] (n = 110) (b) Caterpillar [2] cereal. (n = 110)	Infants 6–12 months of age: 30 g Infants 12–18 months: 45 g				(b.1) 6.9 (b.2) 10.3	*Growth performance* (body weight recovery) *Metabolic traits* (blood parameters)	Stunting prevalence, no differences were observed between (a,b) (NS). Fe: no differences were observed between (a,b) (NS). Hb increased in (b) compared to (a) anemia decreased in (b) compared to (a) (S).

Table 3. Cont.

Author, Year, Country	Type of Study	Subjects, Sample Size (Male/Female), Age	Duration (Days)	Insect	Intervention	Daily Food Portion of Intervention with Insects	Insect Inclusion Level of CFP (g/100 g Expressed in %)	Insect Inclusion of CFP (Expressed in g) for Each Age Group	Protein Inclusion Level of CFP: g/100 g (Expressed in %)	Protein of CFP Per Day (Expressed in g).	Variables/Outcomes	Results
Nirmala et al., 2017 (Indonesia) [45]	Non-randomized controlled trial	Infants, 23 (12/11), 1–5 years	45	*Rhynchophorus ferrugineus*	(a) Usual diet (n = 10) (b) Sago worm inclusive diet (n = 13)	2 pieces of 50 g			(b) 9.70%	(a) 3.9 ±1.7 (b) 5.9 ± 1.7	Growth performance (body weight)	Weight and height no changes were observed between (a) and (b) (NS)
Stull et al., 2018 (USA) [46]	Double-blinded randomized crossover trial	Healthy adults, 20 (9/11), 18–65 years	14	*Gryllodes sigillatus*	(a) Control breakfast meal (n = 10) (b) Cricket breakfast meal (n = 10)	Shake + pumpkin muffin (160 g)	(b) 14.9% Shake; 9.37% Muffin		(b) 14.78%	(a) 9 (b) 21.67	Gut microbiome composition Metabolic traits (inflammatory indicators)	Bifidobacterium animalis increased 5.7 more in (b) compared to (a) (S) Plasma TNF-α decreased b) compared to (a) (S).
Vangsoe et al. A 2018 (Denmark) [47]	Randomized, controlled, single-blinded trial	Healthy young adults, 18(18/-), 18–30 years	56	*Alphitobius diaperinus*	(a) Isocaloric carbohydrate bar (n = 9) (b) Insect protein bar (n = 9)	2 bars a day	(b) 0.04% [3]			(a) 7.2 (b) 8	Changes in muscle mass composition and strength	Morphological adaptations such as hypertrophy or muscle strength show no changes in (a) compared to (b) (NS).
Vangsoe et al. B 2018 (Denmark) [48]	Randomized, cross-over study	Healthy young adults,6 (6/-), 18–30 years	1	*Alphitobius diaperinus*	(a) Drink placebo (water) (b) Drink whey isolate (c) Drink soy isolate (d) Drink insect isolate	400 mL per day	(d) 7.6% [4]	(d) 30.5 g isolate powder		(b) 25 g (c) 25 g (d) 25 g	Crude protein digestibility	Blood concentrations of EAA, BCAA and leucine increased in (b–d) compared to (a) over a 120 min period (S). Slowly digested (d) compared to (b,c) (S).

[1] Severe malnutritior; [2] stunning rates; [3] isolated powder 82% protein; [4] 30.5 g/400 mL; S: significant NS: non-significant; CFP: complementary food product; WF: win food; WF-L: win food lite; CSB: corn soy blends; FFM: fat free mass; sTfr: soluble transferrin receptor; Fe: iron; Hb: hemoglobin; TNF-α: plasma tumor necrosis factor-alpha; AA: amino acid; EAA: essential amino acids; BCAA: branched-chain amino acids.

Table 4. Effect on environmental indicators of edible insects consumed as animal feed and human food.

Insect	Animal Feed Consumption (kg Edible Protein)						Non Waste Insects					Human Food Consumption (kg De Protein)				
	Waste-Feed Insects															
	Author, Year, Country	Land Use (m²)	GHG (Kg CO₂ eq)	Energy Use (MJ)			Author, Year, Country	Land Use (m²)	GHG (Kg CO₂ eq)	Energy Use (MJ)		Author, Year, Country	Water Footprint (m³)	Land Use (m²)	GHG (Kg CO₂ eq)	Energy Use (MJ)
Tenebrio molitor larvae							Thévenot et al., 2018 (France) [F,J] [53]	6.35	5.77	217.37		Oonincx et al., 2012 (USA) [F] [7]		17.68	13.16	167.23
												Miglietta et al., 2015 (Italy) [F,J] [55]	23			
Musca domestica larvae	Van Zanten et al., 2015 (Netherlands) [A,J] [50]	0.07	1.43	18.98												
Hermetia illucens larvae	Salomone et al., 2016 (Italy) [B,I] [51]	0.05	2.1	15.1												
	Muys et al. 2014 (UK) [C,J] [52]	0.06 [D] / 0.19 [E]	2.1	15.1												
Acheta domesticus	Halloran et al., 2017 (Denmark) [F,J] [54]							3.97 [G] / 2.63 [H]								

A: Poultry manure; B: food waste; C: brewery waste; D: manual harvest; E: automatic harvest; F: mixed diet; G: current situation; H: future scenario; system boundaries: (I: from cradle to farm and J: from cradle to meal).

3.2. Health Outcomes in Animal Studies

Study outcomes were related to **appetite control** [32], **growth performance** [34,35,38,39,49], **metabolic traits** [32–36,38–42], **crude protein digestibility** [36,38], and/or **intestinal morphology** [35,37,38]. The following seven edible insects were investigated as a supplement in animal studies: *TM* [33,37,38,40], *Hermetia illucens (HI)* [35,36,38], *Gryllodes sigillatus (GS)* [34,49], *Gryllodes bimaculatus (GB)* [41,42], *Allomyrina dichotoma* larvae *(ALLD)* [32], *Rhynchophorus phoenicis fabricius (RF)* [39], and *AD* [39]. Nine studies used whole insects and three used insect components such as chitin [42], chitosan [49], or glycosaminoglycan [41,42] (Table 2).

3.2.1. Appetite Control

Kim et al. [32] studied the effect of 10 mg/mL of ethanol extract of *ALLD* larvae on the anorexigenic and endoplasmic reticulum (ER) and the stress-reducing effects of *ALLD* on the hypothalamus of previously diet-induced obese mice. Intraventricular cannulation was used to infuse 1 µL of 20% dimethyl sulfoxide (DMSO) and 1 µL of *ALLD* extract (10 mg/mL). Results showed that administration of *ALLD* extract significantly reduced food intake and body weight via appetite-related neuropeptide regulation for 24 h compared to DMSO, which was evident at 2 h after infusion and consistent after 24 h.

3.2.2. Growth Performance

Dabbou et al. [35] evaluated the effects of increasing levels of partially defatted *HI* larva meals on growth performance in 256 male broiler chickens over 35 days. The diets included increasing levels of *HI* larva meal (0, 5, 10, and 15%; *HI*0, *HI*5, *HI*10, and *HI*15, respectively), with *HI*0 as control diet. Increasing levels of dietary *HI* meal administration (5% to 15%, expressed as insect inclusion level of CFP) significantly improved the growth performance (live weight and daily feed intake) of birds by up to 10% in the starter period. The same outcome was reported by Gasco et al. [38] and later studies with replacement meals of *HI* and *TM*. Gasco et al. replaced soybean oil with *HI* and *TM* to meet the growth requirements of 200 36-day-old crossed rabbits for 41 days. Five interventions were tested, with a control diet of 1.5% soybean oil, the partial (50%) or total (100%) substitution of soy-bean oil by *HI* (*HI*50 and *HI*100, respectively) or by *TM* (*TM*50 and *TM*100, respectively). *HI* and *T* fats are suitable sources of dietary lipid in rabbit diets to replace soybean oil and have no detrimental effect on growth performance. A study by Agbemafle et al. [39] analyzed the effect of edible insect powder (*AD* and *RF*) on the nutritional status of malnourished rats using the hemoglobin/protein repletion method in 66 21-day-old male rats for 35 days. Malnutrition was induced by feeding the rats with a 5% protein and ~2 ppm Fe diet for 21 days. Results showed similar increases in weight, bone mineral content, and lean and fat mass in the *AD* + *Solanum torvum*, *AD*, and *RF* groups in comparison to the protein-Fe sufficient group. Bergmans et al. [34] examined the impact of protein-malnutrition and subsequent recovery on body weight and selected inflammatory biomarkers in a study of 65 3-week-old mice for 66 days. Protein malnutrition was induced by administration of an isocaloric hypoprotein diet (5% protein calories) in young male mice for two weeks, followed by a six-week recovery period using a cricket- (*GS*), peanut-, or milk-based diet. The cricket-based diet performed as well as peanut- and milk-based diets in body weight recovery (34%, 39%, and 32%, respectively). In relation to growth performance, Lokman et al. [49] used parts of the insects, evaluating and comparing the effect of dietary chitin and chitosan from cricket and shrimp on growth performance, carcass quality, and organ characteristics in 150 broiler chickens. The authors observed that cricket chitin at 0.5 g/kg significantly improved growth performance, carcass quality, and organ characteristics of broilers in comparison to the chitosan and control diets, which produced a comparatively greater accumulation of fat.

3.2.3. Metabolic Traits

In relation to the **body weight gain achieved with** edible insects, Seo et al. [33] investigated the lipid accumulation and anti-obesity effects of whole powder of *TM* larvae with a diet that simultaneously induced obesity in 35 male mice. In this intervention, five treatment conditions were assigned for 6 weeks The body weight gain of the mice was significantly reduced by up to 19% with the oral administration of 100 mg/kg *TM* larvae and by 25% with 3000 mg/kg *TM* larvae in comparison to mice fed with high-fat-diet (HFD) alone. Ahn et al. [42] investigated the effect of glycosaminoglycan from *GB* (*GbG*) on antiatherosclerotic and antilipidemic effects (including weights of abdominal and epididymal fat) in 50 14-week-old male rats. The rats were acclimated for 1 week with an HFD (60% fat) and then segregated into five treatment groups (control, 5 mg/kg *GbG*, 10 mg/kg *GbG*, 2 mg/kg Pravastatin, and 10 mg/kg chitosan) of 10 rats each. Each group was maintained on the HFD for 1 month. Abdominal fat weight and epididymal fat were significantly decreased in comparison to controls by 16% and 18%, respectively.

In terms of the effects of edible insects on **inflammation**, Ahn et al. [42] also investigated the effect of *GbG* on serum C-reactive protein (CRP) levels. Significant decreases in CRP levels (mg/L) of the *GbG*-treated groups were observed *versus* controls. Furthermore, Bergmans et al. [34] analyzed the gene expression of several inflammatory (TLR4, TNFα, IL-1β, and IFNγ) and anti-inflammatory (IL-4) markers in spleen tissue, observing a similar expression of inflammatory genes in mice on cricket- and milk-based diets to that in mice on a control diet. Both articles by Ahn et al. [41,42] showed that treatment with 5 mg/kg *GbG* reduced glucose levels *versus* controls. Serum aspartate transaminase (AST) and alanine transaminase (ALT) levels were also reduced after *GbG* treatment [41,42]. *TM* larvae also significantly decreased the accumulation of hepatic lipid droplets and levels of plasma ALT and AST in comparison to mice fed with HFD [33]. In another study, the inclusion of insect lipids in rabbit diets did not influence serum AST, ALT, or alkaline phosphatase (ALP) enzyme activities [38].

The **antioxidant** effect of edible insect intake has been addressed by various authors [35,41]. Dabbou et al. [35] observed increasing plasma glutathione peroxidase (GPX) activity in the *HI* groups, which showed a linear response ($p = 0.002$) to an increasing percentage of *HI* meal up to 15%. Ahn et al. [41] studied the antioxidative effects of field cricket *GbG* on two types of male diabetic mice at 12 weeks of age: heterozygous (db/+) (DB-Hetero, normal) and homozygous (db/db) (DB-Homo, diabetes) animals. Results showed that the intake of 5 mg/Kg *GbG* significantly increased the anti-oxidative activities of catalase, superoxide dismutase (SOD), and GPX in the *GbG*-treated group *versus* controls (DB-Homo), observing a reduction in hepatocellular biomarkers after 5 mg/kg of *GbG* treatment. Levels of antioxidative enzymes and activities of catalase, GPX, glutathione-s-transferase, and SOD were also increased by the *GbG* treatment. In this way, hepatocellular oxidative stress triggered by free radical damage was attenuated by these antioxidant enzymes. In the db mice experiment, 5 mg/Kg *GbG* increased catalase activity by 114.9%, GPX by 248.1%, GST by 117.6%, and SOD by 125.7%. In terms of blood cell oxidative damage, protein oxidative damage was also reduced by these GAGs (CaG5 by 18.5%; 5 mg/Kg *GbG* by 18.5%; and Metformin10 by 7.0%), based on the blood neutrophil carbonyl content.

In terms of the effects of edible insects on **blood pressure**, Pessina et al. [40] studied the effects of the protein obtained from the larval stage of *TM* on 24 male spontaneously hypertensive rats (SHRs) and 18 male age-matched rats of the normotensive Wistar Kyoto strain (WKY). Results showed that both the standard diet supplemented with *TMs* and Captopril significantly reduced systolic blood pressure, heart rate, and coronary pressure in SHRs compared with the standard diet. Ahn et al. [42] observed no statistically significant differences in blood pressure (systolic blood pressure and heart rate) between the 5 or 10 mg/kg *GbG* treated groups and controls.

Regarding the effect of edible insect intake on the **blood lipid profile**, Bovera et al. [36] studied the effect of replacing 25% or 50% of soybean content with *HI* larvae meal on 162 16-week-old laying hens for 140 days. A reduction in serum cholesterol and triglyceride levels was observed in both insect-meal fed groups. In a mouse study, Bergmans et al. [34], observed that a recovery diet with cricket (*GS*) for 6 weeks reduced serum levels of triglycerides by 47% in comparison to the control diet. Ahn et al. found a reduction in total serum cholesterol after *GbG* treatment *versus* controls [42] in one study and an inhibition of serum LDL-cholesterol levels after *GbG5* treatment in another [41].

In terms of **other relevant blood parameters**, Agbemafle et al. [39] studied the effects of protein-Fe supplementation on hemoglobin in rats. Hemoglobin iron did not significantly differ among protein-Fe sufficient, *AD*, and *RF* groups. Hemoglobin iron was lowest for the *Solanum torvum* and low protein-Fe groups but highest for the control group. Hemoglobin iron was similar among the low protein-Fe, cricket + *Solanum torvum*, and *RF* groups. Out of all supplemented groups, the cricket + *Solanum torvum* evidenced the greatest change in hemoglobin iron, although this did not differ from the *RF* or protein-Fe sufficient groups. Both studies by Ahn et al. [41,42] showed that treatment with 5 mg/kg *GbG* reduced glucose levels *versus* controls.

3.2.4. Crude Protein Digestibility

Gasco et al. [38] studied crude protein digestibility in rabbits. The addition of *HI* and *T* fats did not influence protein digestibility. In a study of hens, Bovera et al. [36] showed that dry matter, organic matter, and crude protein digestibility coefficients were lower after the *HI*50 diet than after the HI25 diet, probably due to the negative effect of chitin. The dry matter consisted of all nutrients, whereas the organic matter consisted of all nutrients except ash. The crude protein digestibility coefficient is expressed as % of g protein digested per Kg dry matter [36].

3.2.5. Intestinal Morphology

Biasato et al. [37] evaluated the effects of *TM* meal for 43 days on the intestinal microbiota, morphology, and mucin composition of 70 female free-range chickens. Chickens received a corn-soybean gluten meal-based control diet or a 75 g/kg *TM* diet in complete substitution of corn gluten meal. Inclusion of the *TM* dietary meal had no effect on intestinal morphometric indices of the free-range chickens ($p > 0.05$) or on mucin staining intensity of intestinal villi but had a significant effect on gut segment and villus fragment histochemistry ($p < 0.001$ and $p < 0.01$, respectively). Gasco et al. [38] observed that villi height and crypt depth ratio were similarly affected after the dietary inclusion of *HI* and *T* fats *versus* controls. In another study, Dabbou et al. [35] found a lower villus height and greater crypt depth in groups receiving meals with 15% *versus* 0–10% *HI* inclusion rates.

3.3. Health Outcomes in Human Studies

The outcomes of studies were classified as **growth performance** [43–45], **metabolic traits** [43,44,46], **gut microbiota composition** [46], *changes in muscle mass composition and strength* [47], and **crude protein digestibility** [48]. Five different edible insects were investigated in human studies, including *AD* [47,48], *Haplopelma species* (HP) [43], Caterpillar (CT) [44], *Rhynchophorus ferrugineus* (RF) [45], and *Gryllodes sigillatus* (GS) [46]. A parallel design was used by four studies, a randomized design by three [43,44,47] and a non-randomized trial by one [45], while two were cross-over randomized trials [46,48]. Skau et al., 2015, Bauserman et al., 2015, and Nirmala et al., 2017 use the whole edible insect whereas Stull et al., 2018 and Vangsoe et al., A 2018 used powdered form and Vangsoe et al., B 2018 used an isolated protein form.

3.3.1. Growth Performance

Skau et al. [43], used a single-blinded parallel design to study the effect of two rice-based complementary food products (one containing edible spiders) for 9 months on body composition fat-free mass (FFM) and linear growth in 419 six-month-old Cambodian infants. No significant differences were found in FFM or anthropometric changes (weight, height, knee–heel length) between locally produced products (WF and WF-L) and the CSBs. In a cluster randomized controlled trial, Bauserman et al. [44] assessed the efficacy of a cereal made from caterpillars, a micronutrient-rich, locally available alternative animal-source food, to reduce stunting and anemia in 222 infants. Using a non-randomized controlled trial, Nirmala et al. [45] investigated the effect of sago worm *RF* consumption as a component of complementary feeding *versus* a control diet without sago worms for 45 days on the weight and height of 23 infants aged 1–5 years old. No between-group differences in weight or height were observed in the last two studies [44,45].

3.3.2. Metabolic Traits

The effects on metabolic traits were studied by Skau et al. [43], who observed no significant differences in iron status (plasma ferritin, soluble transferrin receptor (sTfR), or hemoglobin concentration) between locally produced products (WF and WF-L) and corn-soy blends. In another study by Bauserman et al. [44], higher Hb concentrations were found in infants in the *caterpillar* cereal group than in the control group (10.7 vs. 10.1 g/dL, $p = 0.03$), and fewer infants were anemic (26% vs. 50%). In a double-blinded randomized crossover study, Stull et al. [46] investigated the effects of 25 g/day of whole cricket powder in 20 healthy adults aged 18–65 years. Participants were randomized into two study arms and consumed either cricket-containing or controlled breakfast foods for 14 days, followed by a washout period and assignment to the opposite treatment. Blood and stool samples were collected at baseline and after each treatment period to assess liver function and microbiota changes. Results evidenced an association between cricket consumption and reduced plasma tumor necrosis factor-alpha (TNF-α).

3.3.3. Gut Microbiota Composition

Results of the aforementioned study by Stull et al. [46] showed that consuming 25 g/day of whole cricket powder supported the growth of probiotic bacterium, *Bifidobacterium animalis*, which underwent a 5.7-fold increase.

3.3.4. Changes in Muscle Mass Composition and Strength

The effect of insect protein as a dietary supplement on muscle mass and strength during prolonged resistance training was assessed in healthy young men using a randomized, controlled, single-blinded trial [47]. Vangsoe et al. [47] studied the effect of insect protein as a dietary supplement to increase muscle hypertrophy and strength gain during prolonged resistance training in 18 healthy young men. Supplementation with insect protein isolates enhanced muscle mass and strength gains in young men during progressive resistance training, without observing significant differences with those consuming an isocaloric carbohydrate supplement.

3.3.5. Crude Protein Digestibility

In a second study, Vangsoe et al. [48] investigated whether their previous observation of no effect of insect protein on muscle mass gain during training [47] could be explained by the bioavailability, digestibility, and amino acid (AA) profile of the insect protein. Participants received three different protein supplementations (25 g of crude protein from whey, soy, insect) or placebo with water on four separate days. Blood samples were collected at 0, 20, 40, 60, 90, and 120 min during each intervention day. Ingestion of whey, soy, or insect protein isolate was found to produce a significant increase in EAA, branched-chain amino acids (BCAAs), and leucine in comparison to placebo. However, ingestion of whey protein isolate led to significantly higher concentrations of AAs compared with soy or insect protein. Insect protein intake showed a tendency towards higher AA concentrations beyond the 120 min period, suggesting that differences in blood AA concentrations between soy and insect protein may be attributable to a slower digestion of the latter. Furthermore, serum insulin concentrations were significantly increased after ingestion of whey and soy protein but were not changed to the same degree after ingestion of insect protein [48].

3.4. Environmental Impacts of Edible Insects

Seven articles assessed the environmental impact of producing insect-based food products for human consumption [7,55] and animal feed; distinguishing between so-called waste-feed insects [50–52] and non-waste-feed insects [53,54]. Regarding the type of insects, three articles investigated *TM* larvae [7,53,55], two *HI* larvae [51,52], one *AD* [54], and one *Musca domestica (MD)* [50].

All seven studies applied the life cycle assessment (LCA) methodology to estimate the potential impacts of producing larvae meals. The most common environmental impacts reported were GHG, LU, and EU, with only one article assessing WFP [55]. Table 4 exhibits the environmental impacts per kg of edible protein from the selected studies. In articles that did not report the environmental impacts per kg of edible protein, these were estimated according to the method of Oonincx et al. [7]. First, kg of fresh product was multiplied by the average dry matter (DM) content of the species and the average content of crude protein in the DM. This value was then multiplied by the edible portion, which was considered to be 100% of edible insects. These environmental impacts were also related to the insect production, meaning that the system boundaries of these studies are from cradle-to-insect farm gate [7,51,52,54,55]. Only Thévenot et al. [53] and Van Zanten et al. [50] reported values up to the mill gate.

The highest EUs between cradle and farm gate were related to heating and air-conditioning systems [51]. When the system boundary was extended to the mill gate, the EU increased by around 5–7% [50,53]. LU was related to the land needed for animal farming as well as for crop cultivation to feed the insects. This parameter was minimized in vertically grown insects. LU and GHG emissions are also lower for waste-feed insects than for non-waste feed insects. With regard to water use, cleaning measures were responsible for the largest fraction, and it was also related to process-specific inputs such as substrate rewetting or water provision for drinking, EU (through the water requirements of power plants), and infrastructure construction [50].

Van Zanten et al. [50] explored the environmental impact of using larvae of the common housefly grown on poultry manure and food waste as livestock feed. Likewise, Salomone et al. [51] applied the LCA to a system of mass-rearing of *HI* grown on food waste [51], while Muys et al. [52] used brewery wastes. Thévenot et al. [53] and Halloran et al. [54] used a mixed diet in the group of non-waste-feed insects. In both studies, all LCA indicators were increased in comparison to non-waste feed insects. In particular, Halloran et al. [54] pointed towards a future, more efficient, cricket farming scenario in which environmental impacts could be reduced (e.g., by around 34% for GHG emissions). Oonincx et al. [7] conducted an LCA study on mealworm production for human food in which GHG production, EU, and land use were quantified and compared to conventional sources of animal protein. All parameters were increased in comparison to insect farming for animal feed and especially waste-feed insect farming [50–52]. Miglietta et al. [55] evaluated the WFP of the production of edible insects, focusing on the water consumption associated with protein content to allow comparison with other animal protein sources. The results showed a decrease of around > 50% in this resource in comparison to beef and pork and of around < 15% in comparison to chicken.

4. Discussion

Food systems are currently facing unprecedented challenges. Rapid depletion of natural resources, climate change, and biodiversity loss further threaten future food systems [56]. Global reports emphasize the need for fundamental transformations of food systems for planetary health [8,57].

At first, insects were mainly appreciated for their nutritional composition. Their newly discovered bioactive compounds may promote animal and human health and position insects beyond the 'simple' protein concept [58].

With regards to the health dimension, weight-control animal studies found that the inclusion of 1 g/mL ethanol extract to *ADLL* larvae [59,60] reduced food intake and body weight compared with vehicle control (evident at 2 h after infusion and consistent after 24 h) and could be a novel potential treatment option for anorexigenic function in high-fat-induced obese mice via reduction of ER stress.

Many edible insect species convert organic substrates into protein- and energy-rich products, contributing to circular economy principles [61]. Malnutrition is a major consequence of fragility and is associated with increased mortality, poor cognitive and motor development, impaired physical performance, reduced income in adulthood, and lower birth weight of offspring [44]. Micronutrient deficiencies are a prevalent problem in low-income countries, responsible for 3.1 million deaths annually in children aged <5 years [62], and could be solved in an accessible manner by insect supplementation containing proteins, essential fatty acids, and micronutrients such as riboflavin, pantothenic acid, biotin, and in some cases, folic acid, copper, iron, magnesium, manganese, phosphorus composition, selenium, and zinc, improving growth and nutritional status during childhood [63]. There are two main reasons for using insects in low-income countries: one is to fight malnutrition, and the other is to improve micronutrient iron deficiency and consequently low values of serum hemoglobin and ferritin. As an example, a study by Agbemafle et al. [39] in rats showed an increase in hemoglobin and ferritin concentrations after an *AD* and *RP* diet compared with a normal diet of casein and ferrous sulfate. Superior results were observed in the groups supplemented with the edible insect *AD* with 23.3% protein CFP *versus* controls receiving only a low-protein and iron supplement and the *Solanum torvum* group, which included 8.8% protein. In a study by Skau et al. [43], supplementation for 18 months with cereals containing insect flour (23%) increased plasma hemoglobin levels in children aged 6 months and lowered the rate of anemia in comparison to the usual diets for this age. Regarding changes in growth, studies have been performed replacing the usual diets of animals with edible insects such as *HI* [35,36,38] and *GS* [49], measuring their fattening and weight increase, and two of them reported significant changes in weight gain [35,49]. Meanwhile, human studies [43–45] showed no significant differences in weight gain improvements between children treated with edible insects and children treated with cereals. This lack of improvement might be associated with the age of participants (<5 years) and various external factors, including difficulties in administering the food and poor adherence to treatment [45,63]. According to social development goals (SDGs), European countries are making efforts towards more sustainable alternative proteins and, in terms of accessibility, edible insects can offer new opportunities to underdeveloped countries [64].

Nutritional assessment of the fat contained in edible insects can play a positive role in feeding, given that they are rich in unsaturated fatty acids, especially polyunsaturated fatty acids (PUFAs) [65] and are especially low in cholesterol [66]. Edible insects contain n-3 PUFA. The increased demand for the omega-3 fatty acids eicosapentaenoic acid (EPA) and docosahexaenoic acid (DHA) has led science and industry to seek alternative methods to sustainably produce these essential fatty acids without relying on over-exploited wild fisheries [67], and edible insects may play a key role. Moreover, a diet that is mainly based on plant food products (common beans, wheat, soybeans, rice, and maize) could increase the risk of deficiencies in vitamin B12, EPA, and DHA [68]. Edible insects can be used to enrich diets, especially plant-based diets based on cereal proteins poor in essential AAs such as lysine, threonine, and tryptophan [69]. In addition, edible insects can be an alternative to proteins from traditional livestock (pork and beef), which have been directly related to increased cardiovascular and stroke risks. In animal studies, the positive effects of edible insect intake have been associated with a decrease in hepatic lipid droplets [33], a reduction [33] or non-increase [38,42] in plasma inflammatory biomarkers (ALT, AST, ALP) [33,38,42], decreases in plasma TNF-l levels [46], blood triglycerides [34,36], blood total cholesterol [36], and blood pressure [40], and an increase in blood serum hemoglobin levels [36,39]. *GbG* intake was found to have a positive effect on plasma glucose levels [41,42] and to reduce LDL-cholesterol and hepatocellular serum biomarkers [41,42]. Therefore, *GbB* can be used as a natural antioxidant, anti-lipidemic, functional food, and in the treatment of diabetes [41]. The therapeutic role of bioactive peptides (BAPs), may in part explain some physiological effects described in our review [70]. BAPs have been identified as edible insect protein hydrolysates/peptides, and their presence has been shown to be similar or higher than that of other dietary proteins in plants and animals. Further research on the BAPs derived from edible insects may reveal novel peptide sequences that may be more potent and/or bioavailable in comparison to BAPs from more conventional dietary proteins [70]. The interest of further pursuing research in the area of BAPs derived from edible insects may lead to the discovery of novel peptide sequences which may be more potent and/or more bioavailable than BAPs generated from more conventional dietary proteins. According to other reviews [71,72], research with insects tested in vivo and in cellular models displayed radical scavenging or metal ion chelation properties as well as the ability to modulate glutathione S-Transferase and catalase. It has been proposed that these activities, which are concentration-dependent, have beneficial antioxidant effects.

Insect protein has the potential to be an ecological, high-quality solution to meet future protein demands, and some insect proteins have proven equivalent or superior to soy protein in terms of nutritional value [47]. Gasco et al. [38] and Bovera et al. [36] described similar or better crude protein digestibility coefficients for diets with edible insect substitution (*HI* and *TM*) than for a soybean-based control diet. In human studies, edible insects showed high amounts of essential nutrients, and 77–98% of edible insect protein has been found to have high digestibility, depending on the species [73]. Protein is an essential macronutrient that is highly important for the structure of skeletal muscle, providing nitrogen and AAs [74]. In general, the availability of AAs stimulates muscle protein synthesis, which is necessary for the creation of skeletal muscle mass [75]. One study in humans [47] reported that supplementation with *AD* (insect inclusion rate of 6.25%) increased concentrations of blood EAA, BCAA, and leucine, similar to the effects of corn soybean meal. Animal protein supplementation was found to produce greater gains in muscle mass and strength compared to other plant sources such as soybean meal [48]. A protein intake of 0.8–1.6 g/kg/day is necessary to maintain protein balance and prevent muscle mass loss [76] in most individuals, but especially in older adults with a low daily energy intake. Older adults tend to consume less than the recommended amount of protein, often due to hyporexia, increasing their risk of fragility [77].

Insects also contain relevant levels of insoluble fiber derived from the exoskeleton, mainly in the form of chitin, which could have a positive impact on gastrointestinal health [78]. This insoluble fiber has been shown to exert antimicrobial, antioxidant, anti-inflammatory, anti-cancer, and immunostimulatory activities [79]. The chitin and chitosan content is between 4.3–7.1% and 2.4–5.8%, respectively, of the dry weight of whole crickets [80]. Supplementation with *TM* flour (inclusion level of 7.5%) had positive effects on intestinal microbiota growth (*Clostridium, Oscillospira, Ruminococcus, Coprococcus,* and *Sutterella*) and improved intestinal health in chickens [37]. In humans, *GS* flour intake resulted in a 5.7% increase in probiotic bacteria (*Bifidobacterium animalis*) in comparison to the same diet without this edible insect [46].

Studies have been published on allergic reactions to different insects and their components and on their cross-reactivity with crustaceans [81]. The main insect allergens were reported to be tropomyosin and arginine kinase, and this reactivity could not be eliminated by thermal treatment or digestion [81]. For instance, Barennes et al. [82] described allergic symptoms in 7.6% of frequent insect consumers, including individuals with allergies to dust mites and/or crustaceans, mainly attributed to the chitin from the exoskeleton [14].

Insects can appear as processed foods, serve as a supplement in animal feed or be used in human food to replace traditional ingredients, as in the case of margarine, milk, or burgers among others [83,84]. Pilot scale processing trials identified the potential of classical margarine technologies to transform insect lipids (*HI* and *TM*) into spreadable products with high fat content (more than 80%) and appropriate product coloring (yellowish) [83]. Substitution of 75% lipids in margarine resulted in a product with an environmental impact that was higher in comparison to conventional margarine, but lower in comparison to butter [85]. Other researchers developed an alternative to bovine milk from *TM* [84] that contained 5.76% fats and 1.19% proteins and represented 59.1% of the environmental burden of standardized bovine milk [84]. The addition of 10% cockroach flour in white bread formulation led to a protein increase of 133% (from 9.7% to 22.7%) and a fat reduction of 64.53%. Megido et al. [86] prepared different formulations of hamburger (beef hamburger, lentil hamburger, and lentil and beef hamburger with 50% insects (*TM*)). Other applications in the insect food industry are as emulsifiers. Higher emulsifying activity index (EAI) values *versus* other proteins and improved functional properties demonstrate the potential of cricket protein hydrolysates as a source of functional alternative proteins in food ingredient formulations [85]. The edible insect market is an emerging economic sector driven by strong market demand and supported by academic research and innovation in private sectors (from processing to selling).

Two aspects should be considered in the comparison of studies in the health dimension. First, consensus is required on the terminology used to facilitate the understanding of results when comparing different studies. Second, more long-term interventions are needed in humans to elucidate the effects on health, given that the average length of interventions is 2 months in animals and 5 months in humans (>2 months in only 2 of the 6 human studies). Regarding the terminology, the four indicators used in this systematic review can be recommended for human studies on the effect of insect intake: (a) the daily food portion used in interventions with insects, (b) insect inclusion level CFP, (c) protein inclusion level of CFP, and (d) protein of CFP per day. The insect inclusion level (g insect/100 g of product) is provided in four of the human studies [43,46–48], with inclusion levels of 1.8% and 9.37–14.9%, respectively, in two of these [43,46]. Vangsoe et al. [47,48] used lower insect inclusion levels of 0.04–7.6% in the form of isolated protein, which has a higher protein content than edible insect powder [81]. Hence, it is crucial to specify whether flour or isolate is used to avoid errors in comparisons. The way in which edible insects are administered is relevant because it may have an impact on the protein digestibility. The term "insect inclusion level" is widely used in animal studies, and 11 of the 12 studies described values ranging between 0.01% and 28.3% for whole edible insect powder and between 0.0005% and 0.05% for the edible insect components glycosaminoglycan [41,42] and chitin/chitosan [49]. The protein quantity of the CFP per day describes the amount of protein provided in the intervention, and this information would be even more valuable if it included the amount of protein provided in the CFP from insects, given that the amount of insect in many CFP compositions is very low compared to other ingredients [43,44]. The protein inclusion level has the potential to allow calculation of the percentage of insect protein with respect to the amount of protein in the CFP.

With regards to the environmental dimension, the increasing need for food production is hampered by the shortage of land for agricultural production for land [87]. Humans currently consume around 40% of the biomass on land and coastlines, and the massive demand for animal proteins, recognized as one of the leading causes of climate change, has created the need for protein alternatives to protect the welfare of future generations [88]. The high nutritional value of edible insects and their protein content make them excellent alternatives to conventional protein sources for animal feed [89]. The environmental impact of current protein sources is very high, contaminating surface waters, spreading pathogenic microorganisms and chemical pollutants, emitting GHG, and causing deforestation [90]. In contrast, insect farming reduces the environmental footprint [91] and the use of pesticides and water [92], and it offers more efficient food conversion. For example, cattle and pigs are considered responsible for 18% of all GHGs, with a major impact on global warming. In terms of sustainability, the waste generated in insect farms is minimal in comparison to that produced by stockbreeding, which is responsible for around 10% of GHG emissions in Europe [93]. The WFP is 79% lower for the production of edible insects than for raising cattle [55], and its LU requirements are 61% lower in comparison to traditional livestock production [93]. The food conversion ratio, i.e., the kg of food needed to make 1 kg of edible weight, is also much lower for edible insects than for pigs, chickens, and cattle [11,94]. Therefore, insects could be a more environmentally and economically sustainable source of protein. As an example, the harvested and processed black soldier fly larvae, valued at around US$200 per ton, can also be more economically transported than manure (valued at USD 10–20 per ton) [95]. In the present systematic review, we highlight the importance of edible insects as food, feed, or waste utilization farming, comparing four environmental impacts (LU, GHG, EU, and WFP) with the FU per kg edible protein and comparing these indicators to those for more traditional proteins, such as those from livestock. Van Raamsdonk et al. [96] discussed the issues related to insects as feed material and showed that insect farming offered a smaller environmental footprint, reduced pesticide use, more efficient food conversion, and a lesser water requirement in comparison to traditional livestock. Furthermore, the conversion efficiency of ingested food was estimated to be 58–85% lower in edible insects *versus* pork and beef and 17% lower *versus* poultry [96] (Table 5).

Table 5. Environmental indicators of traditional livestock animals for food.

Animal	Author, Year, Country	Traditional Livestock Animals for Food (kg de Protein)			
		Water Food Print (m³)	Land Use (m²)	GHG (Kg CO₂ eq)	Energy Use (MJ)
Pork	Vries and de Boer. 2010 (Netherlands) F [97]		47–64	21–53	95–236
	Miglietta et al. 2015 (Italy) F [55]	57			
Chicken	Vries and de Boer. 2010 (Netherlands) F [97]		42–52	18–36	80–152
	Miglietta et al. 2015 (Italy) F [55]	34			
Beef	Vries and de Boer. 2010 (Netherlands) F [97]		144–258	75–170	177–273
	Miglietta et al. 2015 (Italy) F [55]	112			

F: Mixed diet.

A better environmental performance is obtained with waste-fed insects [50,52] than with non-waste-fed insects [53,54]. For human food consumption, the edible insect farm uses a mixed diet (oats, carrots, wheat) that almost doubles LU and GHG values [97]. However, the waste generated in an insect farm is minimal in comparison to that produced by stockbreeding, which is responsible for around 10% of GHG emissions in Europe [94].

The production of edible insects for human consumption is responsible for around 95% less GHG emissions and LU and 62% less EU in comparison to beef production [93]. The environmental benefits of insects are much higher compared with other livestock (pork and poultry), achieving reductions of 90% in GHG, 61% in LU, and 56% in EU [93] (Figure 2).

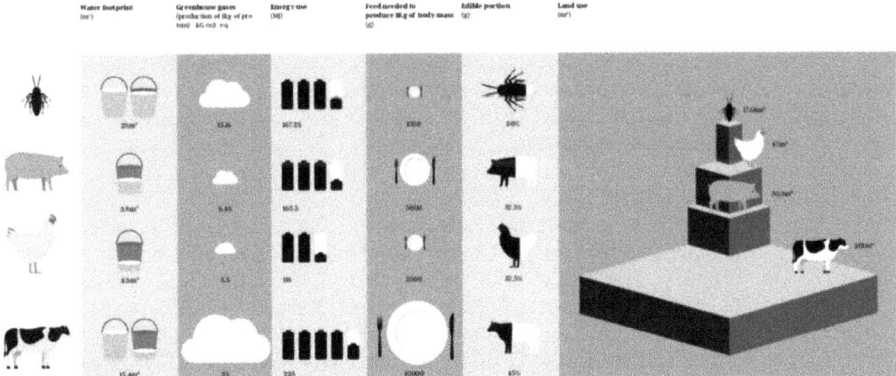

Figure 2. Resource use and environmental impact parameters of insect farming *versus* the production of other livestock (Data on resource use and environmental obtained from Tables 3 and 4).

Further research is needed on EU. For example, EU and related GHG emission may be lesser if insects are used for composting [98]. EU per kg of protein is currently higher for insect meal than for soybean or fish meal [53]. It is recommended to lower EU by using more efficient heating and air-conditioning devices and by adequately insulating production facilities, besides designing automated measures for the separation of pupae and residue substrates [52]. Reducing WFP requires challenging research to conceive and design alternative cleaning measures and/or rearing vessels with a more favorable volume/surface area ratio [52]. Implementing innovative and sustainable food production strategies such as insect farming may contribute to several SDGs, which are themselves interconnected [64], given the importance in food sustainability as defined by Béné et al. [99] (Figure 3).

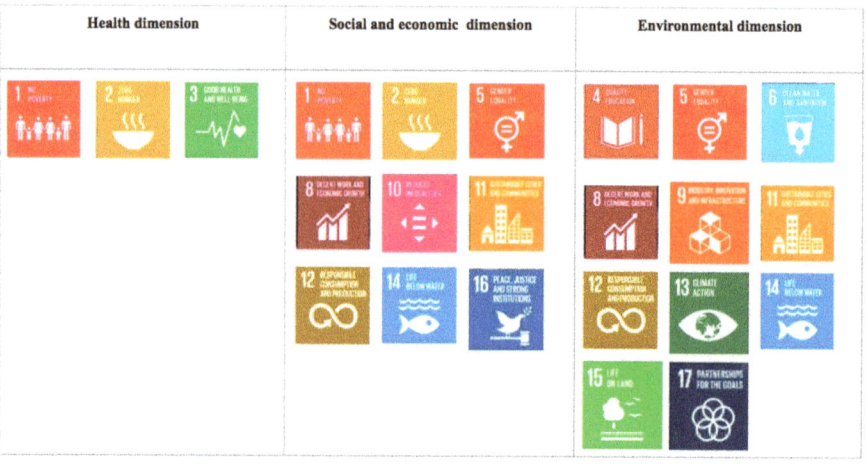

Figure 3. Edible insects and Sustainable Development Goals according to the three dimensions of food sustainability.

Other considerations to be taken as part of the drive towards food sustainability are the acceptability, accessibility, and affordability of edible insect products, which are key to their introduction into the dietary habits of Western societies [99]. In developed countries, entomophagy has been considered a primitive behavior and relegated to rural environments [82], and industrialized populations associate insects with fear and disgust [100]. The exclusion of entomophagy is above all a cultural issue, and it is hard to persuade individuals to accept the practice [101]. The acceptability by populations of food products with edible insects may be difficult in countries where they are not traditionally consumed [102]. It is therefore necessary to search for attributes that could support their popularization [103,104].

5. Conclusions

This systematic review contributes specific information on the potential health benefits offered by edible insects. In animal and human studies, doses up to 7% of edible insect inclusion level significantly improved the live weight, reduced levels of triglycerides, cholesterol, and blood glucose, and increased microbiota diversity (*versus* control diet) in animals, and significantly improved gut health, reduced systemic inflammation (*versus* control diets), increased blood concentrations of essential and branched-chain amino acids, and slowed digestion (*versus* whey treatment) in humans. Comparisons among studies could be facilitated if researchers consistently use three nutritional composition indicators (insect inclusion level, insect protein inclusion level, and total protein inclusion level). Environmental indicators (land use, water footprint, and greenhouse gas emissions) were

40–60% lower for the feed and food of edible insects than for traditional animal livestock, thereby diminishing the carbon footprint. Edible insects contribute to the circular economy because they can use the food and feed waste generated by animals and humans, adding value to these waste products. However, edible insect farming should be more efficient in terms of EU and the need to introduce renewable energy. An important future goal would be to increase the percentage of insect inclusion level in human and animal studies, to make a significant contribution to its application as novel supplementation for health. Moreover, the doses should be comparable to those more widely used for vegetable or animal protein sources. It is essential to increase the social acceptability of edible insects, the main barrier to their introduction into Western diets. Long-term studies are required to elucidate the effect of edible insects on human health, and more data are needed on environmental indicators of the use of edible insects for human food consumption. Food systems should explore alternative sources of proteins, and edible insects are an opportunity for the food industry to improve environmental indicators, with the associated economic benefits, social impact, and global enhancement of planetary health.

Funding: This work was supported by the elBullifoundation private foundation.

Acknowledgments: The authors thank the Spanish Ministry of Science and Competitiveness for their support via the KAIROS-BIOCIR Project PID2019-104925RB-C33 (AEO/FEDER, UE). The authors are responsible for the choice and presentation of information contained in this paper as well as for the opinions expressed therein, which are not necessarily those of UNESCO and do not commit this Organization. The authors express gratitude to Edmon de Haro for his contribution in the design of Figure 3.

Conflicts of Interest: The authors declare no conflict of interest.

References

1. Panel, G. *Future Food Systems: For People, our Planet, and Prosperity*; Global Panel on Agriculture and Food Systems for Nutrition: London, UK, 2020.
2. Steffen, W.; Richardson, K.; Rockström, J.; Cornell, S.E.; Fetzer, I.; Bennett, E.M.; Biggs, R.; Carpenter, S.R.; De Vries, W.; De Wit, C.A.; et al. Planetary boundaries: Guiding human development on a changing planet. *Science* **2015**, *347*, 1259855. [CrossRef] [PubMed]
3. Sterner, T.; Barbier, E.B.; Bateman, I.; Bijgaart, I.V.D.; Crépin, A.-S.; Edenhofer, O.; Fischer, C.; Habla, W.; Hassler, J.; Johansson-Stenman, O.; et al. Policy design for the Anthropocene. *Nat. Sustain.* **2019**, *2*, 14–21. [CrossRef]
4. Gerten, D.; Heck, V.; Jägermeyr, J.; Bodirsky, B.L.; Fetzer, I.; Jalava, M.; Kummu, M.; Lucht, W.; Rockström, J.; Schaphoff, S.; et al. Feeding ten billion people is possible within four terrestrial planetary boundaries. *Nat. Sustain.* **2020**, *3*, 200–208. [CrossRef]
5. Hunter, M.C.; Smith, R.G.; Schipanski, M.E.; Atwood, L.W.; Mortensen, D.A. Agriculture in 2050: Recalibrating targets for sustainable intensification. *Bioscience* **2017**, *67*, 386–391. [CrossRef]
6. Gu, D.; Andreev, K.; Dupre, M.E. Major trends in population growth around the world. *China CDC Wkly.* **2021**, *3*, 604. [CrossRef] [PubMed]
7. Oonincx, D.G.; de Boer, I.J. Environmental impact of the production of mealworms as a protein source for humans-a life cycle assessment. *PLoS ONE* **2012**, *7*, e51145. [CrossRef]
8. Willett, W.; Rockström, J.; Loken, B.; Springmann, M.; Lang, T.; Vermeulen, S.; Murray, C.J. Food in the Anthropocene: The EAT–Lancet Commission on healthy diets from sustainable food systems. *Lancet* **2019**, *393*, 447–492. [CrossRef]
9. Salter, A.M.; Lopez-Viso, C. Role of novel protein sources in sustainably meeting future global requirements. *Proc. Nutr. Soc.* **2021**, *80*, 186–194. [CrossRef]
10. Weindl, I.; Ost, M.; Wiedmer, P.; Schreiner, M.; Neugart, S.; Klopsch, R.; Kühnhold, H.; Kloas, W.; Henkel, I.M.; Schlüter, O.; et al. Sustainable food protein supply reconciling human and ecosystem health: A Leibniz Position. *Glob. Food Secur.* **2020**, *25*, 100367. [CrossRef]
11. Van Huis, A.; Van Itterbeeck, J.; Klunder, H.; Mertens, E.; Halloran, A.; Muir, G.; Vantomme, P. *Edible Insects: Future Prospects for Food and Feed Security*; Food and Agriculture Organization of the United Nations: Rome, Italy, 2013.
12. Nuță, D. New legal requirements regarding the placing of novel foods on the European Union market. *Annals. Food Sci. Technol.* **2017**. [CrossRef]
13. Turck, D.; Castenmiller, J.; De Henauw, S.; Hirsch-Ernst, K.I.; Kearney, J.; Maciuk, A.; Knutsen, H.K. Safety of dried yellow mealworm (Tenebrio molitor larva) as a novel food pursuant to Regulation (EU) 2015/2283. *EFSA J.* **2021**, *19*, e06343. [PubMed]
14. Committee, E.S. Risk profile related to production and consumption of insects as food and feed. *EFSA J.* **2015**, *13*, 4257. [CrossRef]
15. Turck, D.; Castenmiller, J.; De Henauw, S.; Hirsch-Ernst, K.I.; Kearney, J.; Knutsen, H.K. Safety of frozen and dried formulations from migratory locust (Locusta migratoria) as a Novel food pursuant to Regulation (EU) 2015/2283. *EFSA J.* **2021**, *19*, e06667.

16. Turck, D.; Bohn, T.; Castenmiller, J.; De Henauw, S.; Hirsch-Ernst, K.I.; Knutsen, H.K. Safety of partially defatted house cricket (Acheta domesticus) powder as a novel food pursuant to Regulation (EU) 2015/2283. *EFSA J.* **2022**, *20*, e07258. [PubMed]
17. Turck, D.; Castenmiller, J.; De Henauw, S.; Hirsch-Ernst, K.I.; Knutsen, H.K. EFSA NDA Panel (EFSA Panel on Nutrition, Novel Foods and Food Allergens), 2019. *Sci. Opin. Saf. Phenylcapsaicin A Nov. Foodpursuant Regul.* **2015**, *2283*. [CrossRef]
18. Van Huis, A.; Oonincx, D.G. The environmental sustainability of insects as food and feed. A review. *Agron. Sustain. Dev.* **2017**, *37*, 43. [CrossRef]
19. Payne, C.L.R.; Scarborough, P.; Rayner, M.; Nonaka, K. Are edible insects more or less 'healthy' than commonly consumed meats? A comparison using two nutrient profiling models developed to combat over- and undernutrition. *Eur. J. Clin. Nutr.* **2016**, *70*, 285–291. [CrossRef]
20. Da Silva Lucas, A.J.; de Oliveira, L.M.; Da Rocha, M.; Prentice, C. Edible insects: An alternative of nutritional, functional and bioactive compounds. *Food Chem.* **2020**, *311*, 126022. [CrossRef]
21. Hlongwane, Z.T.; Slotow, R.; Munyai, T.C. Nutritional Composition of Edible Insects Consumed in Africa: A Systematic Review. *Nutrients* **2020**, *12*, 2786. [CrossRef]
22. Weru, J.; Chege, P.; Kinyuru, J. Nutritional potential of edible insects: A systematic review of published data. *Int. J. Trop. Insect Sci.* **2021**, *41*, 2015–2037. [CrossRef]
23. Bertola, M.; Mutinelli, F. A Systematic Review on Viruses in Mass-Reared Edible Insect Species. *Viruses* **2021**, *13*, 2280. [CrossRef] [PubMed]
24. Ayensu, J.; Annan, R.A.; Edusei, A.; Lutterodt, H. Beyond nutrients, health effects of entomophagy: A systematic review. *Nutr. Food Sci.* **2018**, *49*, 2–17. [CrossRef]
25. D'Antonio, V.; Battista, N.; Sacchetti, G.; Di Mattia, C.; Serafini, M. Functional properties of edible insects: A systematic review. *Nutr. Res. Rev.* **2021**, 1–54. [CrossRef] [PubMed]
26. Testa, M.; Stillo, M.; Maffei, G.; Andriolo, V.; Gardois, P.; Zotti, C.M. Ugly but tasty: A systematic review of possible human and animal health risks related to entomophagy. *Crit. Rev. Food Sci. Nutr.* **2017**, *57*, 3747–3759. [CrossRef] [PubMed]
27. Ribeiro, M.S.; Ayllón, T.; Malirat, V.; Câmara, D.C.P.; Dias, C.M.G.; Louzada, G.; Fernandes-Ferreira, D.; Medronho, R.D.A.; Acevedo, R.C. High Prevalence of a Newly Discovered Wutai Mosquito Phasivirus in Mosquitoes from Rio de Janeiro, Brazil. *Insects* **2019**, *10*, 135. [CrossRef] [PubMed]
28. Page, M.J.; McKenzie, J.E.; Bossuyt, P.M.; Boutron, I.; Hoffmann, T.C.; Mulrow, C.D.; Moher, D. The PRISMA 2020 statement: An updated guideline for reporting systematic reviews. *Syst. Rev.* **2021**, *10*, 89. [CrossRef]
29. Hall, H.; Fitches, E.; Smith, R. *Insects as Animal Feed: Novel Ingredients for Use in Pet, Aquaculture and Livestock Diets*; CABI: Wallingford, UK, 2021.
30. Hooijmans, C.R.; Rovers, M.M.; de Vries, R.; Leenaars, M.; Ritskes-Hoitinga, M.; Langendam, M.W. SYRCLE's risk of bias tool for animal studies. *BMC Med. Res. Methodol.* **2014**, *14*, 43. [CrossRef]
31. Higgins, J.P.T.; Altman, D.G.; Gøtzsche, P.C.; Jüni, P.; Moher, D.; Oxman, A.D.; Savović, J.; Schulz, K.F.; Weeks, L.; Sterne, J.A.C.; et al. The Cochrane Collaboration's tool for assessing risk of bias in randomised trials. *BMJ* **2011**, *343*, d5928. [CrossRef]
32. Kim, J.; Yun, E.-Y.; Park, S.-W.; Goo, T.-W.; Seo, M. Allomyrina dichotoma larvae regulate food intake and body weight in high fat diet-induced obese mice through mTOR and Mapk signaling pathways. *Nutrients* **2016**, *8*, 100. [CrossRef]
33. Seo, M.; Goo, T.W.; Chung, M.Y.; Baek, M.; Hwang, J.S.; Kim, M.A.; Yun, E.Y. Tenebrio molitor larvae inhibit adipogenesis through AMPK and MAPKs signaling in 3T3-L1 adipocytes and obesity in high-fat diet-induced obese mice. *Int. J. Mol. Sci.* **2017**, *18*, 518. [CrossRef]
34. Bergmans, R.S.; Nikodemova, M.; Stull, V.J.; Rapp, A.; Malecki, K.M.C. Comparison of cricket diet with peanut-based and milk-based diets in the recovery from protein malnutrition in mice and the impact on growth, metabolism and immune function. *PLoS ONE* **2020**, *15*, e0234559. [CrossRef] [PubMed]
35. Dabbou, S.; Gai, F.; Biasato, I.; Capucchio, M.T.; Biasibetti, E.; Dezzutto, D.; Meneguz, M.; Plachà, I.; Gasco, L.; Schiavone, A. Black soldier fly defatted meal as a dietary protein source for broiler chickens: Effects on growth performance, blood traits, gut morphology and histological features. *J. Anim. Sci. Biotechnol.* **2018**, *9*, 49. [CrossRef] [PubMed]
36. Bovera, F.; Loponte, R.; Pero, M.E.; Cutrignelli, M.I.; Calabrò, S.; Musco, N.; Vassalotti, G.; Panettieri, V.; Lombardi, P.; Piccolo, G.; et al. Laying performance, blood profiles, nutrient digestibility and inner organs traits of hens fed an insect meal from Hermetia illucens larvae. *Res. Veter. Sci.* **2018**, *120*, 86–93. [CrossRef] [PubMed]
37. Biasato, I.; Ferrocino, I.; Biasibetti, E.; Grego, E.; Dabbou, S.; Sereno, A.; Gai, F.; Gasco, L.; Schiavone, A.; Cocolin, L.; et al. Modulation of intestinal microbiota, morphology and mucin composition by dietary insect meal inclusion in free-range chickens. *BMC Veter. Res.* **2018**, *14*, 383. [CrossRef]
38. Gasco, L.; Dabbou, S.; Trocino, A.; Xiccato, G.; Capucchio, M.T.; Biasato, I.; Dezzutto, D.; Birolo, M.; Meneguz, M.; Schiavone, A.; et al. Effect of dietary supplementation with insect fats on growth performance, digestive efficiency and health of rabbits. *J. Anim. Sci. Biotechnol.* **2019**, *10*, 4. [CrossRef]
39. Agbemafle, I.; Hanson, N.; Bries, A.E.; Reddy, M.B. Alternative Protein and Iron Sources from Edible Insects but Not Solanum torvum Improved Body Composition and Iron Status in Malnourished Rats. *Nutrients* **2019**, *11*, 2481. [CrossRef] [PubMed]

40. Pessina, F.; Frosini, M.; Marcolongo, P.; Fusi, F.; Saponara, S.; Gamberucci, A.; Dreassi, E. Antihypertensive, cardio-and neuroprotective effects of Tenebrio molitor (Coleoptera: Tenebrionidae) defatted larvae in spontaneously hypertensive rats. *PLoS ONE* **2020**, *15*, e0233788. [CrossRef]
41. Ahn, M.Y.; Kim, B.J.; Kim, H.J.; Jin, J.M.; Yoon, H.J.; Hwang, J.S.; Lee, B.M. Anti-diabetic activity of field cricket glycosaminoglycan by ameliorating oxidative stress. *BMC Complement. Med. Ther.* **2020**, *20*, 1–10. [CrossRef]
42. Ahn, M.Y.; Hwang, J.S.; Kim, M.-J.; Park, K.-K. Antilipidemic effects and gene expression profiling of the glycosaminoglycans from cricket in rats on a high fat diet. *Arch. Pharmacal Res.* **2016**, *39*, 926–936. [CrossRef]
43. Skau, J.K.H.; Touch, B.; Chhoun, C.; Chea, M.; Unni, U.S.; Makurat, J.; Filteau, S.; Wieringa, F.T.; Dijkhuizen, M.A.; Ritz, C.; et al. Effects of animal source food and micronutrient fortification in complementary food products on body composition, iron status, and linear growth: A randomized trial in Cambodia. *Am. J. Clin. Nutr.* **2015**, *101*, 742–751. [CrossRef]
44. Bauserman, M.; Lokangaka, A.; Gado, J.; Close, K.; Wallace, D.; Kodondi, K.-K.; Tshefu, A.; Bose, C. A cluster-randomized trial determining the efficacy of caterpillar cereal as a locally available and sustainable complementary food to prevent stunting and anaemia. *Public Health Nutr.* **2015**, *18*, 1785–1792. [CrossRef] [PubMed]
45. Nirmala, I.; Pramono, M.S. Sago worms as a nutritious traditional and alternative food for rural children in Southeast Sulawesi, Indonesia. *Asia Pac. J. Clin. Nutr.* **2017**, *26*, s40–s49. [PubMed]
46. Stull, V.J.; Finer, E.; Bergmans, R.S.; Febvre, H.P.; Longhurst, C.; Manter, D.K.; Patz, J.A.; Weir, T.L. Impact of Edible Cricket Consumption on Gut Microbiota in Healthy Adults, a Double-blind, Randomized Crossover Trial. *Sci. Rep.* **2018**, *8*, 10762. [CrossRef]
47. Vangsoe, M.T.; Joergensen, M.S.; Heckmann, L.-H.L.; Hansen, M. Effects of insect protein supplementation during resistance training on changes in muscle mass and strength in young men. *Nutrients* **2018**, *10*, 335. [CrossRef] [PubMed]
48. Vangsoe, M.T.; Thogersen, R.; Bertram, H.C.; Heckmann, L. H.L.; Hansen, M. Ingestion of Insect Protein Isolate Enhances Blood Amino Acid Concentrations Similar to Soy Protein in A Human Trial. *Nutrients* **2018**, *10*, 1357. [CrossRef] [PubMed]
49. Lokman, I.H.; Ibitoye, E.B.; Hezmee, M.N.M.; Goh, Y.M.; Zuki, A.B.Z.; Jimoh, A.A. Effects of chitin and chitosan from cricket and shrimp on growth and carcass performance of broiler chickens. *Trop. Anim. Health Prod.* **2019**, *51*, 2219–2225. [CrossRef]
50. Van Zanten, H.H.; Mollenhorst, H.; Oonincx, D.G.; Bikker, P.; Meerburg, B.G.; de Boer, I.J. From environmental nuisance to environmental opportunity: Housefly larvae convert waste to livestock feed. *J. Clean. Prod.* **2015**, *102*, 362–369. [CrossRef]
51. Salomone, R.; Saija, G.; Mondello, G.; Giannetto, A.; Fasulo, S.; Savastano, D. Environmental impact of food waste bioconversion by insects: Application of life cycle assessment to process using Hermetia illucens. *J. Clean. Prod.* **2017**, *140*, 890–905. [CrossRef]
52. Muys, B.; Roffeis, M. Life cycle assessment of proteins from insects. In Proceedings of the Insects to feed the world: 1st International Conference, Wageningen, The Netherlands, 14–17 May 2014.
53. Thévenot, A.; Rivera, J.L.; Wilfart, A.; Maillard, F.; Hassouna, M.; Senga-Kiesse, T.; LE Feon, S.; Aubin, J. Mealworm meal for animal feed: Environmental assessment and sensitivity analysis to guide future prospects. *J. Clean. Prod.* **2018**, *170*, 1260–1267. [CrossRef]
54. Halloran, A.; Roos, N.; Eilenberg, J.; Cerutti, A.; Bruun, S. Life cycle assessment of edible insects for food protein: A review. *Agron. Sustain. Dev.* **2016**, *36*, 57. [CrossRef]
55. Miglietta, P.P.; De Leo, F.; Ruberti, M.; Massari, S. Mealworms for food: A water footprint perspective. *Water* **2015**, *7*, 6190–6203. [CrossRef]
56. Fan, S.; Headey, D.; Rue, C.; Thomas, T. Food Systems for Human and Planetary Health: Economic Perspectives and Challenges. *Annu. Rev. Resour. Econ.* **2021**, *13*, 131–156. [CrossRef]
57. Gill, S.R.; Benatar, S.R. Reflections on the political economy of planetary health. *Rev. Int. Politi. Econ.* **2020**, *27*, 167–190. [CrossRef]
58. Gasco, L.; Józefiak, A.; Henry, M. Beyond the protein concept: Health aspects of using edible insects on animals. *J. Insects Food Feed* **2021**, *7*, 715–741. [CrossRef]
59. Ozcan, L.; Tabas, I. Role of endoplasmic reticulum stress in metabolic disease and other disorders. *Annu. Rev. Med.* **2012**, *63*, 317–328. [CrossRef]
60. Yoshida, T.; Yoshida, J. Simultaneous analytical method for urinary metabolites of organophosphorus compounds and moth repellents in general population. *J. Chromatogr. B Anal. Technol. Biomed Life Sci.* **2012**, *880*, 66–73. [CrossRef] [PubMed]
61. Gasco, L.; Biasato, I.; Dabbou, S.; Schiavone, A.; Gai, F. Animals Fed Insect-Based Diets: State-of-the-Art on Digestibility, Performance and Product Quality. *Animals* **2019**, *9*, 170. [CrossRef] [PubMed]
62. Olson, R.; Gavin-Smith, B.; Ferraboschi, C.; Kraemer, K. Food fortification: The advantages, disadvantages and lessons from sight and life programs. *Nutrients* **2021**, *13*, 1118. [CrossRef]
63. Owino, V.O.; Skau, J.; Omollo, S.; Konyole, S.; Kinyuru, J.; Estambale, B.; Owuor, B.; Nanna, R.; Friis, H. WinFood data from Kenya and Cambodia: Constraints on field procedures. *Food Nutr. Bull.* **2015**, *36*, S41–S46. [CrossRef]
64. Moruzzo, R.; Mancini, S.; Guidi, A. Edible Insects and Sustainable Development Goals. *Insects* **2021**, *12*, 557. [CrossRef]
65. Rumpold, B.A.; Schlüter, O.K. Nutritional composition and safety aspects of edible insects. *Mol. Nutr. Food Res.* **2013**, *57*, 802–823. [CrossRef] [PubMed]
66. Kinyuru, J.N.; Kenji, G.M.; Njoroge, S.M.; Ayieko, M. Effect of processing methods on the in vitro protein digestibility and vitamin content of edible winged termite (*Macrotermes subhylanus*) and grasshopper (*Ruspolia differens*). *Food Bioprocess Technol.* **2010**, *3*, 778–782. [CrossRef]

67. Hixson, S.M. Fish nutrition and current issues in aquaculture: The balance in providing safe and nutritious seafood, in an environmentally sustainable manner. *J. Aquac. Res. Dev.* **2014**, *5*. [CrossRef]
68. Parodi, A.; Leip, A.; De Boer, I.J.M.; Slegers, P.M.; Ziegler, F.; Temme, E.H.M.; Herrero, M.; Tuomisto, H.L.; Valin, H.; Van Middelaar, C.E.; et al. The potential of future foods for sustainable and healthy diets. *Nat. Sustain.* **2018**, *1*, 782–789. [CrossRef]
69. Woolf, P.J.; Fu, L.L.; Basu, A. vProtein: Identifying optimal amino acid complements from plant-based foods. *PLoS ONE* **2011**, *6*, e18836. [CrossRef] [PubMed]
70. Lee, S.H.; Park, D.; Yang, G.; Bae, D.-K.; Yang, Y.-H.; Kim, T.K.; Kim, D.; Kyung, J.; Yeon, S.; Koo, K.C.; et al. Silk and silkworm pupa peptides suppress adipogenesis in preadipocytes and fat accumulation in rats fed a high-fat diet. *Eur. J. Nutr.* **2012**, *51*, 1011–1019. [CrossRef] [PubMed]
71. Wu, Q.; Jia, J.; Yan, H.; Du, J.; Gui, Z. A novel angiotensin-I converting enzyme (ACE) inhibitory peptide from gastrointestinal protease hydrolysate of silkworm pupa (Bombyx mori) protein: Biochemical characterization and molecular docking study. *Peptides* **2015**, *68*, 17–24. [CrossRef]
72. Yi, L.; Lakemond, C.M.; Sagis, L.M.; Eisner-Schadler, V.; van Huis, A.; van Boekel, M.A. Extraction and characterisation of protein fractions from five insect species. *Food Chem.* **2013**, *141*, 3341–3348. [CrossRef]
73. Dobermann, D.; Swift, J.A.; Field, L.M. Opportunities and hurdles of edible insects for food and feed. *Nutr. Bull.* **2017**, *42*, 293–308. [CrossRef]
74. Becker, N.S.; Margos, G.; Blum, H.; Krebs, S.; Graf, A.; Lane, R.S.; Castillo-Ramírez, S.; Sing, A.; Fingerle, V. Recurrent evolution of host and vector association in bacteria of the Borrelia burgdorferi sensu lato species complex. *BMC Genom.* **2016**, *17*, 734. [CrossRef]
75. Tang, J.E.; Perco, J.G.; Moore, D.; Wilkinson, S.B.; Phillips, S. Resistance training alters the response of fed state mixed muscle protein synthesis in young men. *Am. J. Physiol. Regul. Integr. Comp. Physiol.* **2008**, *294*, R172–R178. [CrossRef] [PubMed]
76. Candow, D.G.; Chilibeck, P.D.; Facci, M.; Abeysekara, S.; Zello, G.A. Protein supplementation before and after resistance training in older men. *Eur. J. Appl. Physiol.* **2006**, *97*, 548–556. [CrossRef] [PubMed]
77. Baum, J.I.; Kim, I.Y.; Wolfe, R.R. Protein consumption and the elderly: What is the optimal level of intake? *Nutrients* **2016**, *8*, 359. [CrossRef] [PubMed]
78. Nowakowski, A.C.; Miller, A.C.; Miller, M.E.; Xiao, H.; Wu, X. Potential health benefits of edible insects. *Crit. Rev. Food Sci. Nutr.* **2020**, *62*, 3499–3508. [CrossRef] [PubMed]
79. Liaqat, F.; Eltem, R. Chitooligosaccharides and their biological activities: A comprehensive review. *Carbohydr. Polym.* **2018**, *184*, 243–259. [CrossRef]
80. Finke, M.D. Complete nutrient composition of commercially raised invertebrates used as food for insectivores. *Zoo Biol. Publ. Affil. Am. Zoo Aquar. Assoc.* **2002**, *21*, 269–285. [CrossRef]
81. De Gier, S.; Verhoeckx, K. Insect (food) allergy and allergens. *Mol. Immunol.* **2018**, *100*, 82–106. [CrossRef]
82. Barennes, H.; Phimmasane, M.; Rajaonarivo, C. Insect consumption to address undernutrition, a national survey on the prevalence of insect consumption among adults and vendors in Laos. *PLoS ONE* **2015**, *10*, e0136458. [CrossRef]
83. Smetana, S.; Leonhardt, L.; Kauppi, S.-M.; Pajic, A.; Heinz, V. Insect margarine: Processing, sustainability and design. *J. Clean. Prod.* **2020**, *264*, 121670. [CrossRef]
84. Tello, A.; Aganovic, K.; Parniakov, O.; Carter, A.; Heinz, V.; Smetana, S. Product development and environmental impact of an insect-based milk alternative. *Future Foods* **2021**, *4*, 100080. [CrossRef]
85. Hall, F.G.; Jones, O.G.; O'Haire, M.E.; Liceaga, A.M. Functional properties of tropical banded cricket (Gryllodes sigillatus) protein hydrolysates. *Food Chem.* **2017**, *224*, 414–422. [CrossRef] [PubMed]
86. Megido, R.C.; Alabi, T.; Nieus, C.; Blecker, C.; Danthine, S.; Bogaert, J.; Haubruge, A.; Francis, F. Optimisation of a cheap and residential small-scale production of edible crickets with local by-products as an alternative protein-rich human food source in Ratanakiri Province, Cambodia. *J. Sci. Food Agric.* **2016**, *96*, 627–632. [CrossRef] [PubMed]
87. Spiertz, H. Food production, crops and sustainability: Restoring confidence in science and technology. *Curr. Opin. Environ. Sustain.* **2010**, *2*, 439–443. [CrossRef]
88. Abbasi, T.; Abbasi, S. Biomass energy and the environmental impacts associated with its production and utilization. *Renew. Sustain. Energy Rev.* **2010**, *14*, 919–937. [CrossRef]
89. Gravel, A.; Doyen, A. The use of edible insect proteins in food: Challenges and issues related to their functional properties. *Innov. Food Sci. Emerg. Technol.* **2020**, *59*, 102272. [CrossRef]
90. Springmann, M.; Clark, M.; Mason-D'Croz, D.; Wiebe, K.; Bodirsky, B.L.; Lassaletta, L.; de Vries, W.; Vermeulen, S.J.; Herrero, M.; Carlson, K.M.; et al. Options for keeping the food system within environmental limits. *Nature* **2018**, *562*, 519–525. [CrossRef]
91. Yen, A.L. Entomophagy and insect conservation: Some thoughts for digestion. *J. Insect Conserv.* **2009**, *13*, 667–670. [CrossRef]
92. Birch, A.N.E.; Begg, G.S.; Squire, G.R. How agro-ecological research helps to address food security issues under new IPM and pesticide reduction policies for global crop production systems. *J. Exp. Bot.* **2011**, *62*, 3251–3261. [CrossRef]
93. De Vries, M.; de Boer, I.J. Comparing environmental impacts for livestock products: A review of life cycle assessments. *Livest. Sci.* **2010**, *128*, 1–11. [CrossRef]
94. Flachowsky, G.; Meyer, U.; Südekum, K.-H. Land Use for Edible Protein of Animal Origin-A Review. *Animals* **2017**, *7*, 25. [CrossRef]

95. Tomberlin, J.K.; Sheppard, D.C. Lekking behavior of the black soldier fly (Diptera: Stratiomyidae). *Fla. Entomol.* **2001**, *84*, 729. [CrossRef]
96. Van Raamsdonk, L.W.D.; Van Der Fels-Klerx, H.J.; De Jong, J. New feed ingredients: The insect opportunity. *Food Addit. Contam. Part A* **2017**, *34*, 1384–1397. [CrossRef]
97. Smith, L.G.; Kirk, G.J.D.; Jones, P.J.; Williams, A.G. The greenhouse gas impacts of converting food production in England and Wales to organic methods. *Nat. Commun.* **2019**, *10*, 4641. [CrossRef]
98. Ayilara, M.S.; Olanrewaju, O.S.; Babalola, O.O.; Odeyemi, O. Waste management through composting: Challenges and potentials. *Sustainability* **2020**, *12*, 4456. [CrossRef]
99. Béné, C.; Prager, S.D.; Achicanoy, H.A.; Toro, P.A.; Lamotte, L.; Bonilla, C.; Mapes, B.R. Global map and indicators of food system sustainability. *Sci. Data* **2019**, *6*, 279. [CrossRef] [PubMed]
100. Jensen, N.H.; Lieberoth, A. We will eat disgusting foods together–Evidence of the normative basis of Western entomophagy-disgust from an insect tasting. *Food Qual. Prefer.* **2019**, *72*, 109–115. [CrossRef]
101. Gullan, P.J.; Cranston, P.S. *The Insects: An Outline of Entomology*; John Wiley & Sons: New York, NY, USA, 2014.
102. Verbeke, W.; Spranghers, T.; De Clercq, P.; De Smet, S.; Sas, B.; Eeckhout, M. Insects in animal feed: Acceptance and its determinants among farmers, agriculture sector stakeholders and citizens. *Anim. Feed Sci. Technol.* **2015**, *204*, 72–87. [CrossRef]
103. Melgar-Lalanne, G.; Hernández-Álvarez, A.-J.; Salinas-Castro, A. Edible insects processing: Traditional and innovative technologies. *Compr. Rev. Food Sci. Food Saf.* **2019**, *18*, 1166–1191. [CrossRef]
104. Onwezen, M.C.; Bouwman, E.P.; Reinders, M.J.; Dagevos, H. A systematic review on consumer acceptance of alternative proteins: Pulses, algae, insects, plant-based meat alternatives, and cultured meat. *Appetite* **2021**, *159*, 105058. [CrossRef]

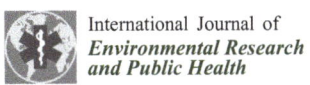

Article

Consumers' Acceptability and Perception of Edible Insects as an Emerging Protein Source

Marta Ros-Baró [1], Violeida Sánchez-Socarrás [1], Maria Santos-Pagès [1], Anna Bach-Faig [2,3,4] and Alicia Aguilar-Martínez [2,3,*]

1. Faculty of Health Sciences, Open University of Catalonia (UOC), 08018 Barcelona, Spain
2. FoodLab Research Group, Faculty of Health Sciences, Open University of Catalonia (UOC), 08018 Barcelona, Spain
3. Unesco Chair on Food, Culture and Development, Open University of Catalonia (UOC), 08018 Barcelona, Spain
4. Food and Nutrition Area, Barcelona Official College of Pharmacists, 08009 Barcelona, Spain
* Correspondence: aaguilarmart@uoc.edu

Abstract: In recent years in Western Europe, studies on entomophagy have drawn the attention of many researchers interested in identifying parameters that could improve the acceptability of insect consumption in order to introduce insects as a sustainable source of protein into the future diet. Analysing the factors involved in consumer acceptability in the Mediterranean area could help to improve their future acceptance. A cross-sectional study was conducted using an ad-hoc questionnaire in which 1034 consumers participated. The questionnaire responses allowed us to study the areas relevant to acceptance: neophobia, social norms, familiarity, experiences of consumption and knowledge of benefits. Only 13.15% of participants had tried insects. Disgust, lack of custom and food safety were the main reasons for avoiding insect consumption. Consequently, preparations with an appetising appearance need to be offered, with flours being the most accepted format. The 40–59-year-old age group was the one most willing to consume them. To introduce edible insects as food in the future, it is important to inform people about their health, environmental and economic benefits because that could increase their willingness to include them in their diet.

Keywords: edible insects; food preferences; entomophagy; nutrition surveys; food choice; food neophobia

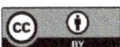

1. Introduction

The substantial improvements in people's health status, hygiene conditions and life expectancy, in the majority of countries over the past 50 years, means that the world population is predicted to increase considerably by 2050 [1]. The rising cost of animal protein production and the increasing environmental pressure on agriculture and livestock farming [2] necessitate the search for productive alternatives and innovative techniques for food production which take into account the nutritional, environmental and sociocultural dimensions of food sustainability [3,4].

The use of insects as human food could meet these demands and prove to be a valid strategy for improving global food security FAO [5]. Compared to conventional livestock, insect production has a higher conversion rate to food. Insects can grow in organic waste (thereby acting as bioconverters), occupy less production space and produce less greenhouse gases [6–8]. For example, when compared to beef production, Ros-Baró et al. [9] found that insect production was responsible for around 95% less greenhouse gas emissions, land and water use, and 62% less energy use. Regarding their nutritional composition, edible insects have bioactive compounds that are beneficial to health: they have the ability to improve intestinal microbiota and are claimed to have not only antioxidant properties, but also to improve some blood parameters [9]. Although nutritional composition depends on the type of insect, its stage of growth and its food, all insects generally have high levels of essential amino acids [10] and highly soluble proteins capable of forming gels or emulsions with a digestibility rate of 78–98%. They contain unsaturated fatty acids [11], micronutrients (riboflavin, pantothenic acid, biotin, thiamine, Vitamin B12, iron, zinc and calcium) and dietary fibre [12–15]. Despite these advantages, including new foods in a diet is a complex issue that requires consumer acceptance and finding a place for them in the culinary system [16,17].

Neophobia, or the refusal—in this case—to try new foods, is one of the main factors influencing the acceptability of edible insects [18–21]. According to Faccio et al. [22,23], people with food neophobia are also more reluctant to try insects. The degree of rejection is related to dislike or disgust, and to a belief that their consumption is associated with cultures from distant and generally low-income countries [17,24]. The refusal to consume insects is based on cultural reasons, since they are considered unpleasant and, in some cases, harmful, or on doubts about the feasibility and viability of farming them safely [24,25].

Entomophagy was a common practice among our ancestors and has been acknowledged as an important role in human development [26,27]. Numerous references to this practice have been found in the literature and history of the ancient peoples of China and the peoples of the Roman Empire, as well as in the sacred writings of Christianity, Judaism and Islam [27]. In Western countries, entomophagy was abandoned many years ago [28].

Providing information about, having positive experiences of, and—at a gastronomical level—incorporating insects into usual recipes together allow their consumption to be endowed with familiarity and proximity [18,29]. Preparations that can make their appearance more appetising will influence their acceptance and, most likely, their consumption as novel foods [30–32].

To date, insects have been very much off the menu in Western cuisine. China, Thailand, Japan, Colombia, Mexico, Peru, Brazil and several African nations are the countries with the greatest tradition of insect consumption [33,34]. The most eaten insects include saturniid caterpillars, beetles, ants, termites, crickets, grasshoppers and palm weevil larvae [35]. In Europe, they appear to be better accepted in Austria, Belgium, Holland and France due to their wider introduction into the food industry as a novel food [36]. However, the edible insect industry is progressing rapidly in order to meet the demand for insects as a food ingredient [36] and is also gaining interest in Western countries [37,38], so more studies in different populations are needed to provide information on factors that may favour the acceptance of insects as food for human consumption.

The aim of this study is to explore the opinions of consumers in Mediterranean Europe of insect consumption. Based on questionnaire responses, the study aims to show the differences between the sociodemographic groups surveyed; to identify which type of insect authorised by the European Food Safety Authority (EFSA) is the most consumed, and in what context; to explore the reasons for refusing to consume them; and to identify which presentations are considered to be the most attractive and what factors might influence potential marketing or consumption to improve the acceptability of insect protein as food for humans in the future.

2. Materials and Methods

2.1. Study Design

An observational, descriptive, cross-sectional study was conducted to collect data on the consumption of insects and the potential factors influencing their acceptance as a new source of alternative protein in a Spanish population sample. The data collection tool was an ad-hoc questionnaire created from a review of previous studies [17–21]. The survey was prevalidated by researchers from the FoodLab group to assess the relevance and appropriateness of the questions. The process of administering the survey was then piloted with a small sample of known persons. After analysing the responses, changes were made to the initial questionnaire used. The final version consisted of 18 questions relating to the potential factors influencing the acceptance of insect consumption, such as neophobia, social and cultural norms, familiarity, perceived benefits or visual characteristics of the preparation or presentation. Nine questions had a binary Yes/No response option, and nine had multiple options to choose from. The questionnaire also included sociodemographic data, such as the respondents' gender, age and place of residence.

2.2. Participants

The study population comprised adults who mainly resided in Catalonia (Spain) and who voluntarily agreed to answer the questionnaire.

2.3. Administration of the Questionnaire

The questionnaire was created on the Qualtrics platform which specialises in online surveys, and was distributed via social media in September 2022. The first screen contained general information about the study. Prior to completing the questionnaire, each participant had to give consent to participate. To ensure the confidentiality of the results obtained, the questionnaires were anonymous and participants could not be identified.

The study was conducted in compliance with the ethical principles for research involving human beings and the processing of personal data contained in the Declaration of Helsinki and was approved by the Ethics Committee of the Open University of Catalonia, CE22-PR28.

2.4. Data Analysis

All responses were analysed using the SPSS version 15.0 for Windows. Yes/No responses were considered nominal and dichotomous categorical variables. Pearson's χ^2 test, which considers a non-parametric test to measure the differences between an observed distribution and a theoretical one, allowed the relationship between these dichotomous variables to be analysed. In the descriptive analysis of data, demographic characteristics and questions with multiple options were expressed as absolute and relative frequencies. For all calculations, a 95% confidence interval was used and relationships of $p < 0.005$ were deemed statistically significant. The results obtained are shown in descriptive tables for the demographic characteristics of the sample, tables of the relationship between the dichotomous variables and their distribution by the participants' gender and age group and descriptive tables of the preferred consumption formats or contexts.

3. Results

The survey was answered by a total of 1034 participants, of whom 68.85% were women and 66% were over 40 years of age. Table 1 shows the sociodemographic characteristics of the participants by gender, age and province of residence. The participants were mainly distributed between the two most populated provinces of Catalonia (Spain).

While most participants (79.8%) expressed interest in trying new foods or being innovative with their cooking, only 48.2% reported that they had tried new foods in the past year. Of these, quinoa and plant-based foods for vegetarians or vegans were the most widely chosen options. Sushi or soya were also among the most frequently mentioned foods. In terms of insect consumption, 86.9% of participants indicated that they had not consumed them and were unwilling to cook them (71%) or to include them in their usual diet (82.2%). Disgust, followed by lack of custom, and safety concerns were the main reasons given by the participants to justify their lack of interest in consuming insects. However, flour-based preparations were the most attractive option in the event of having to consume them (23.5%), followed by biscuits and bars (around 6%). Of those in "Others" ($N = 162$) and on which information was available, the most preferred options, in descending order, were the following: powders, flakes, sweets, burgers and meatballs. Among those who stated that they had eaten insects, the most consumed one was the cricket (5.2%), followed by mealworms (4.8%). Table 2 shows the distribution of participants' responses to the questionnaire.

Table 1. Sample characteristics.

	N	%
Gender		
Female	712	68.86
Male	321	31.04
Non-binary	1	0.1
Age		
18–24	160	15.47
25–39	191	18.47
40–49	274	26.5
50–59	341	32.98
60 or over	68	6.58
Resident in Catalonia		
Tarragona	498	48.16
Barcelona	420	40.62
Girona	50	4.83
Lleida	24	2.32
Resident outside Catalonia	42	4.06

Table 2. Distribution of participants' responses to the questionnaire.

	N	%
When it comes to cooking, do you like trying new things or being innovative with how you prepare your food?		
Yes	825	79.78
No	209	20.22
In the past year, have you introduced new foods into your diet?		
Yes	498	48.16
No	536	51.84
If so, select the foods introduced into the diet		
Tropical fruits	50	4.83
Kefir	79	7.64
Tofu	56	5.41
Seaweed	61	5.89
Sushi	94	9.09
Quinoa	143	13.82
Oats	98	9.47
Soya	74	7.15
Shiitake	43	4.15
Foods for vegetarians or vegans	112	10.83
Others	135	13.05
Have you ever eaten insects?		
Yes	136	13.15
No	898	86.85
If so, what insects have you eaten?		
Crickets	54	5.22
Grasshoppers	39	3.77
Mealworms	50	4.83
Others	39	3.77

Table 2. Cont.

	N	%
Main reasons for not consuming insects		
Disgust	395	38.2
Doubts about safety	98	9.47
It seems to me to be a primitive practice	3	0.29
It seems to me to be an option only for societies with few economic resources	6	0.58
Lack of knowledge	17	1.64
Lack of custom	159	15.37
Cultural reasons	68	6.57
Others	118	11.41
Would you include insects in your usual diet?		
Yes	171	16.54
No	850	82.2
No response	13	1.26
Would you be willing to cook insects at home?		
Yes	290	28.05
No	735	71.08
No response	9	0.87
Would you offer insect-based dishes in a restaurant?		
Yes	259	25.04
No	764	73.89
No response	11	1.06
Do you think insect-based dishes would be welcomed by the general public?		
Yes	170	16.44
No	846	81.82
No response	18	1.74
Would knowing that insect consumption has the potential to be a sustainable food practice encourage you to consume them?		
Yes	511	49.42
No	499	48.25
No response	24	2.33
Do you think insect consumption might become a common practice in the future?		
Yes	603	58.32
No	403	38.97
No response	28	2.71
In what preparations do you think insects would be more attractive?		
If their natural appearance cannot be seen	722	69.82
If their natural appearance can be seen	102	9.87
No response	210	20.31
Which presentations do you find more attractive?		
Flours	243	23.5
Bars	60	5.8
Gels	1	0.09
Jellies	5	0.48
Biscuits	63	6.09
Pills	24	2.32
Smoothies	23	2.22
Others	162	15.66

Analysis of the responses by gender showed significant differences ($p < 0.001$) between men and women regarding their willingness to consume insects, with women being less willing to cook and include them in their diet in a usual manner (Supplementary material, Supplementary Table S1). Likewise, men were more willing than women to consume them in preparations where the whole insect could be seen.

Significant differences were observed in insect consumption by age (Supplementary material, Supplementary Table S2), with those over 60 years of age reporting lower consumption of insects and less intention to consume them. Similarly, they were less willing to try new foods. The age group that was most familiar with insect consumption was the 40–59-year-old one, at 7.2%. These results contrast with the perception, expressed by respondents, of a greater acceptance by adolescents. They considered adolescents to be the age group that would be the most willing to welcome insect consumption, and older adults to be the one least willing to do so.

The context or circumstances in which insects were introduced proved to be different from that of the consumption of other foods.

When the respondents were asked in what context or circumstances they usually introduced new foods into their usual diet, differences regarding insect consumption were found. Participants who reported having consumed insects (13.15%) had done so mostly while on holiday (53.77%). Regarding the other foods, most acknowledged that they had introduced them after consuming them at someone else's home (19.87%) or for health reasons (19.27%) (Figure 1). Although the response to the general question about whether insect-based dishes would be welcomed by the general public was negative, the possibility of offering them in restaurants was more plausible since it decreased negativity by 3.4% compared to the previous question.

Although the majority of study participants would not include insects in their usual diet (82.2%), they were much more positive about their future incorporation (58.3% considered insect eating to possibly be a usual practice in the future). Furthermore, knowing their potential benefits for sustainability improved their willingness to consume them. As the results in Table 3 show, when relating respondents' willingness to include insects in their usual diet, it was found that while 51.9% responded that they would not try them, 56.17% would do so because they were a sustainable protein. The relationship between dichotomous variables was statistically significant ($p = 0.001$).

Table 3. Relationship between willingness to include insects in the usual diet and willingness to include them knowing that doing so has the potential to be a sustainable practice.

Insects Usual Diet	Contribution to Sustainability No N (%)	Contribution to Sustainability Yes N (%)	Total
No	301 (60.32)	224 (43.83)	525 (51.98)
Yes	198 (39.68)	287 (56.17)	485 (48.02)
Total	499 (100)	511 (100)	1010 (100)

Pearson's Chi^2 (1) = 26.3751 p = 0.0013. Excludes no response to each item

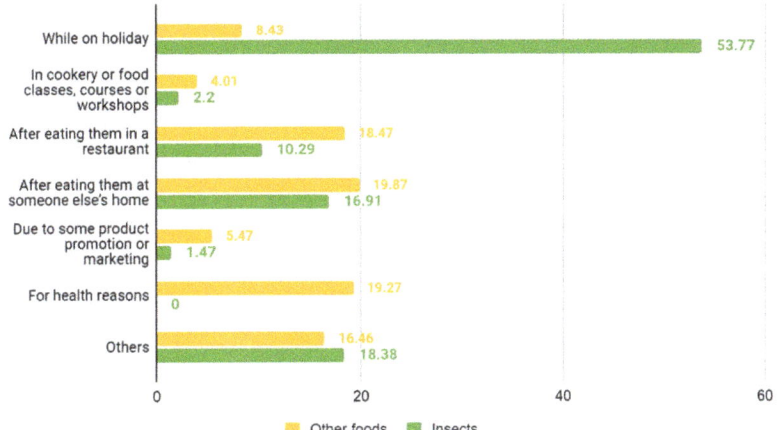

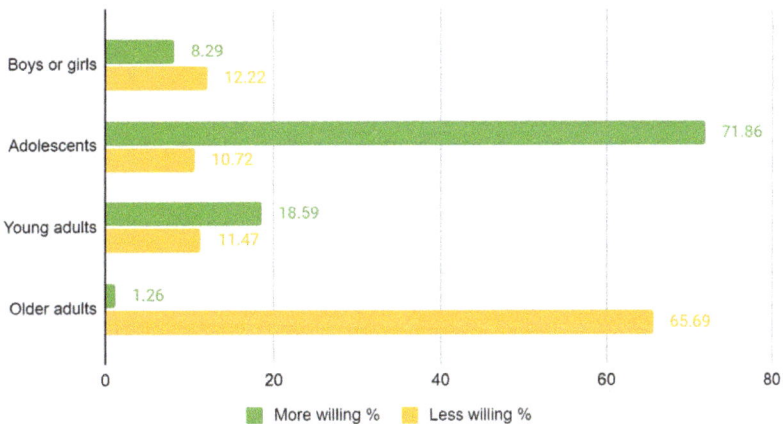

Figure 1. Distribution of food introduction contexts and level of reception by population group. (**a**) Context or circumstances of introduction of new foods into the diet. (**b**) Population group and willingness to welcome insect consumption.

4. Discussion

This study investigated consumer perception of the inclusion of edible insects in human food and showed their poor acceptance by the studied population. Consistent with the studies by [17,18], neophobia was found to be a key obstacle to the acceptance of such products, despite the fact that more and more people appear to be willing to incorporate new foods into the food pattern of the Mediterranean diet, which is typical of the study population [38]. The respondents' mentions of quinoa, sushi or soya as foods recently introduced into the diet reflect the effects of market globalisation on food. Similarly, other recently incorporated products were foods for vegetarians and vegans (10.8%), which is consistent with the observed increase in this trend in society [39,40]. Insect consumption was low, as only 13.1% of respondents mentioned that they had consumed them. This is a higher percentage than that obtained in previous studies, such as the one by Verbeke et al. [17].

Some previous studies have suggested that young people may be more attracted to insect consumption and, for that reason, their degree of neophobia of trying new foods is lower than other age groups, such as young adults or older adults Verbeke et al. [17]. However, contrary to the findings of Verbeke et al. [17], this study found that the 40–49-year-old group was more willing to accept insect consumption, unlike the findings of Hartman et al. [20] where age was not associated with willingness to eat insects.

Consistent with other studies [18], male respondents in this study appeared to have a lower degree of neophobia and were more willing to cook insects and to introduce them into the usual diet than female respondents were.

According to the results obtained from the survey, insects were mostly consumed during a trip to countries where there was a tradition of eating them. While such an experience may be an initial opportunity to try the product and then to incorporate it if the experience is positive [41], in many cases the first experience is of preparations that include whole insects, and this may give rise to even more neophobia among the Western population [42,43]. In addition, there is a marked difference between eating raw and cooked insects, and the incorporation of other ingredients and cooking processes can improve their acceptance at multiple levels [44]. The results of this study show that 69.8% of participants would prefer preparations where the natural appearance could not be seen, which is consistent with other studies [3,20,45–47] which assert that consumers in Western cultures are more willing to eat a processed product than a whole one. Besides the visual characteristics, the willingness to consume new products is favoured by a familiarity with them [20]. In this sense, flour was the preferred format for respondents, so its incorporation into foods such as bread or biscuits may determine better acceptability and a lower degree of neophobia given their familiarity to the Mediterranean population. In addition, it has been reported that personal participation in culinary preparations reduces the degree of disgust felt [8,48]. The use of insect flour as an ingredient would be easy to incorporate into multiple recipes of the cultures of Mediterranean Europe [49,50]. In the quest for strategies or presentations that disguise the presence or shape of insects to meet consumer demand [51], the food industry has identified their potential use in seasoning powders for soups instead of commercial products made from pork or chicken, margarines, milk or burgers [52–55] and also as an emulsifier [45]. Strategies introducing the partial replacement of meat with sustainable protein sources, such as vegetables and insect flours, were successfully employed in food product formulations containing less animal protein [56]. Likewise, Spence et al. [52] have described the application of techniques used in haute cuisine.

Social and cultural norms are also factors that determine food customs and the incorporation of foods [53]. Social acceptance is a significant predictor of the willingness to eat insects, since entomophagy is deemed a primitive practice [25,48] or a source of nutrients in times of economic scarcity [57]. In this study, however, neither the consideration of insect eating as a primitive practice nor the relationship to low economic resources appeared to be important barriers to consumption. While insect preparations might be considered delicacies in Western countries, they are considered a food for basic use, or for use during food emergencies, in other parts of the world [58]. The lack of custom or doubts about insect safety seem to have the greatest impact on the food choice and, after disgust, they are the main reasons for rejection. There are also concerns about the possible presence of pathogenic organisms and heavy metals, and about the potential allergic reactions to their consumption [8,37,59,60]. At every stage of edible insect processing (from farm to fork), control measures and hazard analysis and critical control points (HACCPs) are needed to reduce the risk of foodborne propagation [44,60,61]. In this sense, the positive opinion issued in 2021 by the EFSA—a trusted institution for Western societies—on the safety of the mealworm (*Tenebrio molitor larva*) [62], the migratory locust (*Locusta migratoria*) [63] and the cricket (*Acheta domesticus*) [64] as novel foods (Roma 2020) under Regulation (EU) 2015/2283 [65] could help to dispel doubts about the potential risk to human safety [66] and contribute to a greater willingness to consume them [21]. Globally, there are few legal instruments that treat insects as food [67], so greater sensitisation and awareness-raising would be needed to inform people about the benefits and safety of authorised insects if the aim is to introduce them into the diets of populations that do not have a tradition of entomophagy.

The nutritional benefits of insects and their value as a more sustainable source of protein are of great interest to Western society [12]. These benefits may be of particular interest to groups where protein needs are greater due to their life situation (older adults, athletes, etc.) [13], to societies where protein alternatives are sought due to the scarcity of traditional ones [8] or to raise awareness of the environmental impact of alternative sources due to the risk of surpassing planetary limits [68,69]. In any case, to take advantage of the benefits of insects as an alternative protein source, the proportion of insect proteins included in products must be comparable to that of other common protein sources [9].

Information on the benefits associated with insect consumption influences their acceptance [70]. The results of our study confirm a greater willingness to consume insects when people are informed of the potential sustainability benefits of doing so, increasing the possible acceptability thereof by 36.3%. The connection with the sustainability and well-being of the planet is a social trend that could favour the introduction of insects into the diet [1]. Insect farming for human consumption appears to offer several environmental benefits [71]. These include the use of organic waste, its added value and the reduction of environmental pollution. In addition, it leads to a reduction in greenhouse gas emissions [72], lower water consumption and higher food conversion efficiency [7].

While the study does not mention any potential health benefits of insect consumption, health was one of the most common reasons given for including other novel foods by those who had already done so. This suggests that informing people of the potential health benefits of insect consumption could also improve the willingness to consume insects, as is the case with sustainability.

The implementation of novel, sustainable food production strategies, as is the case with insects, may help to meet several United Nations sustainable development goals as defined by Moruzzo et al. [73]. However, the marketing and consumption of insects as food must strike a balance between regulation, environmental impact, social and market demands and public health needs and prospects [74]. Likewise, culinary preparation procedures and techniques adapted to the sociocultural context must be developed [75]. The market for edible insects is an emerging economic sector supported by academic research and innovation in the private sector (from processing to selling) [21], and it is an easily accessible and economical product [76]. Nevertheless, to boost future lines of production, more pilot tests of acceptability are needed with products that are more familiar to Western society, and more positive experiences need to be generated.

One of the potential limitations of this study is that the convenience sampling method used may have led to a bias relating to the participation of people who were more interested in or motivated by the subject, or who had a higher educational level. Another aspect to consider is that the majority of the responses belonged to the binary Yes/No option. No acceptance scales were used and no account was taken of whether respondents were following any kind of diet. Finally, the survey uses the term insect, which evokes an association with visible and whole insects [77], so perception may have influenced response. Despite these limitations, the study provides valuable information on the main factors that could improve the acceptability of insect consumption in order to introduce insects as a sustainable source of protein into the future diet. The data were drawn from the responses given by 1034 participants, a large number that exceeds other studies on the perception of insects as food in Mediterranean countries. Likewise, conducting a survey in a Mediterranean environment allows a broader view of Western consumer opinion, unlike previous surveys [15–19] whose focus was on consumer opinions in Northern and Central Europe.

5. Conclusions

In the near future, edible insects may appear in Western food in response to the need to look for new and more sustainable sources of alternative protein within the framework of sustainable development goals. Our data corroborate the low consumer acceptance of the inclusion of edible insects in human food through areas relevant to acceptance: neophobia, social norms, familiarity, experiences of consumption and knowledge of benefits. Disgust, lack of custom and food safety are the main reasons for neophobia. Neophobia has previously been studied in other populations, but not in a large sample of the Mediterranean population until now. At the gender level, men are more willing to consume insects, and so too are those in the 40–59-year-old age group.

The environmental and nutritional benefits of this type of product can open the door to the consumption of this novel food, which has been accepted by the EFSA in Europe. Informing people of such benefits for the health of the planet can improve their perception of insects and encourage them to consume them. However, the need to go further and offer products that make edible insects more familiar to Western society is identified. Producing commonly used flour-based products (bread, biscuits, bars, etc.) and offering culinary preparations closer to regional culture are ways to do that.

Supplementary Materials: The following supporting information can be downloaded at: https://www.mdpi.com/article/10.3390/ijerph192315756/s1, Table S1: Distribution of questionnaire responses by the participants' age (95% CI); Table S2: Distribution of questionnaire Distribution of questionnaire responses by the participants' gender (95% CI) responses by the participants' age (95% CI).

Author Contributions: Conceptualization, V.S.-S., M.S.-P., A.A.-M., A.B.-F. and M.R.-B.; methodology, V.S.-S., A.A.-M., A.B.-F. and M.R.-B.; data collection, M.S.-P. and M.R.-B.; formal analysis, V.S.-S.; writing—original draft preparation, M.R-B., A.A.-M., A.B.-F. and V.S-S.; writing—review and editing, V.S. S., A.A.-M., A.B.-F., M.R.-B. and M.S.-P.; supervision, A.A.-M. and A.B.-F. All authors have read and agreed to the published version of the manuscript.

Funding: This research received no external funding.

Institutional Review Board Statement: The study was conducted in accordance with the Declaration of Helsinki, and approved by the Ethics Committee of the Open University of Catalonia, CE22-PR28.

Informed Consent Statement: Informed consent was obtained from all subjects involved in the study.

Conflicts of Interest: The authors declare no conflict of interest.

References

1. Panel, G. *Future Food Systems: For People, Our Planet, and Prosperity*; Global Panel on Agriculture and Food Systems for Nutrition: London, UK, 2020.
2. Gerten, D.; Heck, V.; Jägermeyr, J.; Bodirsky, B.L.; Fetzer, I.; Jalava, M.; Kummu, M.; Lucht, W.; Rockström, J.; Schaphoff, S.; et al. Feeding ten billion people is possible within four terrestrial planetary boundaries. *Nat. Sustain.* **2020**, *3*, 200–208. [CrossRef]
3. Siegrist, M.; Hartmann, C. Consumer acceptance of novel food technologies. *Nat. Food* **2020**, *1*, 343–350. [CrossRef]
4. Salter, A.M.; Lopez-Viso, C. Role of novel protein sources in sustainably meeting future global requirements. *Proc. Nutr. Soc.* **2021**, *80*, 186–194. [CrossRef]
5. Van Huis, A.; Van Itterbeeck, J.; Klunder, H.; Mertens, E.; Halloran, A.; Muir, G.; Vantomme, P. *Edible Insects: Future Prospects for Food and Feed Security*; Food and Agriculture Organization of the United Nations: Rome, Italy, 2013.
6. Abbasi, T.; Abbasi, S. Reducing the global environmental impact of livestock production: The minilivestock option. *J. Clean. Prod.* **2016**, *112*, 1754–1766. [CrossRef]
7. Oonincx, D.G.; De Boer, I.J. Environmental impact of the production of mealworms as a protein source for humans—A life cycle assessment. *PLoS ONE* **2012**, *7*, e51145. [CrossRef]
8. Imathiu, S. Benefits and food safety concerns associated with consumption of edible insects. *NFS J.* **2020**, *18*, 1–11. [CrossRef]
9. Ros-Baró, M.; Casas-Agustench, P.; Díaz-Rizzolo, D.A.; Batlle-Bayer, L.; Adrià-Acosta, F.; Aguilar-Martínez, A.; Medina, F.-X.; Pujolà, M.; Bach-Faig, A. Edible Insect Consumption for Human and Planetary Health: A Systematic Review. *Int. J. Environ. Res. Public Health* **2022**, *19*, 11653. [CrossRef]
10. Bukkens, S.G. The nutritional value of edible insects. *Ecol. Food Nutr.* **1997**, *36*, 287–319. [CrossRef]
11. Finke, M.D. Complete nutrient composition of commercially raised invertebrates used as food for insectivores. *Zoo Biol.* **2002**, *21*, 269–285. [CrossRef]

12. Rumpold, B.A.; Schlüter, O.K. Nutritional composition and safety aspects of edible insects. *Mol. Nutr. Food Res.* **2013**, *57*, 802–823. [CrossRef]
13. Nowakowski, A.C.; Miller, A.C.; Miller, M.E.; Xiao, H.; Wu, X. Potential health benefits of edible insects. *Crit. Rev. Food Sci. Nutr.* **2020**, *62*, 3499–3508. [CrossRef]
14. Ojha, S.; Bekhit, A.E.D.; Grune, T.; Schlüter, O.K. Bioavailability of nutrients from edible insects. *Curr. Opin. Food Sci.* **2021**, *41*, 240–248. [CrossRef]
15. Chinarak, K.; Chaijan, M.; Panpipat, W. Farm-raised sago palm weevil (*Rhynchophorus ferrugineus*) larvae: Potential and challenges for promising source of nutrients. *J. Food Compos. Anal.* **2020**, *92*, 103542. [CrossRef]
16. Medina, F.X. Reflexiones sobre el patrimonio y la alimentación desde las perspectivas cultural y turística. In *Anales de Antropología*; Elsevier: Amsterdam, The Netherlands, 2017; pp. 106–113.
17. Verbeke, W. Profiling consumers who are ready to adopt insects as a meat substitute in a Western society. *Food Qual. Prefer.* **2015**, *39*, 147–155. [CrossRef]
18. Modlinska, K.; Adamczyk, D.; Maison, D.; Goncikowska, K.; Pisula, W. Relationship between Acceptance of Insects as an Alternative to Meat and Willingness to Consume Insect-Based Food—A Study on a Representative Sample of the Polish Population. *Foods* **2021**, *10*, 2420. [CrossRef]
19. Gere, A.; Székely, G.; Kovács, S.; Kókai, Z.; Sipos, L. Readiness to adopt insects in Hungary: A case study. *Food Qual. Prefer.* **2017**, *59*, 81–86. [CrossRef]
20. Hartmann, C.; Shi, J.; Giusto, A.; Siegrist, M. The psychology of eating insects: A cross-cultural comparison between Germany and China. *Food Qual. Prefer.* **2015**, *44*, 148–156. [CrossRef]
21. Schlup, Y.; Brunner, T. Prospects for insects as food in Switzerland: A tobit regression. *Food Qual. Prefer.* **2018**, *64*, 37–46. [CrossRef]
22. Faccio, E.; Guiotto Nai Fovino, L. Food Neophobia or Distrust of Novelties? Exploring consumers' attitudes toward GMOs, insects and cultured meat. *Appl. Sci.* **2019**, *9*, 4440. [CrossRef]
23. La Barbera, F.; Verneau, F.; Amato, M.; Grunert, K. Understanding Westerners' disgust for the eating of insects: The role of food neophobia and implicit associations. *Food Qual. Prefer.* **2018**, *64*, 120–125. [CrossRef]
24. Van Huis, A.; Dicke, M.; van Loon, J.J. Insects to feed the world. *J. Insects Food Feed* **2015**, *1*, 3–5. [CrossRef]
25. van Huis, A. Potential of insects as food and feed in assuring food security. *Annu. Rev. Entomol.* **2013**, *58*, 563–583. [CrossRef] [PubMed]
26. Costa-Neto, E.M. Anthropo-entomophagy in Latin America: An overview of the importance of edible insects to local communities. *J. Insects Food Feed* **2015**, *1*, 17–23. [CrossRef]
27. Durán-Galdo, R.; Saavedra-Garcia, L. Entomofagia,¿ Una potencial alternativa para la seguridad alimentaria?: Una revisión narrativa. *Rev. Española Nutr. Comunitaria* **2022**, *28*, 14.
28. Fleta Zaragozano, J. Entomofagia:¿ una alternativa a nuestra dieta tradicional? *Sanid. Mil.* **2018**, *74*, 41–46.
29. Modlinska, K.; Adamczyk, D.; Goncikowska, K.; Maison, D.; Pisula, W. The Effect of Labelling and Visual Properties on the Acceptance of Foods Containing Insects. *Nutrients* **2020**, *12*, 2498. [CrossRef]
30. Birch, A.N.E.; Begg, G.S.; Squire, G.R. How agro-ecological research helps to address food security issues under new IPM and pesticide reduction policies for global crop production systems. *J. Exp. Bot.* **2011**, *62*, 3251–3261. [CrossRef]
31. De Vries, M.; de Boer, I.J. Comparing environmental impacts for livestock products: A review of life cycle assessments. *Livest. Sci.* **2010**, *128*, 1–11. [CrossRef]
32. Flachowsky, G.; Meyer, U.; Südekum, K.H. Land Use for Edible Protein of Animal Origin-A Review. *Animals* **2017**, *7*, 25. [CrossRef]
33. Gahukar, R.T. Edible insects collected from forests for family livelihood and wellness of rural communities: A review. *Glob. Food Secur.* **2020**, *25*, 100348. [CrossRef]
34. Egonyu, J.P.; Kinyuru, J.; Fombong, F.; Ng'ang'a, J.; Ahmed, Y.A.; Niassy, S. *Advances in Insects for Food and Feed*; Springer: Berlin/Heidelberg, Germany, 2021; Volume 41, pp. 1903–1911.
35. Orkusz, A. Edible Insects versus Meat—Nutritional Comparison: Knowledge of Their Composition Is the Key to Good Health. *Nutrients* **2021**, *13*, 1207. [CrossRef] [PubMed]
36. Yi, L.; Lakemond, C.M.; Sagis, L.M.; Eisner-Schadler, V.; van Huis, A.; van Boekel, M.A. Extraction and characterisation of protein fractions from five insect species. *Food Chem.* **2013**, *141*, 3341–3348. [CrossRef] [PubMed]
37. Lange, K.; Nakamura, Y. Edible insects as a source of food bioactives and their potential health effects. *J. Food Bioact.* **2021**, *14*. [CrossRef]
38. Serra-Majem, L.; Tomaino, L.; Dernini, S.; Berry, E.M.; Lairon, D.; Ngo de la Cruz, J.; Bach-Faig, A.; Donini, L.M.; Medina, F.-X.; Belahsen, R.; et al. Updating the mediterranean diet pyramid towards sustainability: Focus on environmental concerns. *Int. J. Environ. Res. Public Health* **2020**, *17*, 8758. [CrossRef] [PubMed]
39. Janssen, M.; Busch, C.; Rödiger, M.; Hamm, U. Motives of consumers following a vegan diet and their attitudes towards animal agriculture. *Appetite* **2016**, *105*, 643–651. [CrossRef]
40. Kopplin, C.S.; Rausch, T.M. Above and beyond meat: The role of consumers' dietary behavior for the purchase of plant-based food substitutes. *Rev. Manag. Sci.* **2022**, *16*, 1335–1364. [CrossRef]
41. Wassmann, B.; Siegrist, M.; Hartmann, C. Correlates of the willingness to consume insects: A meta-analysis. *J. Insects Food Feed* **2021**, *7*, 909–922. [CrossRef]

42. Gumussoy, M.; Macmillan, C.; Bryant, S.; Hunt, D.F.; Rogers, P.J. Desire to eat and intake of 'insect'containing food is increased by a written passage: The potential role of familiarity in the amelioration of novel food disgust. *Appetite* **2021**, *161*, 105088. [CrossRef]
43. Hwang, J.; Kim, H.; Choe, J.Y. The Role of Eco-Friendly Edible Insect Restaurants in the Field of Sustainable Tourism. *Int. J. Environ. Res. Public Health* **2020**, *17*, 4064. [CrossRef]
44. Melgar-Lalanne, G.; Hernández-Álvarez, A.J.; Salinas-Castro, A. Edible insects processing: Traditional and innovative technologies. *Compr. Rev. Food Sci. Food Saf.* **2019**, *18*, 1166–1191. [CrossRef]
45. Caparros Megido, R.; Alabi, T.; Nieus, C.; Blecker, C.; Danthine, S.; Bogaert, J.; Haubruge, É.; Francis, F. Optimisation of a cheap and residential small-scale production of edible crickets with local by-products as an alternative protein-rich human food source in Ratanakiri Province, Cambodia. *J. Sci. Food Agric.* **2016**, *96*, 627–632. [CrossRef]
46. Gmuer, A.; Guth, J.N.; Hartmann, C.; Siegrist, M. Effects of the degree of processing of insect ingredients in snacks on expected emotional experiences and willingness to eat. *Food Qual. Prefer.* **2016**, *54*, 117–127. [CrossRef]
47. Jensen, N.H.; Lieberoth, A. We will eat disgusting foods together–Evidence of the normative basis of Western entomophagy-disgust from an insect tasting. *Food Qual. Prefer.* **2019**, *72*, 109–115. [CrossRef]
48. Looy, H.; Dunkel, F.V.; Wood, J.R. How then shall we eat? Insect-eating attitudes and sustainable foodways. *Agric. Hum. Values* **2014**, *31*, 131–141. [CrossRef]
49. Capdevila, I.; Cohendet, P.; Simon, L. Establishing New Codes for Creativity through Haute Cuisine. The Case of Ferran Adrià and elBulli. *Technol. Innov. Manag. Rev.* **2015**, *5*, 25–33. [CrossRef]
50. Baker, M.A.; Legendre, T.S.; Kim, Y.W. Edible insect gastronomy. In *The Routledge Handbook of Gastronomic Tourism*; Routledge: London, UK, 2019; pp. 412–419.
51. Hamerman, E.J. Cooking and disgust sensitivity influence preference for attending insect-based food events. *Appetite* **2016**, *96*, 319–326. [CrossRef] [PubMed]
52. Spence, C.; Hobkinson, C.; Gallace, A.; Fiszman, B.P. A touch of gastronomy. *Flavour* **2013**, *2*, 14. [CrossRef]
53. Nischalke, S.; Wagler, I.; Tanga, C.; Allan, D.; Phankaew, C.; Ratompoarison, C.; Razafindrakotomamonjy, A.; Kusia, E. How to turn collectors of edible insects into mini-livestock farmers: Multidimensional sustainability challenges to a thriving industry. *Glob. Food Secur.* **2020**, *26*, 100376. [CrossRef]
54. Chaijan, M.; Panpipat, W. Techno-biofunctional aspect of seasoning powder from farm-raised sago palm weevil (*Rhynchophorus ferrugineus*) larvae. *J. Insects Food Feed* **2021**, *7*, 187–195. [CrossRef]
55. Tello, A.; Aganovic, K.; Parniakov, O.; Carter, A.; Heinz, V.; Smetana, S. Product development and environmental impact of an insect-based milk alternative. *Future Foods* **2021**, *4*, 100080. [CrossRef]
56. Talens, C.; Llorente, R.; Simó-Boyle, L.; Odriozola-Serrano, I.; Tueros, I.; Ibargüen, M. Hybrid Sausages: Modelling the Effect of Partial Meat Replacement with Broccoli, Upcycled Brewer's Spent Grain and Insect Flours. *Foods* **2022**, *11*, 3396. [CrossRef]
57. Yen, A.L. Entomophagy and insect conservation: Some thoughts for digestion. *J. Insect Conserv.* **2009**, *13*, 667–670. [CrossRef]
58. Raheem, D.; Carrascosa, C.; Oluwole, O.B.; Nieuwland, M.; Saraiva, A.; Millán, R.; Raposo, A. Traditional consumption of and rearing edible insects in Africa, Asia and Europe. *Crit. Rev. Food Sci. Nutr.* **2019**, *59*, 2169–2188. [CrossRef]
59. van Huis, A. Edible insects are the future? *Proc. Nutr. Soc.* **2016**, *75*, 294–305. [CrossRef]
60. Mézes, M. Food safety aspect of insects: A review. *Acta Aliment.* **2018**, *47*, 513–522. [CrossRef]
61. Caparros Megido, R.; Desmedt, S.; Blecker, C.; Béra, F.; Haubruge, É.; Alabi, T.; Francis, F. Microbiological Load of Edible Insects Found in Belgium. *Insects* **2017**, *8*, 12. [CrossRef] [PubMed]
62. Turck, D.; Castenmiller, J.; De Henauw, S.; Hirsch-Ernst, K.I.; Kearney, J.; Maciuk, A.; Knutsen, H.K. Safety of dried yellow mealworm (*Tenebrio molitor* larva) as a novel food pursuant to Regulation (EU) 2015/2283. *EFSA J.* **2021**, *19*, e06343.
63. Turck, D.; Castenmiller, J.; De Henauw, S.; Hirsch-Ernst, K.I.; Kearney, J.; Knutsen, H.K. Safety of frozen and dried formulations from migratory locust (*Locusta migratoria*) as a Novel food pursuant to Regulation (EU) 2015/2283. *EFSA J.* **2021**, *19*, e06667.
64. Turck, D.; Bohn, T.; Castenmiller, J.; De Henauw, S.; Hirsch-Ernst, K.I.; Knutsen, H.K. Safety of partially defatted house cricket (*Acheta domesticus*) powder as a novel food pursuant to Regulation (EU) 2015/2283. *EFSA J.* **2022**, *20*, e07258. [PubMed]
65. Belluco, S.; Halloran, A.; Ricci, A. New protein sources and food legislation: The case of edible insects and EU law. *Food Secur.* **2017**, *9*, 803–814. [CrossRef]
66. Turck, D.; Bohn, T.; Castenmiller, J.; De Henauw, S.; Hirsch-Ernst, K.I.; Knutsen, H.K. Safety of frozen and dried formulations from whole house crickets (*Acheta domesticus*) as a Novel food pursuant to Regulation (EU) 2015/2283. *EFSA J.* **2021**, *19*, e06779. [PubMed]
67. Grabowski, N.T.; Tchibozo, S.; Abdulmawjood, A.; Acheuk, F.; M'Saad Guerfali, M.; Sayed, W.A.; Plötz, M. Edible insects in Africa in terms of food, wildlife resource, and pest management legislation. *Foods* **2020**, *9*, 502. [CrossRef] [PubMed]
68. Ordoñez-Araque, R.; Egas-Montenegro, E. Edible insects: A food alternative for the sustainable development of the planet. *Int. J. Gastron. Food Sci.* **2021**, *23*, 100304. [CrossRef]
69. de Boer, J.; Aiking, H. Prospects for pro-environmental protein consumption in Europe: Cultural, culinary, economic and psychological factors. *Appetite* **2018**, *121*, 29–40. [CrossRef] [PubMed]
70. Sogari, G.; Menozzi, D.; Mora, C. Sensory-liking expectations and perceptions of processed and unprocessed insect products. *Int. J. Food Syst. Dyn.* **2018**, *9*, 314–320.
71. Schlüter, O.; Rumpold, B.; Holzhauser, T.; Roth, A.; Vogel, R.F.; Quasigroch, W.; Vogel, S.; Heinz, V.; Jäger, H.; Bandick, N.; et al. Safety aspects of the production of foods and food ingredients from insects. *Mol. Nutr. Food Res.* **2017**, *61*, 1600520. [CrossRef]

72. Foley, J.A.; Ramankutty, N.; Brauman, K.A.; Cassidy, E.S.; Gerber, J.S.; Johnston, M.; Mueller, N.D.; O'Connell, C.; Ray, D.K.; West, P.C.; et al. Solutions for a cultivated planet. *Nature* **2011**, *478*, 337–342. [CrossRef]
73. Moruzzo, R.; Mancini, S.; Guidi, A. Edible Insects and Sustainable Development Goals. *Insects* **2021**, *12*, 557. [CrossRef]
74. Committee, E.S. Risk profile related to production and consumption of insects as food and feed. *EFSA J.* **2015**, *13*, 4257. [CrossRef]
75. Deroy, O.; Reade, B.; Spence, C. The insectivore's dilemma, and how to take the West out of it. *Food Qual. Prefer.* **2015**, *44*, 44–55. [CrossRef]
76. Roos, N.; Van Huis, A. Consuming insects: Are there health benefits? *J. Insects Food Feed* **2017**, *3*, 225–229. [CrossRef]
77. Evans, J.; Alemu, M.H.; Flore, R.; Frøst, M.B.; Halloran, A.; Jensen, A.B.; Maciel-Vergara, G.; Meyer-Rochow, V.B.; Münke-Svendsen, C.; Olsen, S.B.; et al. 'Entomophagy': An evolving terminology in need of review. *J. Insects Food Feed* **2015**, *1*, 293–305. [CrossRef]

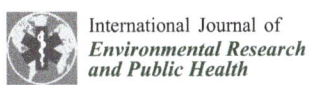

Article

Quality Food Products as a Tourist Attraction in the Province of Córdoba (Spain)

Mª Genoveva Dancausa Millán [1] and Mª Genoveva Millán Vázquez de la Torre [2,*]

[1] Department of Statistics, Córdoba University, 14071 Córdoba, Spain
[2] Department of Quantitative Methods, Universidad Loyola Andalucía, 14004 Córdoba, Spain
* Correspondence: gmillan@uloyola.es

Abstract: Traveling to learn about the gastronomy of a destination is becoming increasingly important among tourists, especially in the wake of the pandemic. Quality foods endorsed by protected designations of origin (PDOs) are increasingly in demand, as are experiences related to their production processes. In this study, the seven PDOs in the province of Córdoba (Spain) are analyzed. These PDOs produce olive oil, wine or ham. A field study was performed, whereby 315 gastronomic tourists who visited a gastronomic route or a PDO in Córdoba were surveyed. The objective was to characterize the profile of visiting tourists and to anticipate future demand using ARIMA models. The results indicate that the growth in gastronomic tourism in Córdoba is lower than that in the wider region, and that there are no significant differences among the different profiles (oil tourist, enotourist and ham tourists) due in part to the fact that most tourists travel from nearby regions. The novelty of this study is that three products are analyzed, and strategies are proposed to deseasonalize this type of tourism, for example, by creating a gastronomic brand that represents Córdoba and selling products under that brand (especially in international markets), by highlighting raw materials and prepared dishes and by making gastronomy a complement to heritage tourism in the city and rural tourism in the province.

Keywords: gastronomic routes; Iberian ham; olive oil; wine; Córdoba; ARIMA; food; gastronomic tourism

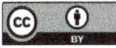

1. Introduction

The gastronomy of a region is part of its culture and identifies food products with the territory [1,2], constituting both a material heritage formed by a raw material and agri-food products, such as cheese, wine, oil, etc., ham, etc., and an intangible heritage shaped by the recipes with which food dishes are prepared, culinary traditions, etc. [3]. This heritage is being increasingly appreciated by people who taste these foods, constituting potential resources that serve as a basis for the growing development of gastronomy because geographical and cultural diversity provides a great variety of foods and ways of preparing them [4], with food being considered an essential good as well as an integral part of the social and cultural heritage [5] that can be exploited not only from the perspective of food but also as a tourist product.

Improvements in gastronomic resources are providing new opportunities to many territories, especially rural ones; gastronomy is becoming not only an identity for the residents of an area but also an attraction for potential tourists who want to learn about it.

Since the beginning of the 21st century, people have become more concerned with having a balanced and healthy diet and spending their leisure time visiting destinations where food is of high quality to learn about how it is produced, especially foods belonging to the Mediterranean diet. The Mediterranean diet is based on various nutrients, including *fats* such as olive oil, that yield vitamins and antioxidants that are very beneficial to human health [6,7]; *meats,* which provide protein, vitamins and minerals (including, among other cured meats, Iberian ham); *fruits*, which are a source of vitamins, fiber, water and minerals; and *vegetables*, which provide fiber, vitamins, minerals and carbohydrates. The great variety of products that comprise the Mediterranean diet are attracting an increasing number of tourists who want to learn about it, with gastronomy being one of the main reasons to visit cultural destinations such as Italy [8] and Greece [9]. This diet has a lower environmental impact because it includes many plant-derived and fewer animal products [10], and it is better for human health [11,12].

Of all the foods mentioned above, in this study, we will analyze Iberian ham, wine and olive oil as elements of Córdoba gastronomy, and from a tourist attraction perspective, to determine the factors that characterize the gastronomic tourist and to estimate potential demand.

Andalusia, an region located in the south of Spain, has a rich gastronomy comprising dishes whose recipes date back more than a thousand years, such as octopus casserole or eggplant almodrote, whose origin stems from the region's Jewish heritage. During the 800 years of coexistence of Jewish and Muslim people in the Iberian Peninsula, there are dishes in which Judo–Christian–Arab culinary traditions have been mixed, creating a fusion of gastronomic elements where culinary traditions are combined, giving rise to the current Andalusian cuisine.

The methods of preparing dishes and the quality of the food elements that constitute typical dishes at a destination are now generating tourism, which is gaining more relevance every day in Andalusia and is becoming the main reason for tourists to visit certain areas of the region.

Córdoba, one of the eight provinces that are part of the Andalusia region, has a continental Mediterranean climate, with temperatures ranging between 9.2 °C in January and 36 °C in July and August. Rainfall varies between 400 to 600 mm per year, concentrated from October to April. Its vegetation is characterized by Mediterranean forest, in which trees of different oak ecotypes and other autochthonous herbaceous plants predominate, forming a landscape called *dehesa*, which is defined by its three functional zones: pasture, arable and mountain. The morphology of the terrain is characterized by shallow, acidic soils with an abundance of granites, gneisses or slates. Such morphology makes these lands agriculturally very unproductive. However, rain-fed crops grow here, as do the olive and the holm oak, whose fruit, the acorn, is the main food of the Iberian pig. The region's capital includes four World Heritage declaration sites and is a heritage city. Cultural tourism is one of the main drivers of its economy, which has been severely affected by the COVID-19 pandemic; however, the province relies mainly on agriculture and livestock, with tourist activity representing complementary income to the fundamental activities of the primary sector.

Rural tourism, active tourism, cultural tourism and gastronomic tourism are among the main tourist activities that an individual can engage in when visiting the province.

Every year, thousands of people visit the province to taste typical Córdoba dishes, such as *flamenquín*, *rabo de toro* (braised oxtails), and *salmorejo*, with recipes from Arab and Jewish heritage that are made with top-quality raw materials, such as olive oil, ham or wine endorsed by protected designations of origin (PDOs) that certify the quality of these products [13].

However, despite having these raw materials, tourist demand is still low compared to that for other gastronomic destinations. What is happening with gastronomic tourism in Córdoba? Why is it still in the takeoff phase despite having seven PDOs and two restaurants that have received Michelin stars (NOOR Restaurant, 2 stars; Choco restaurant, one star)? Would having a restaurant in Córdoba with a green star (green stars indicate restaurants with environmental, resource management and waste disposal initiatives) attract tourists, considering that Córdoba does not currently have such restaurants? What types of gastronomic tourist does Córdoba receive? What are their main characteristics?

To answer these questions, oil, wine and ham PDOs in the province of Córdoba were analyzed, the demand profile and existing supply related to each gastronomic product was investigated, and a gastronomic tourist profile was identified for each product, in case different marketing campaigns are necessary for different tourist profiles.

To analyze the aforementioned, univariate and bivariate descriptive statistics were used to identify the degree of association between variables, and interviews were conducted with owners of restaurants and wineries, oil mills and ham curing facilities with the objective of identifying gastronomic tourist profiles. SARIMA models were applied to predict the future demand of gastronomic tourists for oil, wine and ham, providing a vision of the potential demand. The results obtained indicate that the demand for gastronomic tourism will grow, but not as quickly as rural tourism after the pandemic.

To improve the demand for gastronomic tourism, a series of strategies are proposed so that the growth in demand for gastronomic tourism in Córdoba will be higher than expected.

After this introduction, in the second section, designations of origin in Córdoba are analyzed. The third section contains a brief review of the existing scientific literature in this field. The fourth section presents the methodology used in this study. The fifth section presents the main results of the research. The last two sections provide a discussion and conclusions.

2. Protected Geographical Indications and Designation of Origins as Quality Hallmarks of Agri-Food Products

New trends in consumer habits have led to a growing interest in gastronomic products of higher quality that are differentiated and adapted to the new needs of different groups and market segments [8,14]. This increase in the consumption of differentiated products based on their quality is obtained through geographical indicators of origin and, in particular, PDOs, which integrate in their definition not only geographical origin but also the relevant forms, traditions and specialization involved when producing high-quality products, as well as production regulation and control mechanisms [15]. To increase their competitiveness and expand their market share, agri-food companies try to establish differentiation strategies for their products based on highlighting differences in attributes, materials or characteristics with respect to a competitor's product.

In Spain, there are 199 agri-food product PDOs and 159 PGIs; therefore, Spain has a great variety of quality food products, especially wine (97 PDO), oil (30 PDO) and cheese (27), indicating that Spain is a good gastronomic destination (Table 1).

Table 1. Distribution of agri-food products, wines and spirits with PDOs and PGIs in Spain, Andalusia and Córdoba (July 2022).

Agri-Food Products	PDO			PGI		
	Spain	Andalusia	Córdoba	Spain	Andalusia	Córdoba
Fresh meat (and offal)	-	-	-	22	1	-
Meat products	5	2	1	11	2	-
Cheese	27	-	-	2	-	-
Other animal products (honey)	3	1	-	4	-	-
Oils and fats (31 oils and 2 butters)	30	12	4	3	-	-
Fruits, vegetables and fresh and transformed cereals	26	3	-	36	3	-
Fish, seafood and fresh crustaceans and derived products	1	-	-	4	4	-
Other products (saffron, paprika, tiger nut, hazelnut, vinegar and cider)	9	3	1	-	-	-
Bakery, confectionary, pastry and dessert products	-	-	-	16	4	-
Cochineal	1	-	-	-	-	-
Total PDO and PGI of agri-food products	102	21	6	98	14	0
Wines with designation of origin (DO)	74	7	1	-	-	-
Wines with qualified design of origin (DO Ca)	2	-	-	-	-	-
Quality wines with geographical indication (QW)	10	1	-	-	-	-
Paid wines (PV)	11	-	-	-	-	-

Table 1. *Cont.*

Agri-Food Products	PDO			PGI		
	Spain	Andalusia	Córdoba	Spain	Andalusia	Córdoba
Wines with geographical indication (GI)	-	-	-	41	16	2
Aromatized wines	-	-	-	1	1	-
Total PDO and PGI of Wines	97	8	1	42	17	2
Spirits with PGI	-	-	-	19	1	-
Total PDO and PGI	199	30	7	159	32	0

Source: Prepared by the authors based on information from the Ministry of Agriculture, Food and Environment and the European Commission, Directorate General of Agriculture and Rural Development [16].

The province of Córdoba has seven PDOs, among which oil accounts for four, with one each for wine, Iberian ham and vinegar. The most visited is the wine PDO, with more than 30,000 tourists per year [17]. The PDOs are detailed below:

- Iberian Ham: "Los Pedroches" PDO. Located to the north of the province and encompassing 32 municipalities with an area of 3612 km^2, the predominant climate in the area is Mediterranean but with a certain continental touch and winds from the Atlantic, with cold winters and long, dry and hot summers and with little rainfall. This climate, together with the structure of the soils, is favorable to the growth of oaks and their fruit (acorn), which is the sustenance of the pigs from which the ham is obtained), forming a *dehesas* (savannah-like open woodland), a typical ecosystem in the area.
- Wine: Montilla-Moriles Designation of Origin. This environment encompasses a total of 17 municipalities and more than 5000 hectares of vineyards, and distinguishes an area differentiated by the type of soil, considered "Superior" (approximately 1600 hectares). The main grape types are Pedro Ximénez, Layren, Baladí, Verdejo, Moscatel de Grano Menudo, Moscatel de Alejandría, Torrontés, Chardonnay, Sauvignon Blanc and Macabeo.
- Vinegar: Vinagre de Montilla-Moriles Designation of Origin. These vinegars are obtained exclusively by the acetification of PDO wines and have been produced with PDO wines since 2015.
- Oil: The province of Córdoba is the second largest nationwide in terms of olive oil production, with 317,000 tons of oil produced in the 2020–21 season [18]. It has four designations of origin:
  - Baena Designation of Origin: This was Spain's first agri-food Designation of Origin (1971). It encompasses eight municipalities and covers an area of approximately 60,000 hectares, with an average annual production ranging from 30 to 45 million kilos of oil.
  - Priego de Córdoba Designation of Origin (1995): This Designation of Origin encompasses the municipalities of Almedinilla, Carcabuey, Fuente Tójar and Priego de Córdoba, covers approximately 30,000 hectares, and is located in the southwest of the province of Córdoba, in Sierra Subbética park.
  - Aceite de Lucena Designation of Origin: Located in the south of the province of Córdoba, it encompasses 10 municipalities; it is the newest of the four Designations of Origin (2008) and comprises 73,000 hectares.
  - Montoro—Adamuz Designation of Origin (2007): This Designation of Origin encompasses the municipalities of Montoro, Adamuz, Espiel, Hornachuelos, Obejo, Villaharta, Villanueva del Rey and Villaviciosa de Córdoba, as well as the northern part of the municipality of Córdoba. It contains approximately 55,000 hectares of controlled olive groves.

Three of these products (wine, olive oil and ham) can contribute to directly and indirectly increasing the wealth of the region through business activities such as tourism, but there is a need to raise awareness within the business sector to synergize production activity (agriculture/livestock) and services (tourism). The symbiosis of both activities will allow the creation of a tourism product that makes Córdoba more attractive as an international gastronomic destination.

Figure 1 presents a map of the province of Córdoba, where practically all the municipalities of the province, except the capital, are under some designation of origin, with some included in more than one.

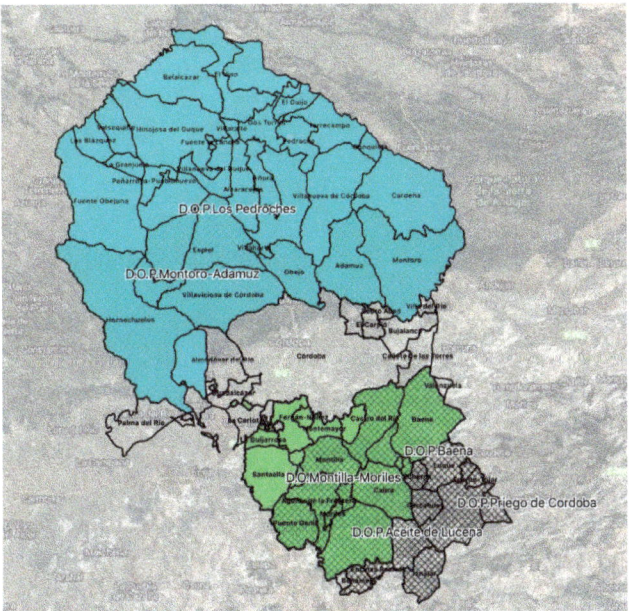

Figure 1. Geographical location of PDOs in the province of Córdoba. Source: own elaboration.

In the figure, blue represents the Pedroches ham PDO; green represents the Montilla-Moriles wine PDO, and the hatched area represents the four olive oil PDOs.

In recent years, there has been greater interest in Córdoban food products and tourism, materializing, on the one hand, with the expansion of restaurants linked to popular cuisine and local quality products endorsed by PDOs and PGIs, and, on the other hand, in the consolidation of the gastronomic tourism area [3,4,19–21], turning this type of tourism into an important dynamic element of the economy and culture of the areas where they are located.

The development of gastronomic tourism in the interior areas of Córdoba contributes to integrating the traditional primary productive function with the specialized tertiary industry, increasing the sources of income, improving the levels of income and employment for the local population, and generating multifunctionality in rural territories.

However, to commercialize gastronomic products from the tourist's point of view, gastronomic routes must be created that include producers, restaurants, shops, etc.; that is, public entities and private companies that work on creating a gastronomic circuit (gastronomic routes), which can solve the difficulties of commercializing regional food products because these circuits are instruments to promote such foods. In this way, the use of geographical quality indicators makes it easy for consumers to recognize the superior and differentiating qualities of each product. Strengthening the origin or provenance attributes of products has thus become an important marketing tool for the commercialization of products and brands, especially if these brands belong to the agri-food sector [22]. The place of origin or provenance of products can become an important source of competitive advantage for companies, capable of influencing consumers when valuing products or brands [23].

Gastronomic routes are defined as itineraries that allow the recognition and enjoyment of the agricultural and industrial production process and the tasting of regional cuisine considered an expression of regional cultural identity. These routes consist of producers who welcome tourists in their establishments and provide them with food services and regional restaurants that showcase traditional dishes based on local primary production and agroindustries in the area. They are organized around a key product or, in some cases, around a basket of products that characterize the route and give it identity; such itineraries are developed using road networks [24].

There can be countless activities related to the products with which a route is identified: visits to producers, who receive tourists in their establishments, showing them the preparation process and allowing them to taste the products; visits to restaurants that offer traditional dishes with local products; and visits to museums that relate product and place, among other activities.

When designing a gastronomic route, public entities and producers should link tourism with food and at no point ignore other attractions that link the food and beverage cluster with tourism, as doing so usually leads to the loss of development and market opportunities for both.

Among the elements that characterize a gastronomic route are (a) the production that distinguishes it from another region, (b) the itinerary developed along a road network, (c) the establishments attached to the route that produce, distribute or advertise the food that highlights the route, (d) a minimum number of participants along each route that justifies its opening, (e) a regulatory norm that regulates the functioning of the participants, (f) a regional menu whose dishes have been prepared with the products that characterize the route, (g) a local organization, association or tourism office that offers information about the gastronomic route, (h) the signage for the route and a map that provides explanatory information about it, and (i) culinary offerings of the product in restaurants and establishments in the area [25].

For gastronomic tourism to be successful, it is necessary, first, to have a quality raw material and, second, to have good dishes prepared from those materials whose recipes are typical of the area, to have a good gastronomic route, which includes not only the places that produce the raw material (vineyards, dehesas, curing facilities, oil mills, wineries, etc.) but also restaurants where tourists can sample the traditional food or customs of the area, accommodation, shops, etc.., and to have a well-structured offering that is part of the gastronomic route. However, if a gastronomic route is not publicized or known, few tourists will visit it. To achieve this, marketing campaigns in specialized magazines, international fairs, etc., are needed to create awareness among potential gastronomic tourists so that they will visit Córdoba and be interested in its gastronomy. These actions will serve as the bases or pillars to attract gastronomic tourists to the gastronomic destination of Córdoba (Figure 2).

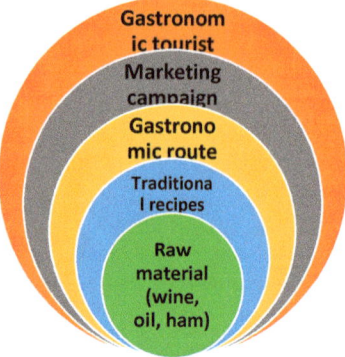

Figure 2. Pillars of gastronomic tourism in the province of Córdoba. Source: own elaboration.

3. Literature Review

Gastronomic tourism is based on a combination of factors such as food, culture, the geography of the destination and the availability of infrastructure to support tourism. Studies have shown that the culture and environmental factors of a destination shape its gastronomic identity. While the geography and climate of a destination determine the type of food that can grow in the area, history and tradition influence the cuisine and eating habits of the destination and thus collectively determine its gastronomic identity [26].

There is a large amount of scientific literature that analyzes gastronomic tourism from different perspectives:

- Territory: Gastronomic tourism has been studied in specific regions or countries, such as France, in which Batat [27] investigated the role of Michelin-starred chefs as change-makers and advocates of tourism activities in both rural and urban areas; Italy, in which Privitera et al. [28] analyzed the opportunities of gastronomic tourism for local development around the Sicily region; Greece, in which Pavlidis & Markantonatou [29] analyzed the promotion of gastronomic tourism in the northern regions of Greece; Singapore, in which Chaney & Ryan [26] described the evolution of gastronomic tourism in Singapore; Malaysia, in which Sanip and Mustapha analized the sustainability of gastronomic tourism in Malaysia [30,31]; Mexico, in which Correa [32] determined the factors that can help restaurants to be more competitive in the face of a health crisis in the state of Zacatecas; and Kenya, in which Josphine [33] carried out a critical review of gastronomic tourism development in Kenya.
- Product: Gastronomic tourism has been investigated based on a specific product, such as cheese, in which Medeiros et al. [34] carried out a study on the artisanal cheese of Serro; wine [17]; olive oil, in which Dancausa et al. [3] analyzed olive oil as a gourmet ingredient in contemporary Andalusian cuisine; ham, in which Millán et al. [35] investigated ham tourism as an opportunity for development in rural areas; tea or coffee, in which Seyitoğlu & Alphan [36] examined the tea and coffee museum experience of travelers from around the world; fish, in which Pratiwi' [37] study aims to develop gastronomic tourism based on fish on the island of Belitung; or prepared dishes [38].
- Motivation: Such studies investigate what motivates tourists to undertake gastronomic tourism [39]. Decrop [40] analyzes the concept of motivation by emphasizing four different components (motives, needs, desires and benefits). Other authors, such as Hernandez & Dancausa [38], distinguish between types of tourist who visit gastronomical destinations, finding that motivation can be a main or secondary factor and classifying gastronomic tourists as follows. Gastronomy connoisseurs (gourmet tourists) are well-versed in gastronomy, and their main motivation for travel is to taste different products or typical dishes of the destinations they visit, as well as to purchase said products and learn in situ. They usually travel continuously throughout the year visiting prestigious restaurants. Gastronomy enthusiasts do not have a high degree of education in gastronomy but know the world of gastronomy relatively well. They typically have a university education, and their main motivation for traveling is to experience firsthand what they have read in different specialized magazines. Individuals interested in gastronomy do not have technical training in gastronomy but are interested in the world of gastronomy. Their main motivation for traveling is to experience typical dishes or products of their destinations, although not exclusively but as a complement to other tourist activities. Gastronomy novices, for various reasons (such as in response to advertising or a desire for new experiences), visit restaurants, wineries, or oil mills despite lacking knowledge regarding gastronomy. Their main motivation for traveling is not related to gastronomy, but they secondarily dedicate a few hours of their journey to gastronomy.

Gastronomy fits well as the main motivation (for gastronomy connoisseurs and enthusiasts, who visit a place specifically to enjoy its culinary offerings) and as a secondary motivation (for example, for those for whom, although their main motivation is not to learn about the gastronomic richness of a destination, do consider gastronomy as a tourism option) for engaging in gastronomic tourism. In turn, as a main or secondary motivation, gastronomy can represent an intensification or extension of daily life. Whatever the motivation, such tourists can experience completely different gastronomy from that of their place of origin [41–44].

- Satisfaction: These studies analyze how satisfied tourists are with the gastronomy of the destination they visit [45–47], investigating how well a destination performs through an analysis of tourist satisfaction, with one of the most important factors when choosing a holiday destination being satisfaction with previous stays [48,49].
- Consumption: Studies investigate gastronomic tourism from the perspective of hedonistic theory, which stipulates that tourists will consume food for the sake of experiencing it and not for hunger, and thus, food consumption is more experiential than functional [50,51].
- Gastronomic tourist profile: These studies analyze gastronomic tourist profiles [52,53] using various techniques, such as neural networks [54], cluster analysis [55], factor analysis [35] and tourism demand forecasting models using ARIMA models [56–58].

Many studies on gastronomy investigate different factors, e.g., motivation, satisfaction, territory, product, etc., all of which are equally relevant, allowing the characterization of tourists to better understand their tastes and preferences, facilitating the construction of a more adequate tourism product adapted to the demand [59].

The novelty of this research is that it analyzes the entire gastronomic products associated with PDOs in Córdoba; existing studies focus on specific raw materials, not all materials, nor do they compare them. In addition, strategies are proposed to improve this tourist segment. The following two hypotheses are tested:

H1: *The profile of gastronomic tourists depends on the product they consume.*

H2: *Gastronomic tourism in the province of Córdoba will expand after the pandemic.*

4. Materials and Methods

The primary data sources of data were obtained through fieldwork that involved surveying a population of tourist consumers who visited one of the seven PDOs in the province of Córdoba in 2021–2022, with the objective of determining which factors influence gastronomic tourists. To this end, a questionnaire was administered to verify its validity as a measurement instrument according to [60,61], and a pre-test was performed with 40 gastronomic tourists to verify that it satisfied the following criteria:

1. Simple, viable and accepted by tourists and researchers (viability).
2. Reliable and accurate, that is, with error-free measurements.
3. Adequate for the problem to be measured.
4. Reflects the underlying theory in the phenomenon or concept to be measured (construct validity). Questionnaires similar to those used by previous gastronomic tourism researchers were used [3,4,13,17,62–66].

A questionnaire consisting of 38 items divided into four blocks (Table 2) was designed. The first block collected personal information (age, gender, level of education, marital status, etc.). The second block collected information about the gastronomic route taken (how the tourist found out about the gastronomic route, if the route met his/her expectations, what would improve the route, purpose for traveling the gastronomic route, etc.). The third block collected information on the motivation for gastronomic tourism (the reason for choosing the gastronomic route) and a self-classification of the tourist's level of gastronomic tourism. The fourth assessment block (on the services received during the route, price of the trip, hospitality and treatment received, etc.) was a questionnaire directed at the population of tourist consumers visiting a gastronomic route/PDO in Córdoba. Access by the investigators to the routes (curers, oil mills, wineries, restaurants, etc.) and permission to conduct interviews with tourists was authorized by the managing body and owner of each PDO.

Table 2. Technical aspects of the survey.

	Demand Survey
Population	Tourists of both sexes over 18 years old who visited a gastronomic route or PDO in Córdoba
Sample size	315
Sampling error	±4.2%
Confidence level	95%; $p = q = 0.5$
Sampling system	Simple random
Date of fieldwork	September 2021–January 2022

Prior to responding to the questionnaire, tourists were informed of the academic purposes of the study and the anonymity of their answers. Verbal consent was obtained prior to administering the questionnaire. At all times, the visitor's anonymity was guaranteed.

With the information obtained in the survey, the following were carried out:

1. A univariate descriptive analysis was conducted to determine the profile of tourists, segmented by product, i.e., wine, oil and ham, with the objective of identifying if there are significant differences between tourists.
2. A bivariate analysis was conducted using contingency tables to identify whether there is an association or independence between two variables, using the χ^2 statistic (where H_0 is that the analyzed variables are independent and H_1 is that the analyzed variables are related). The aim of said analysis was to determine the associations between variables, thus allowing the identification of the profiles of gastronomic tourists.
3. A SARIMA model (used in previous studies of tourists, such as those by Lim [67] to predict tourist demand in Macao after the COVID-19 pandemic; Yang [56] to predict tourist demand in 29 Chinese regions, and Petrevska [57] to predict tourist demand in Macedonia; Zhang [58] to predict tourist occupancy in a hotel) was used to predict the potential demand of gastronomic tourists in Córdoba, based on a sample (61 observations) collected from February 2015 to May 2022. ARIMA models, popularly known as the Box–Jenkins (BJ) methodology, analyze the probabilistic, or stochastic, properties of economic time series themselves [58]. In this case, this was the number of gastronomic tourists in Córdoba.

5. Results

Table 3 provides the characteristics of gastronomic tourists in Córdoba; the data have been categorized by product to determine specific profiles, with the objective of testing Hypothesis 1. The segmentation of the tourist profile by product indicates that there are a series of common variables, such as gender, because the majority of the gastronomic tourists were male, with the highest percentage in oil tourism (58.2%), had a high school/secondary education level (43.8% of ham tourists, 40.1% of enotourists and 38.5% of oil tourists), were married, travelled accompanied and came mainly from Andalusia (58.9% of ham tourists, 43.1% of enotourists and 59.4% of oil tourists). For place of origin, there was a greater than 15-point difference between some products, because enotourism, which is better known internationally, draws a greater number of foreigners than do ham or oil, which are not known as tourist products in international markets. More than 60% of tourists worked for others and used vacations to travel to Córdoba; travel was very seasonal, and they spent less than 24 h in the province of Córdoba. Many classified themselves as excursionists because they spent less than six hours at a destination. Therefore, they did not spend the night, which is a problem for the city. Overnight stays, with respect to the average daily expenditure, are between EUR 66 and 100 for ham tourism and oil tourism, and higher than EUR 100 for enotourism. The average income was between EUR 1500 and 2000 for olive oil tourists and ham tourists, and between EUR 1000–1500 for enotourists. This result is significantly different from those reported in other relevant studies of Andalusia [53–69], where enotourists who visited Andalusia had greater purchasing power (EUR 2500) than ham and oil tourists, because many enotourists are international tourists who visit the Xeres PDO, which receives more than half a million visitors per year, the vast majority of which are foreign tourists with high purchasing power. If similar studies on the profile of oil tourists are analyzed, such as that by Alonso and Northcote [70] in Australia, a similarity is observed in terms of with whom the trip is made, where few tourists make the trip alone. For Córdoba, 2% of oil tourists and 4.7% of enotourists travelled alone, compared with 2% reported in other studies of gastronomic tourism, such as that by Olivera [71]. In Mealhada, Portugal, some variables are similar, such as a higher percentage (56%) of men choosing this type of tourism as well as the level of education of tourists. In a study by Orgaz and Lopez [72] in the Dominican Republic and a study by Huertas et al. [48] in Mocha Canton, Ecuador, the tourists were mostly male (56% and 51%, respectively, in both countries), but the age distribution was different. In Córdoba, approximately 30% of gastronomic tourists were between 50 and 59 years of age (30.5%) with medium purchasing power; in contrast, in the study by Orgaz and Lopez, gastronomic tourists were younger (30 to 39 years old), and in the study by Huertas, such tourists were between 21 and 27 years old (27%), mainly with low purchasing power.

Table 3. Profile of gastronomic tourists in Córdoba (%).

Block	Question	Classification	Percentage of Ham Tourists	Percentage of Enotourists	Percentage of Oil Tourists
Personal characteristics of gastronomic tourists	Age	18–29 years	14.2	23.0	14.4
		30–39 years	27.1	28.4	27.3
		40–49 years	20.3	**32.0**	19.3
		50–59 years	**31.1**	13.2	**30.4**
		Over 60 years	7.3	3.4	8.6
	Education level	No completed studies	9.3	1.0	9.4
		Primary and secondary studies	19.6	32.9	18.6
		Secondary Bachelor	**43.8**	**40.1**	**38.5**
		Higher studies	27.4	26.0	33.5
	Gender	Male	**57.5**	**51.2**	**58.2**
		Female	42.5	49.8	41.8
	Marital status	Single	26.9	35.0	26.9
		Married	**47.7**	**44.0**	**48.2**
		Divorced/separated	25.2	20.3	24.3
		Other	0.2	0.7	0.6
	Monthly income level of the family unit	Less than EUR 1000	19.8	23.9	19.8
		EUR 1001–1500	19.8	47.6	20.0
		EUR 1501–2000	30.3	18.3	30.0
		EUR 2001–2500	20.0	7.4	20.0
		More than EUR 2500	10	2.8	10.2
	Who do you travel with?	Alone	3.2	4.7	2.0
		Accompanied by my partner	48.9	45.6	49.4
		With friends	37.7	32.3	38.4
		With relatives	10.3	17.4	10.2
	Where are you from?	**Andalusia**	**58.9**	**43.1**	**59.4**
		Rest of Spain (except Andalusia)	30.1	34.3	29.8
		European Union (except Spain)	10.0	12.5	10.2
		United States	0.2	0.1	0.2
		Rest of the world (except European Union)	0.7	10	0.5

Table 3. Cont.

Block	Question	Classification	Percentage of Ham Tourists	Percentage of Enotourists	Percentage of Oil Tourists
	Employment situation	Employed by others	**61.4**	**70.1**	**62.2**
		Self-employed	10.2	8.5	10.2
		Retired	17.4	7.4	17.3
		Unemployed	8.3	3.4	8.1
		Student	2.7	10.6	2.2
	Duration of the trip	Less than 24 h	**53.7**	**83.2**	**54.2**
		1–3 days	34.3	9.7	33.3
		More than 3 days	12.0	7.1	12.5
	Daily expenditure	Less than EUR 30	11.2	11.9	11.1
		EUR 30–65	24.0	17.6	23.9
		EUR 66–100	**42.1**	22.4	**43.9**
		More than EUR 100	22.7	**48.1**	21.1

Source: own elaboration. Bold indicates the highest value classification.

Regarding routes (Table 4), this type of tourism is popularized mainly through the internet or social networks (ham tourism, 61.4%; enotourism, 35.8%; and oil tourism, 48.1%). Because ham is a product that is not well known in international markets, social networks and the internet are the best disseminators of information about this tourist product. With respect to the expectations tourists had of routes, almost 80% reported that their expectations were met (ham tourism, 84.2%; oil tourism, 80.6%; and enotourism, 79.2%). The percentage for enotourism may be lower because many enotourists have already experienced other wine routes and draw comparisons, indicating that it is necessary to improve the Montilla-Moriles route, especially the explanation of the route (40.1%) and to improve the enotourism and oil tourism routes in general through better signage (50.6% and 47.7%, respectively). The degree of satisfaction with the three products exceeded 76% for more than 80% of the interviewees, with oil tourists being the most satisfied and those who would be willing to repeat the visit using a similar route (96.6%). This product, unlike wine, can only be found in countries of the Mediterranean basin, where there is a good climate and other tourist activities can be carried out.

The main motivation for gastronomic tourism (Table 5) was to learn the process of making oil (50.3%), wine (65.8%) and ham (50.5%), with wineries, ham curing and oil mills being the main attractions. At the end of the visit, tourists have the opportunity to taste the product and better appreciate the quality of the wines, hams and oils in the area. Among the respondents, 97% agreed with the creation of a combined route of gastronomic products, because they thought that the route would be gastronomically enriched and would be more attractive through the pairing of products, e.g., oil–ham and oil–cheese (Table 5).

The results of Tables 3–5 indicate that Hypothesis 1 was not fulfilled (the profile of gastronomic tourists depends on the product they consume) due to the similarity in the classification of the variables. In Table 3 (personal characteristics of gastronomic tourists) where 10 variables were analyzed, seven of them had the highest classification in the same category, coinciding in 70% (age, education level, gender, who the tourist travelled with, where the tourist was from, employment situation, and duration of the trip). In Table 4 (questions about the visit) where nine variables were analyzed, seven had a similar classification, coinciding in 77.7% (number of people who travelled the route with the tourist; whether the PDO or the gastronomic route met the tourist's expectations; whether the tourist would be interested in receiving more information after the visit; whether the price paid seemed to be consistent with the route; whether the tourist came expressly for this gastronomic route, or if it was offered to them in Andalusia; whether the tourist would repeat the experience using a similar route; degree of satisfaction with the visit), and in Table 5 (motivations) of the three variables analyzed, two of them had the maximum similarity of 66.6% (What were the reasons for the visit?; What would you think about the creation of a combined route of various gastronomic products with theatrical performances?). Therefore, the profile of the gastronomic tourist is similar in terms of ham, olive oil and wine.

Table 4. Univariate results of the survey of gastronomic tourism on Andalusia: questions about the visit.

Block	Question	Classification	Percentage of Ham Tourists	Percentage of Enotourists	Percentage of Oil Tourists
Questions about the visit	Number of people who travelled the route with you	1 person	8.3	15.6	12.2
		2 to 4 people	**76.2**	**70.1**	**66.3**
		More than 4 people	15.5	14.3	21.6
	Has the PDO or the gastronomic route met your expectations?	**Yes**	**84.2**	**79.2**	**80.6**
		No	15.8	20.8	19.4
	What would you improve?	Nothing	0.3	1.3	0.9
		Signage	**50.6**	**38.5**	**47.7**
		Explanation of the route or the PDO	24.8	40.1	39.1
		More audiovisual media	18.3	15.9	11.7
		Other	6	4.2	0.6
	Would you be interested in receiving more information after the visit?	**Yes, if it is free**	**62.3**	**74.3**	**59.7**
		Yes, in any case	17.5	6.2	20.2
		I do not think it's necessary	20.2	19.5	10.2
	Did you come expressly for this gastronomic route, or was it offered to you in Andalusia?	**I came expressly from my place of origin**	**76.1**	**59.7**	49.4
		It was circumstantial; they offered it to me	23.9	40.3	**51.6**
	Does the price paid seem to be consistent with the route?	**Yes**	**92.7**	**90.1**	**96.3**
		No	3.8	9.9	3.8
	How did you learn about the route?	Travel agencies	5.2	14.6	13.9
		Online, through social networks	**61.4**	35.8	**48.1**
		On the recommendation of friends and family	31.3	**45.8**	32.2
		Other media	2.1	3.9	5.8
	I would repeat the experience using a similar route	**Yes**	**82.3**	**87.1**	**96.6**
		No	17.7	12.8	3.4
	Degree of satisfaction with the visit	Less than 25%	6.0	4.4	0.6
		25–50%	4.2	7.9	1.1
		51–75%	8.3	5.4	2.7
		76–99%	**61.4**	**64.2**	**57.0**
		100%	20.1	18.1	38.6

Source: own elaboration Bold indicates the highest value classification.

Figure 3 shows a map of relationships between gastronomic tourist classifications and scores given to gastronomy in Córdoba. The blue circles represent the personal classification variable with respect to gastronomy. The majority of tourists classified themselves as people interested in gastronomy (largest blue circle). They did not have training in gastronomy. Although one of the motivations for traveling to Córdoba is gastronomy, it is not the main reason. These tourists rated gastronomy favorably, with thick blue lines representing the highest scores (7, 8, 9, 10). Gastronomy connoisseurs (gourmet tourists) were the minority (smallest blue circle). They have vast gastronomic training and come to Córdoba expressly for its gastronomy. This type of tourist rated Córdoba food very positively, with scores ranging from 6 to 10 for gastronomy in Córdoba. For tourists who classified themselves as gastronomic novices, their expectations were met the least with respect to Córdoba's food, in part because they did not understand gastronomy and had not visited other gastronomic destinations to appreciate the differences. However, on average, the gastronomy in Córdoba was very well rated, with the largest green circles representing scores of 9 and 10, indicating that Córdoba is a good gastronomic destination; however, this resource is not sufficiently exploited.

Table 5. Univariate results of the survey of gastronomic tourists: motivations.

Block	Question	Classification	Percentage of Ham Tourists	Percentage of Enotourists	Percentage of Oil Tourists
Questions about the motivation for the visit	What were the reasons for the visit?	Learn the culinary tradition of the destination	40.2	31	39.6
		Learn the process of making oil/wine/ham and visit oil mills, ham curing facilities, wineries	50.5	65.8	50.3
		Attend gastronomic festivals	9.3	3.2	10.1
	How do you rate the current situation in terms of tourism management at sites like the ones you have visited?	Good	**49.3**	39.4	**51.6**
		Fine	29.1	**52.8**	27.9
		Bad	21.6	7.8	20.5
	What would you think about the creation of a combined route of various gastronomic products with theatrical performances?	I agree	**98.1**	**99.3**	**96.5**
		I do not agree; I prefer to visit a single gastronomic route and not several	1.9	0.7	3.5

Source: own elaboration. Bold indicates the highest value classification.

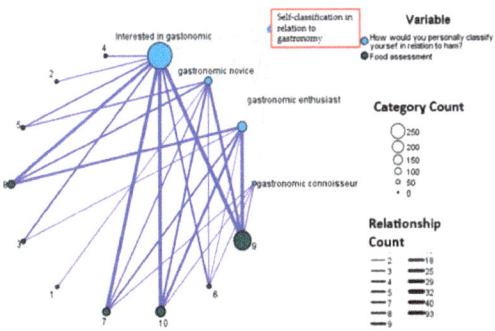

Figure 3. Relationship map. Source: own elaboration.

For a more in-depth analysis of the relationship between the different variables, bivariate analysis was carried out (Table 6). There is a strong relationship between tourist age and motivation to engage in gastronomic tourism ($\chi^2 = 325.71, p \leq 0.001$): the older the tourist, the more positively he/she valued gastronomic tourism. Age also influences knowledge of gastronomy ($\chi^2 = 62.32$): younger tourists' main motivation was to visit oil mills, wineries, ham curing facilities and learn about the production process, and older tourists' (aged over 50 years) main motivation was tasting dishes that feature olive oil, wine or Iberian ham. Additionally, gender was related to satisfaction ($\chi^2 = 11.88$), with women giving lower scores to the degree of satisfaction. Tourists who use oil, wine or ham more often (daily) rated such gastronomic products more positively because they appreciate the raw material more when they use it every day ($\chi^2 = 62.32$). Younger tourists used new technologies, the internet, social networks and tourism websites to learn about tours, while older tourists engaged in tours based on recommendations from friends and family. There is also a strong relationship between the reason for engaging in gastronomic tourism and age.

Table 6. Bivariate analysis.

Associated Variables	χ^2	df	p-Value
Age/Motivation for engaging in gastronomic tourism	325.71	8	<0.001
Satisfaction with visit/gender	11.86	4	0.019
Satisfaction/self-classification regarding gastronomy	62.32	16	<0.001
Satisfaction/Place of origin	241.47	16	<0.001
Satisfaction/Education level	264.89	12	<0.001

χ^2 Chi-square statistic. Related variables, α = 0.05; df = degrees of freedom.

In addition, education level and degree of satisfaction are related: tourists with a higher education level had a somewhat lower degree of satisfaction, either because they believed the explanations about the production process were not very accurate or because they believed that there was a need for more audiovisual media (χ^2 = 264.89).

To forecast the demand for gastronomic tourism in Córdoba, ARIMA models were used in an attempt to quantify the evolution of this type of tourism from January 2015 to June 2022 (Figure 4) and to determine the effect of the COVID-19 pandemic on this tourism segment, with the aim of testing Hypothesis 2.

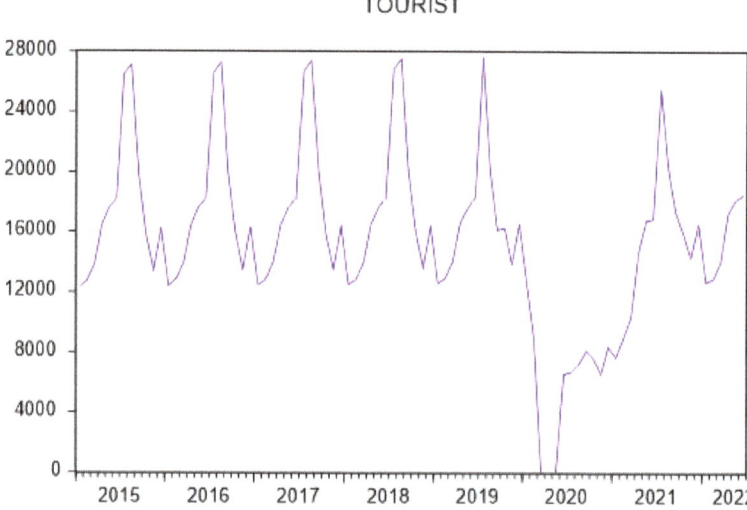

Figure 4. Monthly evolution of the number of gastronomic tourists in Córdoba (January 2015 to June 2022). Source: own elaboration based on information from the Designations of Origin of Córdoba. Vertical axis is thousands of people.

There are few studies that attempt to forecast the demand of gastronomic tourism, hence the importance of this study. To predict this demand, we collected monthly information from January 2015 to July 2022 on the number of gastronomic tourists who visited PDOs/gastronomic festivals in Andalusia. To model the number of gastronomic tourists (tourist), the BJ methodology was used to design a seasonal ARIMA (SARIMA) model (Tables 7 and 8), where a variable is analyzed with reference to its past values.

$$\Phi(B)\,\phi(B)\,(1-B)^d\,(1-B^s)^D\,Y_t^{(\lambda)} = \theta(B)\,\theta(B)\,a_t$$

Table 7. Estimation of the SARIMA model.

Variable	Coefficient	Std. Error	t-Statistic	Prob.
AR (1)	−0.497661	0.101278	−4.913816	0.0000
SMA (12)	−0.942206	0.062879	−14.98443	0.0000

Significant parameters $\alpha = 0.05$.

Table 8. GARCH test.

Variable	Coefficient	Std. Error	z-Statistic	Prob.
	Variance Equation			
C	1.14×10^{-4}	2.47×10^{-5}	4.620412	0.0000
RESID (−1)^2	13.83276	0.962786	14.36743	0.0000
GARCH (−1)	0.114353	0.012500	9.147971	0.0000

Absence of autoregressive conditional heteroscedasticity. Dependent variable: TOURIST. 1. Method: ML—ARCH (Marquardt)—Normal distribution. GARCH = C(1) + C(2) * RESID(−1)^2 + C(3) * GARCH(−1).

The demand for gastronomic tourism in Córdoba, called tourist in the model, is a variable with a nonnormal distribution, which has been corrected with Box–Cox transformation $\lambda = 0.2$ (tourist1 = tourist^0.2), and the mean trend was corrected with two differentiations in mean and 1 seasonal differentiation. This model is estimated to forecast the monthly demand for gastronomic tourism in Córdoba.

$$(1 + 0.497661B)(1 - B)^2 (1 - B^{12}) \text{Tourist}^{0.2} = (1 + 0.942206 B^{12}) a_t$$

Figure 5 shows the evolution of the gastronomic tourist variable (current), the values estimated by the model for those same dates (fitted) and the errors committed by the estimated model (residual), observing that these residuals are normal when between the range of ±2 Sd (standard deviation), except for 2020, when there were months that there was no tourism due to travel restrictions, resulting in abnormal estimates.

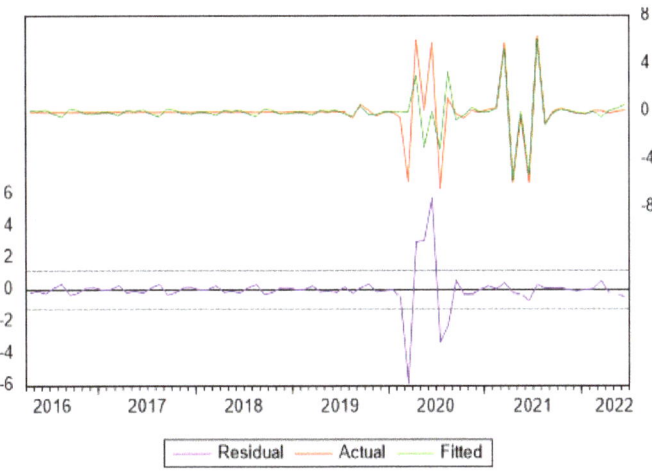

Figure 5. Monthly evolution of the number of gastronomic tourists in Córdoba and estimation errors (January 2015 to June 2022). Source: own elaboration based on ARIMA model estimate.

This model was used to forecast the demand for gastronomic tourism after the pandemic, which indicates that the expected growth will cause this type of tourism to exceed pre-pandemic levels. This may be because tourists seek natural environments as destinations, considering them safer. In fact, this type of tourism is more individualized and usually occurs in small groups; however, it is still considered seasonal tourism [73], distinguishing itself from gastronomic tourists who usually visit the provincial capital in the months from May to September. These tourists want to taste dishes made with quality products from the area; in contrast, gastronomic tourists who visit the province tend to concentrate their travel around the olive harvest (October–January), grape harvest (September and October), and pig slaughter (November–December), when tourists can participate in olive pole-beating (hitting branches to make the olives fall), grape harvesting, or the preparation of pork meat products after slaughter. Thus, although olive groves, vineyards, dehesas, oil mills, wineries and ham curing facilities, as well as olive, wine and ham museums, can be visited throughout the year, demand continues to be seasonal.

Table 9 provides a comparison of the real data for the number of tourists before and after the pandemic in Córdoba. The predictions for the months of July to December 2022 indicate an increase of 13,982 gastronomic tourists compared to the numbers before the pandemic (year 2019), indicating a recovery of this sector with an increase of 12% higher than other types of tourism. This finding suggests that after the pandemic, tourists have preferred to visit inland environments related to nature and seek quality gastronomic products; however, although these figures are positive, the number of gastronomic tourists is still low compared to other Spanish and international gastronomic destinations.

Table 9. Differences in tourist numbers before and after the COVID-19 pandemic in Córdoba.

Year/Month	Tourists	Year/Month	Tourists	Difference	% Variation
2022/07	28,110	2019/07	27,590	520	1.88
2022/08	22,345	2019/08	20,140	2205	10.94
2022/09	17,524	2019/09	16,130	1394	8.64
2022/10	18,132	2019/10	16,240	1892	11.65
2022/11	15,625	2019/11	13,830	1795	12.97
2022/12	22,736	2019/12	16,560	6176	37.29
total	124,472		110,490	13,982	12.65

Source: by authors. Column %Variation = tourists year 2022/tourists year 2019.

From the previous predictions, it can be affirmed that gastronomic tourism is a market niche still to be sufficiently exploited in Córdoba, especially oil tourism and ham tourism, having great potential for development in the province (growth greater than 12%). Therefore, Hypothesis 2 is confirmed, indicating that gastronomic tourism in the province of Córdoba will expand after the pandemic, but that this growth could be greater with adequate promotion given the uniqueness of these gastronomic products, which cannot be found in other places in the world, especially Iberian ham, making Córdoba a special destination.

6. Discussion

Based on research on gastronomic tourism and the results of this study carried out in the province of Córdoba, the profile of tourists can be different; for example, of those who attend the Trujillo Cheese Festival and the Cherry Blossom Festival in the Jerte Valley in Extremadura (Spain), the main tourists are women, 54.4% [74]; however, in the province of Córdoba, men predominate as tourists for all products studied (57.1% ham tourists, 51.2% wine tourists and 58.2% oil tourists), with the percentage of women being lower (42.5% ham tourists, 49.8% wine tourists and 41.8% oil tourists). The education level among tourists is also different; in Extremadura, university students were the predominate respondents (49.5%), and in the study by Mejía et al. [75], 59% of the respondents who engage in gastronomic tourism were university students. In the province of Córdoba, those with a baccalaureate level of education account for 43.8% of ham tourists and 38.5% of oil tourists, with the highest level being almost 20 points lower in Córdoba. However, there is similarity with respect to the origin of tourists; 27.5% are from the Extremadura region, and 24.7% from a nearby region. In Córdoba, more than 43% are from Andalusia, reaching 59.4% for oil tourists. Therefore, gastronomic tourism does not require spending the night, unlike other tourist activities, especially beaches, where gastronomic tourists are mainly foreigners [72]. There is much similarity in the tourist profiles of the three products analyzed. Compared with that for other places or products, the degree of satisfaction exceeds 76% for more than 90% of the respondents, reaching 95.6%, indicating that the tourism products offered based on gastronomy are high quality, similar to the results obtained in the study by Clemente et al. [76] with respect to the profile of gastronomic tourists in Valencia, where 97% of those surveyed considered gastronomy in the area to be good or very good.

Gastronomic tourists in Córdoba are therefore satisfied and would repeat experiences, a finding that is similar to the results reported by Huertas [52] in Canton-Mocha (Ecuador), where more than 91% of tourists would return to that same gastronomic destination. In Córdoba, the high returns for ham tourism (82.3%) and oil tourism (96.6%) are due to the relationship between satisfaction and repeated experience.

In an analysis of products and tourists' personal classification in relation to the products, Córdoba enotourists have an income of EUR 1001 to 1500, which is very different from the tourists who visit the Quinta da Gaivosa wineries in Portugal [77]. These enotourists can be classified in the highest category (Figure 6), wine connoisseurs, indicating that they are great connoisseurs of wine culture, travel expressly for reasons related to wine and earn more than EUR 3000 per month, buying wine in the winery after the visit. This is the type of tourist profile that the Montilla-Moriles route should seek.

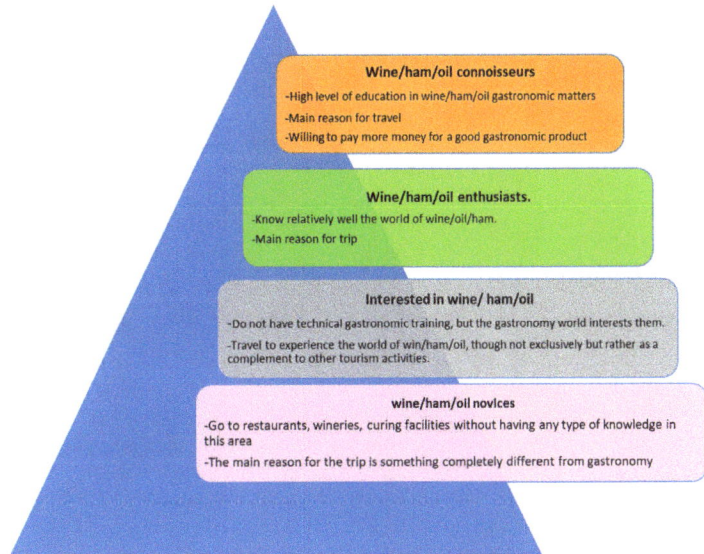

Figure 6. Classification of the gastronomic tourist according to product. Source: own elaboration.

Therefore, the tourists at the top of the pyramid (Figure 6) are the most selective and demanding, but those who travel to a destination know what product they are looking for, are willing to pay more for the gastronomic product and, if the experience is satisfactory, will repeat it, creating loyalty to that destination. A gastronomic destination has a life cycle similar to any tourism product. The basic concept of the life cycle in tourism studies, attributed to Butler [78], refers to the fact that tourist destinations show an evolutionary path formed by different stages: exploration, participation, development, consolidation, stagnation and decline or rejuvenation; for example, within gastronomic tourism destinations, there are some that are emerging, such as oil tourism [79], or are very developed, such as the wine routes in the Napa Valley [80]. To transition Córdoba into a gastronomy reference, tourists who have been introduced to the product must become more familiar with the product, and their advertising of the destination will encourage other tourists to come in the future, with the aim of becoming an exclusive gastronomic destination for gastronomy connoisseurs. Given the quality of the products found in the province of Córdoba, good tourism planning and marketing could turn it into a gastronomic destination similar to France, as indicated by Cunha [81]. Increasingly, there is a need to focus on promoting the values of intangible heritage, such as the gastronomy of a region, both for residents and tourists. Due to interactions with other cultures, gastronomy should always be understood as part of the cultural experience of a country or region. Gastronomic richness must be supported by the competent local, regional and national authorities so that traditions and culinary values are not lost over time. Considering the importance of certified products for the gastronomic identity of a region, it is necessary to combat the extinction of several gastronomic traditions that may lack product certification and/or support from competent authorities. To increase the number of tourists, gastronomic routes should be created, similar to those designed in the Cunha study in the Dão-Lafões region (Portugal), which would encourage the number of overnight stays in Córdoba and would increase the richness of that area.

7. Conclusions

The province of Córdoba has three key materials from a gastronomic point of view, i.e., olive oil, which is part of the Mediterranean diet and present in all Andalusian cuisine; ham, as not only a nutritional element rich in protein, but also part of typical dishes such as *flamenquín;* and wine, as a drink that complements a dish and as a cooking element in typical recipes such as sirloin steak or meat with Pedro Ximénez wine, making Córdoba a high-quality gastronomy region. However, this culinary wealth is not being sufficiently exploited from the tourist's point of view. A brand that identifies Córdoba as a gastronomic destination should be created; this approach will increase the number of tourists, because although tourism will grow by 12%, as determined using an ARIMA model, such growth is lower than that seen in other areas of the interior of the community [82] that have expanded by 147% after the pandemic. It is necessary to develop activities that increase the average expenditure of tourists and increase overnight stays in the city and province. For these two elements, average spending and overnight stays are among the lowest in Andalusia (EUR 68.6 and 2.9 days in Córdoba compared to EUR 72 and 5.1 days in Andalusia) [83].

The differentiated quality of the food products, the cultural tradition and their artisanal preparation make these products tourist attractions, especially considering the changes in tourist consumers' habits (vacations more distributed throughout the year, although they are shorter, weekend trips, the desire for a healthy life, natural landscapes—the current situation, i.e., the pandemic, has contributed to this—environmentalism, etc.). The areas that host these PDOs have seen their wealth increased, and the quality of life of their populations has improved.

Finding tourists with a certain socioeconomic profile requires time. Tourists who have a high income level and a university level of education, want to spend the night in the area, and use the services that are available should be sought; however, for this to occur, these areas must be provided with those services and facilities (hospitality, restaurants, activities, etc.).

There are detractors of tourist activity. Such individuals think that tourism in the province of Córdoba will lead to the destruction of the rural environment they visit as a result of the explosion of services exceeding the carrying capacity of destinations, causing a loss of identity in the area and increasing housing prices, etc., which, although they could occur, are easily avoidable with proper planning.

The availability of unique foods and other gastronomic offerings at destinations must be complemented with a specific strategy for the promotion of gastronomic tourism for it to be successfully developed [33]. Based on our analysis of the three products, Córdoba has a greater potential for attracting ham and oil tourists because wine tourism already has well-established routes, such as those for La Rioja [84], and it will be very difficult to compete with them in the short and medium terms. Therefore, effort should be focused on the development and improvement of ham and oil routes.

Regarding the hypotheses, Hypothesis 2, which refers to growth of the demand for gastronomic tourism, is confirmed, but not at the desired levels, and Hypothesis 1 is not confirmed, because tourist profiles do not differ with respect to the gastronomic products they consume. This is due in part to the fact that tourists are from nearby and their personal characteristics and motivations are very similar.

Based on the obtained results, the following strategies are proposed (using the reference products wine, olive oil and Iberian ham) that could contribute to improving this tourism segment:

- Create plans and/or complementary activities that will encourage overnight stays in the area. These activities can range from festivities, samplings and fairs to tastings, training courses, competitions and stargazing, taking advantage of the low light at night in many of these rural areas, and lasting more than one day to encourage overnight stays.
- The above would make sense as long as a hospitality and catering infrastructure with the capacity to accommodate these types of events is adequately developed. For this, there must be investments in the area as a complement to the production of goods that is already being carried.
- This symbiosis between products with a designation of origin and geographical area, accompanied by corresponding marketing campaigns, would not take long to bear fruit [85].
- Develop signage within the area that encompasses the three products. Adequate signage, as part of street furniture in these rural areas, would contribute, both as publicity (for those who, at that time, are not engaging in tourist activities) and as information for tourists who wish to move from one place to another. Not surprisingly, through our research, lack of signage was identified as an item that need to be improved for designations of origin in the province of Córdoba.
- The seven designations of origin should combine their efforts not only to develop economies of scale that minimize the associated costs of advertising and promotion, but also, as all products are highly recommended both from the gastronomic and nutritional perspectives, to organize routes that cover one, two or all three products. For example, dinners or lunches could be organized between olive producers or vineyards, focusing on products of the land, after a day in which the tourists have visited an oil mill, a ham curing facility and/or a winery. Such events could be accompanied by live performances, if desired.
- Generate awareness of "sharing tourism" among the different designations of origin. That is, to offer a wider variety of activities and products so that potential tourists do not need to leave the area.
- Create an association among the seven PDOs in the province of Córdoba that would support their interests, with campaigns aimed at attracting investments and promoting tourism. The similarity of offerings and the areas in which they are developed make this type of union very viable because conflicting interests are highly unusual.
- All of the above would be much easier with the involvement and cooperation of economic agents and public administration. The management and processing of grants and subsidies, national and international promotion, public events, and the designation of protected areas or natural parks, etc., will be more effective if the highest possible levels of decision-making capacity participate.
- The implementation of these "recommendations" should be made with the supervision of a panel of experts related to different areas of knowledge, for example, economists, lawyers, agronomists, forestry engineers, architects, biologists, landscapers, etc., to minimize the risks that can lead to overcrowding natural landscapes of incalculable beauty as much as possible.

Good management of the gastronomic resources in Córdoba could make this province a well-known destination and valued at the national and international levels.

In conclusion, an increasing number of tourists seek specific learning experiences in which gastronomy plays a predominant and central role [86]. For Córdoba to be an internationally recognized gastronomic destination, it is necessary not only to have good raw materials and exquisite dishes but also to be recognized in international markets. This work serves as a barometer of the situation of this segment, aiming to help public agencies and private companies join forces and address the errors detected. The synergy among all actors will make Córdoba a high-quality gastronomic destination.

One limitation of this study was that it used a joint survey of tourists to the capital and to the province of Córdoba. The survey yielded an average gastronomic tourist profile for each product (wine, olive oil and ham). It would be interesting to differentiate gastronomic tourists visiting the capital from those visiting the province in case there are significant differences.

As future lines of research, it would be interesting to compare profiles of gastronomic products and differentiate between national and foreign tourists to achieve a better segmentation and to compare the gastronomic tourists of Córdoba with those of other World Heritage cities.

Author Contributions: Conceptualization, M.G.D.M. and M.G.M.V.d.l.T.; methodology, M.G.D.M.; software, M.G.D.M.; validation, M.G.D.M. and M.G.M.V.d.l.T.; formal analysis, M.G.D.M. and M.G.M.V.d.l.T.; investigation, M.G.D.M. and M.G.M.V.d.l.T.; resources, M.G.M.V.d.l.T.; data curation, M.G.D.M.; writing—original draft preparation, M.G.D.M. and M.G.M.V.d.l.T.; writing—review and editing, M.G.D.M. and M.G.M.V.d.l.T.; visualization, M.G.D.M.; supervision, M.G.M.V.d.l.T.; project administration, M.G.D.M.; funding acquisition, M.G.M.V.d.l.T. All authors have read and agreed to the published version of the manuscript.

Funding: This research received no external funding.

Institutional Review Board Statement: Not applicable.

Informed Consent Statement: Informed consent was obtained from all subjects involved in the study.

Data Availability Statement: The data presented in this study are available on request from the corresponding author.

Conflicts of Interest: The authors declare they have no conflicts of interest.

References

1. Alfiero, S.; Bonadonna, A.; Cane, M.; Lo Giudice, A. Street food: A tool for promoting tradition, territory, and tourism. *Tour. Anal.* **2019**, *24*, 305–314. [CrossRef]
2. Cohard, J.C.R.; Martínez, J.D.S.; Simón, V.J.G. Valorizando el territorio con alimentos excelentes: Los aceites de alta gama en el sur de España. In *Arethuse: Scientific Journal of Economics and Business Management*; Società Editrice Esculapio: Bologna, Italy, 2013; pp. 75–90.
3. Dancausa, M.G.; Millán, M.G.; Huete, N. Olive oil as a gourmet ingredient in contemporary cuisine. A gastronomic tourism proposal. *Int. J. Gastron. Food Sci.* **2022**, *29*, 100548. [CrossRef]
4. Armesto, X.A.; Gómez, B. Productos agroalimentarios de calidad, turismo y desarrollo local: El caso del Priorat. *Cuad. Geográficos* **2004**, *34*, 83–94.
5. Csurgó, B.; Hindley, C.; Smith, M.K. The role of gastronomic tourism in rural development. In *The Routledge Handbook of Gastronomic Tourism*; Saurabh Kumar Dixit, Ed.; Routledge: Oxford, UK, 2019; pp. 62–69.
6. Guasch-Ferré, M.; Willett, W.C. The Mediterranean diet and health: A comprehensive overview. *J. Intern. Med.* **2021**, *290*, 549–566. [CrossRef]
7. Martínez-González, M.A.; Salas-Salvadó, J.; Estruch, R.; Corella, D.; Fitó, M.; Ros, E.; Predimed Investigators. Benefits of the Mediterranean diet: Insights from the PREDIMED study. *Prog. Cardiovasc. Dis.* **2015**, *58*, 50–60. [CrossRef] [PubMed]
8. Cavicchi, A.; Santini, C. Food tourism and foodies in Italy: The role of the Mediterranean diet between resilience and sustainability. In *Sustainable Tourism Practices in the Mediterranean*; Tüzün, I., Ergül, M., Johnson, C., Eds.; Routledge: New York, NY, USA, 2020; pp. 137–152.
9. Velissariou, E.; Vasilaki, E. Local gastronomy and tourist behavior: Research on domestic tourism in Greece. *J. Tour. Res.* **2014**, *9*, 120–143.

10. Sáez-Almendros, S.; Obrador, B.; Bach-Faig, A.; Serra-Majem, L. Environmental footprints of Mediterranean versus Western dietary patterns: Beyond the health benefits of the Mediterranean diet. *Environ. Health* **2013**, *12*, 118. [CrossRef]
11. Dussaillant, C.; Echeverría, G.; Urquiaga, I.; Velasco, N.; Rigotti, A. Evidencia actual sobre los beneficios de la dieta mediterránea en salud. *Rev. Méd. Chile* **2016**, *144*, 1044–1052. [CrossRef]
12. Bach, A.; Roman, B.; Serra, L. El porqué de los beneficios de la dieta mediterránea. *Jano Med. Humanid.* **2007**, *1648*, 26.
13. De Uña-Álvarez, E.; Villarino-Pérez, M. Linking wine culture, identity, tourism and rural development in a denomination of origin territory (NW of Spain). *Cuad. Tur.* **2019**, *44*, 93–110. [CrossRef]
14. de Pouplana, J.R. Las tendencias del turismo pos-COVID-19. *Tecnohotel Rev. Prof. Hostel. Restauración* **2020**, *485*, 30–31.
15. Márquez, A.M.; Hernández Ortiz, M.J. Cooperación y sociedades cooperativas: El caso de la Denominación de Origen Sierra Mágina. *Rev. Estud. Coop. Revesco* **2001**, *74*, 123–149.
16. Ministerio de Agricultura Pesca y Alimentación. *Datos de las Denominaciones de Origen Protegidas (D.O.P.), Indicaciones Geográficas Protegidas (I.G.P.) y Especialidades Tradicionales Garantizadas (E.T.G.) de Productos Agroalimentarios*; MAPA: Madrid, Spain, 2022.
17. Cava, J.A.; Millán, M.G.; Dancausa, M.G. Enotourism in Southern Spain: The Montilla-Moriles PDO. *Int. J. Environ. Res. Public Health* **2022**, *19*, 3393. [CrossRef] [PubMed]
18. Consejeria de Agricultura. Ganadería, Pesca y Desarrollo Sostenible Junta de Andalucía. 2022. Available online: https://www.juntadeandalucia.es/agriculturaypesca/observatorio/servlet/FrontController?action=RecordContent&table=11114&element=3868182&subsector=&2022 (accessed on 12 June 2022).
19. López-Guzmán, T.; Sánchez-Cañizares, S. Gastronomy, tourism and destination differentiation: A case study in Spain. *Rev. Econ. Financ.* **2012**, *1*, 63–72.
20. Jiménez Beltrán, J.; López-Guzmán, T.; Santa-Cruz, F.G. Gastronomy and tourism: Profile and motivation of international tourism in the city of Córdoba, Spain. *J. Culin. Sci. Technol.* **2016**, *14*, 347–362. [CrossRef]
21. Pérez-Gálvez, J.C.; Medina-Viruel, M.J.; Jara-Alba, C.; López-Guzmán, T. Segmentation of food market visitors in World Heritage Sites. Case study of the city of Córdoba (Spain). *Curr. Issues Tour.* **2021**, *24*, 1139–1153. [CrossRef]
22. Vega, V.; Freire, D.A.; Guananga, N.I.; Garlobo, E.R.; Alarcón, M.R.; Aguilera, P. Gastronomía ecuatoriana y turismo local. *Dilemas Contemp. Educ. Política Valores* **2018**, *6*, 1–17.
23. Agrawal, V. A review of Indian tourism industry with SWOT analysis. *J. Tour. Hosp.* **2016**, *5*, 196–200.
24. Turgarini, D.; Pridia, H.; Soemantri, L.L. Gastronomic Tourism Travel Routes Based on Android Applications in Ternate City. *J. Gastron. Tour.* **2021**, *8*, 57–64. [CrossRef]
25. Franco, A.F.; Martinez, L.F.; Mindiola, L.A. Diseño de una ruta gastronómica de los emprendimientos de comidas típicas en la ciudad de Santo Domingo. *Dilemas Contemp. Educ. Política Valores* **2020**, *48*, 1–12. [CrossRef]
26. Chaney, S.; Ryan, C. Analyzing the evolution of Singapore's World Gourmet Summit: An example of gastronomic tourism. *Int. J. Hosp. Manag.* **2012**, *31*, 309–318. [CrossRef]
27. Batat, W. The role of luxury gastronomy in culinary tourism: An ethnographic study of Michelin-Starred restaurants in France. *Int. J. Tour. Res.* **2021**, *23*, 150–163. [CrossRef]
28. Privitera, D.; Nedelcu, A.; Nicula, V. Gastronomic and food tourism as an economic local resource: Case studies from Romania and Italy. *GeoJournal Tour. Geosites* **2018**, *21*, 143–157.
29. Pavlidis, G.; Markantonatou, S. Gastronomic tourism in Greece and beyond: A thorough review. *Int. J. Gastron. Food Sci.* **2020**, *21*, 100229. [CrossRef] [PubMed]
30. Sanip, M.N.A.M.; Mustapha, R. Sustainability of Gastronomic Tourism in Malaysia: Theoretical Context. *Int. J. Asian Soc. Sci.* **2020**, *10*, 417–425. [CrossRef]
31. Hussin, H. Gastronomy, tourism, and the soft power of Malaysia. *Sage Open* **2018**, *8*, 2158244018809211. [CrossRef]
32. Correa, L.Á. Gastronomic tourism, factors that affect the competitiveness of restaurants in Zacatecas, México. *Tur. Patrim.* **2022**, 49–65. [CrossRef]
33. Josphine, J. A critical review of gastronomic tourism development in Kenya. *J. Hosp. Tour. Manag.* **2021**, *4*, 27–39.
34. Medeiros, M.D.L.; da Cunha, J.A.C.; Passador, J.L. Gastronomic tourism and regional development: A study based on the minas artisanal cheese of Serro. *Cad. Virtual Tur.* **2018**, *18*, 168–189.
35. Millán, M.G.; Sánchez-Ollero, J.L.; Dancausa, M.G. Ham Tourism in Andalusia: An Untapped Opportunity in the Rural Environment. *Foods* **2022**, *11*, 2277. [CrossRef]
36. Seyitoğlu, F.; Alphan, E. Gastronomy tourism through tea and coffee: Travellers' museum experience. *Int. J. Cult. Tour. Hosp. Res.* **2021**, *15*, 413–427. [CrossRef]
37. Pratiwi, Y. Traditional Fish Gangan: An Icon of Gastronomic Tourism from Belitung Island. *Gastron. Tour. J.* **2020**, *7*, 14–19. [CrossRef]
38. Hernandez, R.; Dancausa, M.G. Culinary Tourism. Traditional Gastronomy of Córdoba (Spain). *Estud. Perspect. En Tur.* **2018**, *27*, 413–430.
39. Berbel-Pineda, J.M.; Palacios-Florencio, B.; Ramírez-Hurtado, J.M.; Santos-Roldán, L. Gastronomic experience as a factor of motivation in the tourist movements. *Int. J. Gastron. Food Sci.* **2019**, *18*, 100171. [CrossRef]
40. Decrop, A. Tourists' Decision-Making and Behaviour Processes. In *Consumer Behaviour in Travel and Tourism*; Pizam, A., Mansfeld, Y., Eds.; The Haworth Hospitality Press: Philadelphia, PA, USA, 2000; pp. 103–133.

41. Nicoletti, S.; Medina-Viruel, M.G.; Di-Clemente, E.; Fruet-Cardozo, J.V. Motivations of the Culinary Tourist in the City of Trapani, Italy. *Sustainability* **2019**, *11*, 2686. [CrossRef]
42. González, F.; Moral-Cuadra, S.; López-Guzman, T. Gastronomic Motivations and Perceived Value of Foreign Tourists in the City of Oruro (Bolivia): An Analysis Based on Structural Equations. *Int. J. Environ. Res. Public Health* **2020**, *17*, 3618. [CrossRef]
43. Moral-Cuadra, S.; Acero, R.; Rueda, R.; Salinas, E. Relationship between consumer motivation and the gastronomic experience of olive oil tourism in Spain. *Sustainability* **2020**, *12*, 4178. [CrossRef]
44. Cordova-Buiza, F.; Gabriel-Campos, E.; Castaño-Prieto, L.; Garcia-Garcia, L. The Gastronomic Experience: Motivation and Satisfaction of the Gastronomic Tourist—The Case of Puno City (Peru). *Sustainability* **2021**, *13*, 9170. [CrossRef]
45. Alegre, J.; Garau, J. Tourist satisfaction and dissatisfaction. *Ann. Tour. Res.* **2010**, *37*, 52–73. [CrossRef]
46. Yoon, Y.; Uysal, M. An examination of the effects of motivation and satisfaction on destination loyalty: A structural model. *Tour. Manag.* **2005**, *26*, 4556. [CrossRef]
47. Murphy, P.; Pritchard, M.P.; Smith, B. The destination product and its impact on traveller perceptions. *Tour. Manag.* **2000**, *21*, 43–52. [CrossRef]
48. Kozak, M. Destination benchmarking. *Ann. Tour. Res.* **2002**, *29*, 497–519. [CrossRef]
49. Alegre, J.; Cladera, M. Repeat visitation in mature sun and sand holiday destinations. *J. Travel Res.* **2006**, *44*, 288–297. [CrossRef]
50. Hu, Y.; Min, H.K. Enjoyment or indulgence: What draws the line in hedonic food consumption? *Int. J. Hosp. Manag.* **2022**, *104*, 103228. [CrossRef]
51. Fettahlıoğlu, H.S.; Yıldız, A.; Birin, C. Hedonik Tüketim Davranışları: Kahramanmaraş Sütçü İmam Üniversitesi ve Adıyaman Üniversitesi Öğrencilerinin Hedonik Alışveriş Davranışlarında Demografik Faktörlerin Etkisinin Karşılaştırmalı Olarak Analizi. *Int. J. Soc. Sci.* **2014**, *27*, 307–331.
52. Huertas, T.E.; Suarez, E.S.; Cuetara, L.M. Perfil del cliente gastronómico del cantón Mocha. *Rev. UNIANDES Epistem.* **2016**, *3*, 497–506.
53. Dancausa, M.G.; Millán, M.G.; Hernández, R. Analysis of the demand for gastronomic tourism in Andalusia (Spain). *PLoS ONE* **2021**, *16*, 1–23. [CrossRef]
54. Moral-Cuadra, S.; Solano-Sánchez, M.Á.; Menor-Campos, A.; López-Guzmán, T. Discovering gastronomic tourists' profiles through artificial neural networks: Analysis, opinions and attitudes. *Tour. Recreat. Res.* **2022**, *47*, 347–358. [CrossRef]
55. Menor-Campos, A.; Hidalgo-Fernández, A.; López-Felipe, T.; Jara-Alba, C. Gastronomía local, cultura y turismo en Ciudades Patrimonio de la Humanidad: El comportamiento del turista extranjero. *Investig. Turísticas* **2022**, *23*, 140–161. [CrossRef]
56. Yang, Y.; Zhang, H. Spatial-temporal forecasting of tourism demand. *Ann. Tour. Res.* **2019**, *75*, 106–119. [CrossRef]
57. Petrevska, B. Predicting tourism demand by ARIMA models. *Econ. Res.-Ekon. Istraživanja* **2017**, *30*, 939–950. [CrossRef]
58. Zhang, M.; Li, J.; Pan, B.; Zhang, G. Weekly hotel occupancy forecasting of a tourism destination. *Sustainability* **2018**, *10*, 4351. [CrossRef]
59. Pérez-Priego, M.A.; Garcia-Moreno Garcia, M.B.; Gomez-Casero, G.; Caridad, L. Segmentation based on the gastronomic motivations of tourists: The case of the Costa Del Sol (Spain). *Sustainability* **2019**, *11*, 409. [CrossRef]
60. García de Yébenes, M.J.; Rodríguez, F.; Carmona, L. Validación de cuestionarios. *Reumatol. Clínica* **2009**, *5*, 171–177. [CrossRef] [PubMed]
61. Villavicencio-Caparó, E.; Ruiz-García, V.; Cabrera-Duffaut, A. Validation of questionnaires. *Rev. OACTIVA UC Cuenca* **2016**, *1*, 75–80.
62. López-Guzmán, T.; Cañizares, S.M.S. La gastronomía como motivación para viajar. Un estudio sobre el turismo culinario en Córdoba. *PASOS Rev. Tur. Patrim. Cult.* **2012**, *10*, 575–584. [CrossRef]
63. Millán-Vázquez, G.; Arjona-Fuentes, J.; Amador-Hidalgo, L. Olive oil tourism: Promoting rural development in Andalusia (Spain). *Tour. Manag. Perspect.* **2017**, *21*, 100–108. [CrossRef]
64. Schmidt, M.E.; Steindorf, K. Statistical methods for the validation of questionnaires. *Methods of information in medicine* **2006**, *45*, 409–413. [CrossRef]
65. Kazi, A.M.; Khalid, W. Questionnaire designing and validation. *J. Pak. Med. Assoc.* **2012**, *62*, 514.
66. Cava, J.A.; Millán, G.; Hernandez, R. Analysis of the Tourism Demand for Iberian Ham Routes in Andalusia (Southern Spain): Tourist Profile. *Sustainability* **2019**, *11*, 6047. [CrossRef]
67. Lim, W.M.; To, W.M. The economic impact of a global pandemic on the tourism economy: The case of COVID-19 and Macao's destination-and gambling-dependent economy. *Curr. Issues Tour.* **2022**, *25*, 1258–1269. [CrossRef]
68. Gujarati, D. *Essentials of Ecomnometrics*, 5th ed.; SAGE Publications, Inc.: San Mateo, CA, USA, 2021; pp. 1–632.
69. Millán, G.; Pérez, L.M. Comparación del perfil de enoturistas y oleoturistas en España. Un estudio de caso. *Cuad. Desarro. Rural* **2014**, *11*, 167–188.
70. Alonso, A.D.; Northcote, J. The development of olive tourism in Western Australia: A case study of an emerging tourism industry. *Int. J. Tour. Res.* **2010**, *12*, 696–708. [CrossRef]
71. Oliveira, S. La gastronomía como atractivo turístico primario de un destino: El Turismo Gastronómico en Mealhada—Portugal. *Estud. Y Perspect. En Tur.* **2011**, *20*, 738–752.
72. Orgaz, F.; López, T. Análisis del perfil, motivaciones, y valoraciones de los turistas gastronómicos. El caso de la República Dominicana. *Ara: Rev. Investig. Tur.* **2017**, *5*, 43–52.

73. Martín, J.M.; Salinas, J.A.; Rodriguez, J.A.; Ostos, M.D.S. Analysis of tourism seasonality as a factor limiting the sustainable development of rural areas. *J. Hosp. Tour. Res.* **2020**, *44*, 45–75. [CrossRef]
74. Folgado, J.A.; Hernández, J.M.; Duarte, P.A.O. El perfil del turista de eventos culturales: Un análisis exploratorio. *Cult. Desarro. Nuevas Tecnol. VII Jorn. Investig. Tur.* **2014**, *1*, 57–74.
75. Mejía, M.O.; Franco, W.C.; Franco, M.C.; Flores, F.Z. Perfil y Preferencias de los Visitantes en Destinos Con Potencial Gastronómico: Caso 'Las Huecas' de Guayaquil [Ecuador]. *Rosa Ventos* **2017**, *9*, 200–215. [CrossRef]
76. Clemente, J.S.; Roig, B.; Valencia, S.; Rabadan, M.T.; Martinez, C. Actitud hacia la gastronomía local de los turistas: Dimensiones y segmentación de mercado. *PASOS Rev. Tur. Patrim. Cult.* **2008**, *6*, 189–198. [CrossRef]
77. Coelho, S.; Remondes, J.; Costa, A.P. Estudo do perfil e motivações do enoturista: O caso da quinta da Gaivosa. *Cult. Rev. De Cult. Tur.* **2021**, *15*, 3.
78. Butler, R. The concept of a tourist area cycle of evolution: Implications for management of resources. *Can. Geogr.* **1980**, *24*, 5–12. [CrossRef]
79. Millán-Vázquez, G.; Pablo-Romero, M.; Sánchez Rivas, J. Oleotourism as a Sustainable Product: An Analysis of Its Demand in the South of Spain (Andalusia). *Sustainability* **2018**, *10*, 101. [CrossRef]
80. Scorrano, P.; Fait, M.; Maizza, A.; Vrontis, D. Online branding strategy for wine tourism competitiveness. *Int. J. Wine Bus. Res.* **2019**, *31*, 130–150. [CrossRef]
81. Cunha, S. Turismo gastronómico, un factor de diferenciación. *Millenium* **2018**, *2*, 93–98. [CrossRef]
82. Instituto Nacional de Estadistica. Available online: https://www.ine.es/jaxiT3/Datos.htm?t=1995 (accessed on 1 July 2022).
83. Instituto de Estadística y Cartografía de Andalucía. 2022. Available online: https://www.juntadeandalucia.es/institutodeestadisticaycartografia/badea/informe/datosaldia?CodOper=b3_271&idNode=9801#51246 (accessed on 4 July 2022).
84. Marzo-Navarro, M.; Pedraja-Iglesias, M. Use of a winery's website for wine tourism development: Rioja region. *Int. J. Wine Bus. Res.* **2021**, *33*, 523–544. [CrossRef]
85. Correia, A.; Moital, M.; Oliveira, N.; da Costa, C.F. Multidimensional segmentation of gastronomic tourists based on motivation and satisfaction. *Int. J. Tour. Policy* **2009**, *2*, 37–57. [CrossRef]
86. Jong, A.; Varley, P. Food tourism policy: Deconstructing boundaries of taste and. *Tour. Manag.* **2016**, *60*, 212–222. [CrossRef]

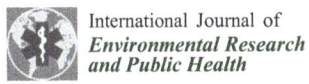

Article

The Evaluation of Rural Outdoor Dining Environment from Consumer Perspective

Mian Yang [1,2], Wenjie Fan [2], Jian Qiu [1,*], Sining Zhang [1] and Jinting Li [2]

[1] Faculty of Architecture, Southwest Jiaotong University, Chengdu 610000, China
[2] Faculty of Art, Sichuan Tourism University, Chengdu 610000, China
* Correspondence: qiujian@home.swjtu.edu.cn; Tel.:+86-139-8185-1328

Abstract: The quality of the environment should be measured by the satisfaction of the public and guided by the issues of public concern. With the development of the internet, social media as the main platform for people to exchange information has become a data source for planning and management analysis. Nowadays, the rural catering industry is becoming increasingly competitive, especially after the pandemic. How to further enhance the competitiveness of the rural catering industry has become a hot topic in the industry. From the perspective of consumers, we explored consumers' preferences in a rural outdoor dining environment through social media data. The research analyzed the social media data through manual collection and object detection, divided the landscape of the rural outdoor dining environment into eight categories with 35 landscape elements, and then used BP (Back Propagation) neural network nonlinear fitting and least square linear fitting to analyze the 11,410 effective review pictures from eight rural restaurants' social media comments in Chengdu. We derived the degree of consumer preference for the landscape quality of the rural outdoor dining environment and analyzed the differences in preference among three different groups (regular customers, customers with children, and customers with the elderly). The study found that agricultural resources are an important factor in the competitiveness of rural restaurant environments; that children's emotions when using activity facilities can positively influence consumers' dining experiences; that safety and hygiene environment are important factors influencing the decisions of parent–child dining; and that older people are more interested in outdoor nature, etc. The research results provide suggestions and knowledge for rural restaurant managers and designers through human-oriented needs from the perspective of consumers, and clarify the preferences and expectations of different consumer groups for rural restaurant landscapes while achieving the goal of rural landscape protection.

Keywords: social media data; outdoor dining environment preference; rural restaurants; human-oriented; rural sustainable development

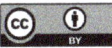

1. Introduction

The catering industry can become the core of destination development, which, in turn, can promote overall economic development to achieve the goal of sustainable development [1]. As an important development strategy put forward by China in recent years, the Rural Revitalization Strategy puts forward higher target requirements for the construction of agriculture, farming, and rural areas. Rural tourism, as an important pathway to rural revitalization, is highly valued at this stage. At the same time, the field of rural tourism research requires more comprehensive research from a wider range of academic disciplines [2]. As an important part of rural tourism, rural catering has ushered in a historic development period under the good momentum of rural tourism development [3]. The rural catering industry is vital to promoting the rural economy and protecting local cultural capital, and can also promote the joint development of urban and rural areas. As an important attraction for rural restaurants, the rural outdoor dining environment (ODE) plays an important role in the development of rural restaurants [4]. As a traditional settlement, the countryside is an important spatial carrier for agricultural production, ecological conservation, and cultural inheritance, and it has irreplaceable functions and status as urban areas [5]. The harmonious integration of "bottom-up" human-oriented needs can enhance the freedom, continuity, and diversity of the development of individual forms of villages, and avoid the "one size fits all" development model of villages caused by planning assumptions lacking human-oriented considerations [6]. Therefore, we believe that the research of rural ODE focusing on consumer needs is very important for rural revitalization and rural sustainable development.

1.1. Rural Outdoor Dining Environment

With the increased interest of urban residents in rural areas, the rural landscape has promoted the development of rural tourism [7] and highlighted its economic value [8]. The properties, leisure infrastructure, culture, and natural landscape of rural tourism sites are all important pull factors for rural tourism [9]. Under scientific tourism development, these resources can be better protected and sustainable development of rural resources can be realized [10]. Food tourism has a very important role in rural tourism, which creates more jobs for local people and promotes economic development [11,12]. A study by Scozzafava et al. [13] found that restaurants that supported local food and organic products positively influenced customers, and that restaurants with local products were three times more likely to be chosen than restaurants without local products. Rinaldi et al. [14] studied the local identity and attractiveness of rural areas and agriculture, and suggested that local dining resources must address and strengthen the link between place (territorial/geographic dimension) and people (cultural dimension). Food, the environment, and novelty value are the main prerequisites for attracting consumers to promote urban and rural co-development [15,16]. It can be seen that the study of the rural dining environment contributes to the development of rural tourism as well as the sustainable development of the rural landscape.

Customers need a unique dining environment to enjoy a different experience (Liu and Jang, 2009) [17]. With the change in lifestyle, dining out in rural areas has become an important social behavior. Auty (2006) found that whereas consumers stated that food type and food quality were the main variables in choosing a restaurant, as consumers' dining needs increased, the environment of the restaurant became the determining factor [18]. Therefore, the physical environment of catering is very important in shaping the image of restaurants and influencing customer behavior [19,20]. Scholars have also studied the relationship between consumers' dining experiences and individual factors. Based on quantitative analysis, Ryu et al. identified a six-factor scale consisting of facility aesthetics, ambiance, lighting, service offerings, layout, and social factors as a procedure to assess DINESCAPE in upscale restaurant environments [21], and found that facility aesthetics, atmosphere, and staff had a significant impact on customer pleasure [22]. Hong and Hsu [23] summarized restaurant interior environments into four dimensions: physical environment (architecture, restaurant name, sign, interior design and decoration, furniture and equipment, layout, lighting, temperature, aroma, and music), product and service (appearance and flavor of food and beverages, plating, the items on and design of the menu, tableware, employees' expressions, employees' physical movement and gestures, employees' introductions, communication, and storytelling), employee's aesthetic traits (appearance, voice, and body odor), and other customers' aesthetic traits (customer appearance, voice, behavior, and etiquette). Yang et al. [4] proposed three ODE dimensions that influence consumer satisfaction with rural restaurants: quality and facilities (uniform, appearance, garnish, table setting, service quality, table placement, illumination, and decorations), image and atmosphere (name, natural sound, signage, and music), and landscape elements (pavement, artificial structure, buildings, and ornamental plants), and found that customers in rural areas tend to prefer to experience natural landscapes, and no other study proposed the ODE dimensions as far as we know. Albright et al. [24] found that women and older adults tend to be more interested in making healthy choices in restaurants. Bai et al. [25] also found that women were more selective in choosing safe restaurant environments to protect themselves. Based on the above, we know that most of the previous studies on the dining environment focused on the building or indoor environment, and few studies focused on the consumer preference of ODE in rural restaurants [4]. The outdoor environment of a rural restaurant differs somewhat from the influencing elements of the indoor environment, and together they affect consumer satisfaction in dining. The outdoor and indoor environment elements, the requirements of different customer groups, and consumer preference for the rural landscape elements of rural restaurants all have some differences, and together affect consumer satisfaction [26]. Therefore, the improvement of the rural ODE is very important to enhance the attractiveness of rural restaurants.

Ayala et al. [27] called for a more microscopic and nuanced look at the interactions of participants in order to understand the interactions of multiple stakeholders in urban construction and the conflicts and risks that arise from them. However, to the best of our knowledge, there is little support for the study of rural ODEs and the refinement of dining environments. This helps to advance the creation of a landscape environment for rural restaurants, thus achieving an improved ODE for rural restaurants. In summary, the refined classification of consumer preferences for rural outdoor dining environments has significant value and can provide theoretical help and advice to restaurant managers and planners in various aspects of planning, design, and management. Therefore, we proposed, for the first time, a refined study of consumer preferences for the quality of the rural ODE from the perspective of social media user-generated content, and argued that the results can help the rural catering industry to improve its competitiveness and the sustainable development of rural areas.

1.2. The Use of Social Media Data in Landscapes

Big data has now shown scientific advantages in tourism research. Humanism and data application will be the two major themes of future urban development [28]. When human behavior and social activities are deeply data-driven, human needs can also be finely measured and predictively analyzed [29]. In recent years, social media user content and other data in urban planning and landscape design have also provided a substantial scientific basis for the study of users' aesthetic preferences, perceptions, activity patterns, and other issues. Guan et al. [30] found significant seasonal variation in park visitation through anonymous phone location data and review content from local review sites, and seasonal fluctuations in park spatial characteristics in relation to seasonal activities, visitor perceptions, and visitation patterns. Using social media photos from Flickr and Panoramio, Tieskens et al. [31] estimated correlations between landscape attributes and landscape preferences, arguing that social media data can serve as evidence of the value of landscape elements, the location of people's interactions with the landscape, and how these interactions characterize the landscape. Li et al. [32] combined visitor ratings obtained from social media with government assessment scores to study visitor preferences for cultural ecosystem services in rural landscapes. Natural landscapes, infrastructure, and services were found to have a significant impact on the public in rural landscapes, and the relationship between different rural landscape features was not consistent across preferences for cultural ecosystem services. The findings enrich the dimension of sensory elements of cultural ecosystems and better support the management, planning, and conservation of rural landscapes. Zhang et al. [33] conducted a thorough complexity, visual scale, and color study of the visual attributes of the landscape for each attraction by evaluating photos posted by Sina Weibo users, based on a fixed-point photography experiment. The mapping relationship between the visual attributes of the landscape space and the perception of the observer was revealed. Huang et al. [34] presented a study on the application of big data in improving landscape plant gardening methods and found that the metrics of big data landscape design outperformed traditional landscape design. Several studies have shown that social media data play an important role in the field of landscape research, even complementing traditional data analysis methods, and exploring the role of landscape elements in management, planning, and conservation from research perspectives such as landscape preference and landscape perception.

Research on restaurant environment evaluation and satisfaction through social media data is also growing in popularity. Qin et al. [35] evaluated the development of the quality of the urban restaurant space at the macro level of the urban environment by using consumer review data in Dianping. Through the quantification of social media data, they found a method that can evaluate a service quality of the restaurant. Jung et al. [36] studied the changes in satisfaction with dining out before and after the pandemic through the content of comments on social media data and concluded that the study of changes in consumer dining needs is an important way to help restaurant companies adapt to the development of social changes and promote sustainable management. Koufie et al. [37] discuss what millennials look for in restaurant reviews and the importance of a restaurant's online word-of-mouth among today's millennial population, and also emphasize that social media should be incorporated into the restaurant's marketing communication strategy in restaurant management. It is evident that the study of user-generated content on social media has important value for restaurant management.

Public policy research should be an integrated innovation based on a human-oriented approach, with interdisciplinary knowledge applied to the areas underlying the assumptions of rational managers [38]. Analysis of the rural outdoor dining environment based on social media data can grasp a large amount of information on consumers' perceptions and feelings [39]. When the information is closely linked, we can provide theoretical support for tourism planning and management from the field of landscape architecture. From the perspective of user-generated content on social media platforms, this paper applies artificial intelligence to identify the sensory perceptions and their associated elements present in user-posted comments through object detection techniques in computer vision. Based on the analysis of the results, to determine consumers' landscape preferences for ODE, to study the impact of landscape quality on consumer decision-making and dining experience in a human-oriented manner. The research purposes of this paper are as follows:

1. Study consumer preferences for the landscape environment of rural ODEs through social media user-generated content.
2. To explore which type of landscape in rural ODEs is most preferred by consumers to improve the quality of rural tourism services.
3. Provide suggestions for the construction of rural ODEs to promote the integrated development of rural culture and tourism, protect rural landscapes, and upgrade the quality of rural tourism.

2. Materials and Methods

2.1. Data Collection

Dianping is the most widely used restaurant search platform in China, providing consumers with information on restaurants, finding dining destinations, sharing dining experiences, making dining plans, and so on. The content shared by users included ratings, text comments, and images of the restaurant, which contained a great deal of information about the environment, such as seating, decor, and service, and served as the main source of data collection for our experiment. As a city with a tourism orientation of "tourism destination dominated by Chinese rural vacation", Chengdu is the origin of Chinese agritainment and the representative of rural tourism development in China. Outdoor dining and recreation are one of the key features of Chinese agritainment tourism. We chose the Taohuaguli scenic area as the research site. It is a famous rural tourist attraction in Chengdu with a focus on gastronomy tourism and agricultural sightseeing, and is known as a "National Famous Town for Special Landscape Tourism". In 2021, the village received 1.83 million tourists and had a tourism income of nearly CNY 200 million [40]. Based on consumer ratings, we have selected the eight highest rated country restaurants in the area for our data collection: Shouhuangjiang (tea and gastronomy, 1288 images), Longquan

Banshan Villa (B&Bs and restaurants, 1515 images), Yunlixiaozuo (Sichuan cuisine, 3927 images), Liangwang (B&Bs and gastronomy, 1490 images), Mo'antaoli (afternoon tea and private kitchen, 1602 images), Dengxian (Sichuan cuisine, 511 images), Creeper (B&Bs and gastronomy, 288 images), and Picnics restaurant (gastronomy, 789 images).

We collect user-generated review images from the rural restaurants through Dianping and use object detection, a statistical method for detecting a certain class of semantic objects in digital images, to analyze and extract statistical information from images instead of manual labor. Object detection is a research hotspot in computer vision and has been widely used in social science research [41]. A total of 11,583 images were obtained, of which 173 sample images were excluded because they were too blurred to identify the landscape elements. A total of 11,410 valid sample images were obtained, with a validity rate of 98.5%.

2.2. Data Classification

Interventionary studies involving animals or humans, and other studies that require ethical approval, must list the authority that provided approval and the corresponding ethical approval code.

In the process of sorting out the image information, we combined the three dimensions proposed by Yang et al. [4] with the ODE landscape elements that frequently appear in the statistics for preliminary classification, and classified the elements into 37 types. Then, we referred to the Delphi method [42] that Bao et al. used to classify wetland landscapes [43]. Three experts (including a professor of rural landscape planning research, an experienced rural landscape planner, and a rural restaurant manager) were invited to conduct a field survey. Considering the functional characteristics and landscape features of each landscape element, the final classification was into eight broad categories and 35 specific landscape elements (Table 1).

Table 1. Classification of landscape elements of ODE.

Classification No.	Category	Landscape No.	Element	Frequency	Landscape No.	Element	Frequency
I	Production landscape	1	Orchard	1289	2	Flower garden	1380
II	Recreation facilities	3	Table	6480	4	Sunshade	4233
		5	Chair	6379	6	Cassette	5488
III	Sanitary facilities	7	Toilet	444	8	Dustbin	1563
		9	Washbasin	342			
IV	Lighting	10	Streetlight	1700	11	Light strip	1722
		12	Lawn light	4438	13	Spotlight	2293
V	Guided tour	14	Art board	1745	15	Billboard	1791
		16	Road sign	1506			
VI	Service	17	Dress code	787	18	Catering decoration	4073
		19	Catering setting	5511			
VII	Children's facilities	20	Slide	1768	21	Swing	1905
		22	Sandpit	1243	23	Seesaw	1118
VIII	Landscape	24	Viewing platform	2430	25	Waterscape	4255
		26	Tree	8340	27	Shrub	7564
		28	Grassland	8751	29	Landscape stone	4917
		30	Rockery	2475	31	Feature wall	1585
		32	Sculpture	4415	33	Railing	4700
		34	Path	3639	35	Flower bowl	4986

To further clarify the target differences in market segments, we classified posts with the keywords "parents, elders" as the elderly dinner group, with 2704 photos screened, and classified the comments with the keywords "children, kids, teenagers" as the parent–child dinner group, with 4141 photos screened, and the overlap between the two groups was double counted and 1323 photos were screened.

2.3. Data Processing

The object detection algorithm has been widely used in the field of image recognition [44,45]. In this research, the Yolo algorithm [46] is used to supervise the object detection network, and a sample set of 35 landscape elements was constructed from the dataset, each containing 20 pictures, a total of 700 images were used to train the object detection model to learn to recognize various landscape elements. We then fed 11,410 images of the rural ODE evaluation comments into the object detection model and counted the elemental information contained in each image, as shown in Figure 1.

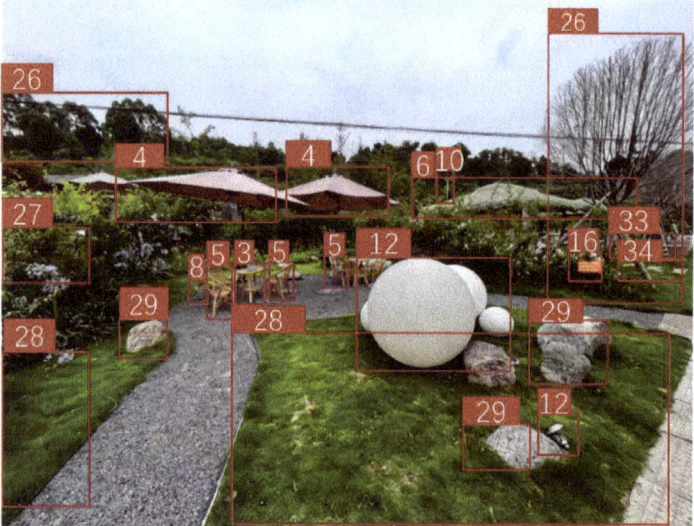

Figure 1. Object detection model data recognition diagram.

The BP neural network model is a multilayer feedforward neural network model trained according to the error backpropagation algorithm with arbitrarily complex pattern classification capability and an excellent ability to map multidimensional functions and fit nonlinear models. The neural network consists of an input layer, an output layer, and a hidden layer with a custom number of layers, which consists of a number of neurons. In the forward transmission process of the BP neural network, the neuron in the latter layer receives the input signals transmitted by the neuron in the previous layer and assigns weights to these signals. The summation result is compared with the threshold value of the current neuron, and then the result is processed by the activation function to obtain the output score [47]. Due to the large amount of data, we chose the ReLu activation function in order to reduce the dependence between parameters, reduce the overfitting rate, and enhance the robustness of the model. The output result as Formula (1):

$$Y_i = ReLu(W_i X_i + b) \quad (1)$$

where X_i is the input value, i.e., 35 elements, 1 for presence and 0 for absence; W_i is the weight and Y_i is the output value. The BP network structure is shown in Figure 2.

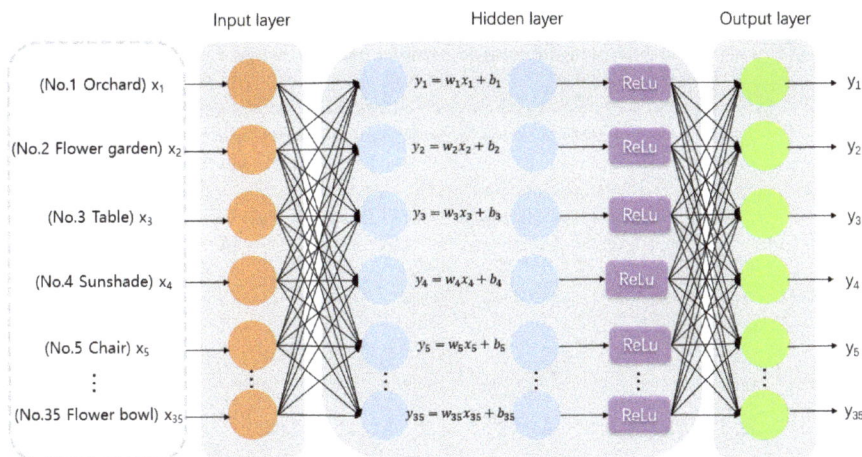

Figure 2. The BP network model.

In the model training process, we extracted 80% of the sample set for BP neural network training, which is used to construct the relationship between landscape elements and restaurant ratings. A total of 20% of the sample set was used for the test set, which is used to verify the effect of the training model. A cross-validation method is used, whereby the training and test sets are randomly divided and averaged over multiple training sessions. The output value of each element is the landscape element score, thus comparing and analyzing consumers' landscape element preferences in the rural ODE, and the research framework is shown in Figure 3.

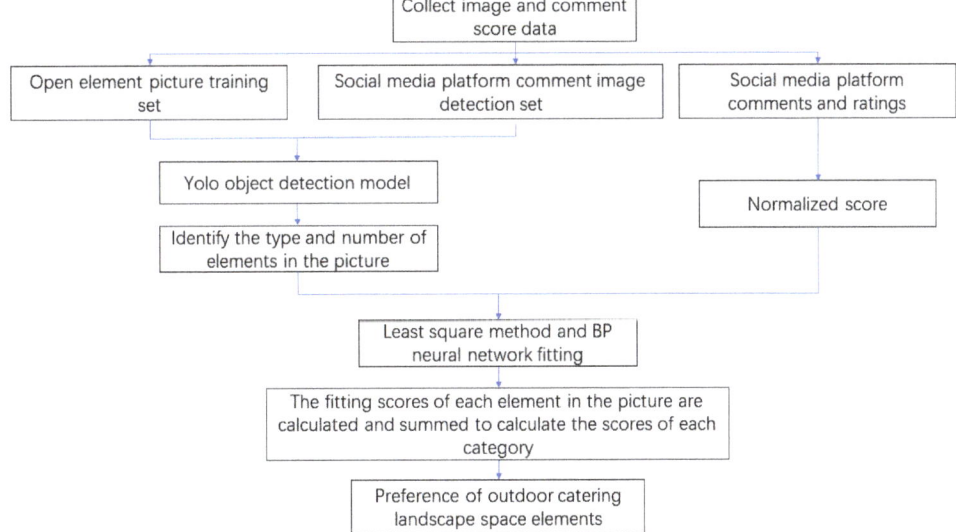

Figure 3. Research framework.

2.4. Validation of the Fitting Effect

The least square method is used for linear fitting, and the BP neural network is used for nonlinear fitting to verify the accuracy of model fitting. Normalize the score so that its range is in the interval [0,1]. Define the ratio of the number of samples with a relative error of ± 0.1 to the number of all samples as the fitting rate as a measure of fitting index. The fitting rate of the BP neural network is 89.579%, while the fitting rate of the least square method is 87.564% (see Figure 4). Although both fitting methods are effective, the BP neural network model has considered certain nonlinear factors, and the generalization effect of the model is better. By extending the batch processing with BP neural networks, adding a regularization module, and setting a small learning rate, the fitting results can be prevented from affecting non-significant data [48], the research findings can be more objective and valid. Therefore, we choose the fitting results of the BP neural network for discussion.

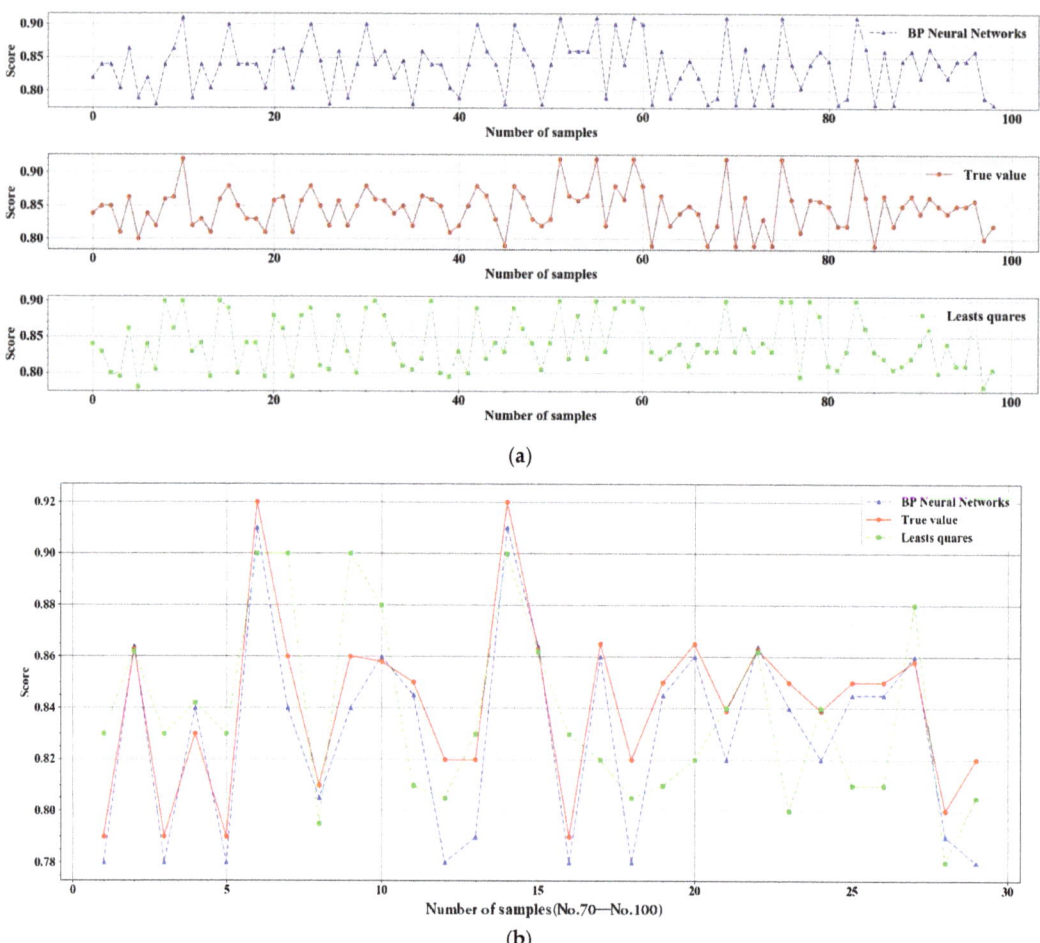

Figure 4. (a) shows the fitting result under each methods of a 100 samples cut; (b) shows the comparison results of fit rates of a 30 samples cut.

3. Results

3.1. Overall Fitting Results

The fitting results of landscape categories and elements are shown in Table 2. From Table 2, the preference ranking of the eight categories of the consumers is children's facilities (0.8740) > service (0.8703) > landscape (0.8670) > lighting (0.8593) > recreation facilities (0.8475) > sanitary facilities (0.8393) > production landscape (0.8275) > guided tour (0.8237).

Table 2. Overall landscape categories and elements preference.

Category	Score	Element	Score	Element	Score
Production landscape	0.8275	Orchard	0.797	Flower garden	0.858
Recreation facilities	0.8475	Table	0.836	Sunshade	0.848
		Chair	0.838	Cassette	0.868
Sanitary facilities	0.8393	Toilet	0.842	Dustbin	0.837
		Washbasin	0.839		
Lighting	0.8593	Streetlight	0.860	Light strip	0.863
		Lawn light	0.856	Spotlight	0.858
Guided tour	0.8237	Art board	0.851	Billboard	0.802
		Road sign	0.818		
Service	0.8703	Dress code	0.872	Catering decoration	0.847
		Catering setting	0.892		
Children's facilities	0.8740	Slide	0.912	Swing	0.842
		Sandpit	0.841	Seesaw	0.901
Landscape	0.8670	Viewing platform	0.892	Waterscape	0.866
		Tree	0.881	Shrub	0.853
		Grassland	0.864	Landscape stone	0.861
		Rockery	0.878	Feature wall	0.894
		Sculpture	0.878	Railing	0.803
		Path	0.859	Flower bowl	0.875

From the preference of landscape elements, we find that slides and seesaws are highly preferred across all. Natural landscapes, such as plant landscapes and the view of the scenery, and artificial landscapes, such as feature walls, sculptures, and flower bowls, are all highly preferred. The preferences of catering decoration, cassette, flower garden, and art board are significantly higher among similar landscapes, while the preference of orchards, railings, and billboards are the opposite.

3.2. Fitting Results of Parent-Child Group

From Table 3, the preference ranking of the eight categories of the parent–child dinner group is children's facilities (0.8985) > sanitary facilities (0.8706) > lighting (0.8567) > recreation facilities (0.8560) > landscape (0.8531) > production landscape (0.8525) > service (0.8473) > guided tour (0.8170).

Table 3. Landscape categories and elements preference of parent–child dining group.

Category	Score	Element	Score	Element	Score
Production landscape	0.8525	Orchard	0.850	Flower garden	0.855
Recreation facilities	0.8560	Table	0.833	Sunshade	0.866
		Chair	0.868	Cassette	0.857
Sanitary facilities	0.8706	Toilet	0.862	Dustbin	0.861
		Washbasin	0.889		
Lighting	0.8567	Streetlight	0.854	Light strip	0.862
		Lawn light	0.861	Spotlight	0.850
Guided tour	0.8170	Art board	0.814	Billboard	0.821
		Road sign	0.816		
Service	0.8473	Dress code	0.852	Catering decoration	0.841
		Catering setting	0.849		
Children's facilities	0.8985	Slide	0.932	Swing	0.912
		Sandpit	0.921	Seesaw	0.929
Landscape	0.8531	Viewing platform	0.834	Waterscape	0.802
		Tree	0.861	Shrub	0.863
		Grassland	0.862	Landscape stone	0.850
		Rockery	0.853	Feature wall	0.864
		Sculpture	0.879	Railing	0.876
		Path	0.837	Flower bowl	0.857

In detail, we find that all the children's facilities, such as slides, seesaws, sandpits, and swings, are highly preferred. Clean sanitary facilities with the preference of washbasins and toilets are highly preferred. Natural landscapes, such as plant landscapes, and artificial landscapes, such as feature walls, sculptures, and railings, are highly preferred. The preference for chairs and sunshades is significantly higher in the recreation facilities. The preference for light strips, flower gardens, and attendant dress code is higher among the similar landscape elements, while the preference for road signs, art boards, and waterscapes is the opposite among similar landscapes.

3.3. Fitting Results of Elder Group

From Table 4, the preference ranking of the eight categories of the elderly dining crowd is from high to low: recreation facilities (0.8840) > landscape (0.8781) > service (0.8680) > production landscape (0.8520) > sanitary facilities (0.8516) > guided tour (0.8213) > children's facilities (0.8090) > lighting (0.8067).

Table 4. Landscape categories and elements preference of elder dining group.

Category	Score	Element	Score	Element	Score
Production landscape	0.8520	Orchard	0.837	Flower garden	0.867
Recreation facilities	0.8840	Table	0.876	Sunshade	0.883
		Chair	0.897	Cassette	0.889
Sanitary facilities	0.8516	Toilet	0.851	Dustbin	0.858
		Washbasin	0.846		
Lighting	0.8067	Streetlight	0.849	Light strip	0.814
		Lawn light	0.797	Spotlight	0.767
Guided tour	0.8213	Art board	0.819	Billboard	0.817
		Road sign	0.828		
Service	0.8680	Dress code	0.868	Catering decoration	0.861
		Catering setting	0.875		
Children's facilities	0.8090	Slide	0.812	Swing	0.802
		Sandpit	0.791	Seesaw	0.831
Landscape	0.8781	Viewing platform	0.903	Waterscape	0.855
		Tree	0.881	Shrub	0.863
		Grassland	0.874	Landscape stone	0.871
		Rockery	0.868	Feature wall	0.889
		Sculpture	0.853	Railing	0.879
		Path	0.832	Flower bowl	0.873

From the preference of landscape elements, we find that chairs, cassettes, sunshades, and tables are highly noted in this group. Natural landscapes, such as plant landscapes and views of the scenery, as well as artificial landscapes, such as feature walls, railings, flower bowls, and landscape stones, are highly preferred. The preference of catering decorations, flower gardens, dustbins, street lights, and road signs is significantly higher among similar landscapes, while the opposite is true for lawn lights, sandpits, and spotlights.

4. Discussion

Rural products with a high degree of localization are the basis for the development of rural tourism. The traditional rural landscape is highly distinctive and can enhance the local tourism brand [49,50]. With eight types of landscape categories and 35 landscape elements summarized through the statistics of 11,410 photos collected from social media data, this is the first study to refine the classification of rural ODEs and is an important contribution to this field of study. We used BP neural network analysis to score the preferences of the landscape types and the landscape elements. In terms of theoretical research, we studied consumers' experiential preferences in rural outdoor dining environments, explored the use of rural landscape elements in rural restaurants, and called for the reasonable protection and utilization of rural resources with positive values. In practice, this paper suggests that planners and managers can take advantage of the localization and seasonal variation of production landscapes, clarify the target positioning of restaurant clientele, and complete the construction of infrastructure services for different groups, including protection of rural resources and the environment (biodiversity and natural and human landscape resources) to promote the competitiveness of rural restaurants and to improve the competitiveness of rural restaurants, while contributing to sustainable rural development.

Different people have different needs and preferences for ODEs of rural restaurants, and understanding the behavioral needs of different groups of people when it comes to outdoor recreation is becoming increasingly important [51]. In terms of overall consumer preference score, consumer preference for children's facilities is significant. When children regard an activity as a game, they show more signs of emotional health [52], and the pleasure soundscape and multitasking of children's play have a positive impact [53]. Therefore, we concluded through our study that the emotional perceptions displayed by children when using the children's facilities in rural ODEs can have a significant positive impact on consumers' dining decisions, yet children's activities are often ignored in research as an element of restaurant attraction. Agriculture and production, as important cultural and natural resources in the traditional countryside, are important pull factors for rural tourism and also influence consumers' preference for rural restaurants. In its landscape planning, rural restaurants should pay attention to both the functional expression of the landscape in terms of cultural, historical, educational, and research values of the agricultural landscape; otherwise consumers will be limited in the experiences they receive and the ways they can participate [54]. The agricultural landscape is the main component of agricultural culture, and they are mutually reinforcing. Rational use of agricultural resources around a rural restaurant is a win-win model for both the restaurant and the rural area. The preference for the seasonal characteristics of agricultural landscapes in the dining experience of rural restaurant consumers and the value of agricultural culture in rural restaurants are also worthy of further study. In this study, the landscape category shows a high preference, and in the planning and design process, more refined design considerations should be made for its specific elements, such as Rossetti et al. [55] suggesting that railings have a positive impact on aesthetics and safety, but they are easy to ignore and lead to inactivity and boredom. Even in our study, as an important landscape element, Zhang et al. [56,57] believe that walls have a comprehensive negative impact, even causing depression and boredom, because they hinder the green landscape or accumulate pollutants. It is clear that functional infrastructure can have a positive impact and appeal if it is well designed. Therefore, in the design of infrastructure, it should also be integrated into local culture for careful design consideration.

In contrast to the needs of different groups of people, children's facilities can meet the needs of interaction between parents and children [58], but also influence the consumption decisions of the family dinner crowd [59]. This study argues for this result, proving that children's activities have a positive impact on consumers of outdoor dining in the rural area, and also finding in the published user-generated data that four types of children's landscape facilities—sandpits, seesaws, slides, and swings—are highly attractive to the parent–child gathering group. The choice of colors, materials and types of children's facilities needs to be studied more finely in relation to different environments and specific groups [60]. This study complements the results of the selection of facility types in a rural ODE. The sanitary environment is also a high concern for family dinner groups in the outdoor environment of country restaurants, especially after the outbreak of the COVID-19 pandemic [61]. Although evolutionary theories of landscape preference suggest that people naturally prefer waterscapes [62], and that the presence of water triggers preference and pleasure, and that it always enhances visual quality [63], in the parent–child group, we found that consumers preferred water features less than other elements. Meanwhile, the parent–child group also has a low preference for environments that are dangerous to children, such as viewing platforms and paths that may blur the borders. Instead, there is a greater preference for elements, such as railings and feature walls, that have a separating and enclosing effect. Therefore, we believe that safety and hygiene are important factors that influence the decision of the parent–child group to ODEs in rural restaurants. The kinds of children's play spaces in a rural ODE that can better allay parents' concerns about safety in order to improve consumer satisfaction with the environment are subject to further research. Moreover, children are extremely sensitive to the physical environment, especially the light environment [64]. A reasonably good light environment can elicit positive emotions and a desire to explore, [65] has similar findings to our study, and we believe that suitable restaurant lighting environment has a certain appeal and competitive advantage for parent–child groups. Those dining with their elders are more interested in the leisure and landscape categories, and it can be argued that elderly people prefer to eat and relax outdoors in good environments [66]. Therefore, restaurant managers could create a leisurely and beautiful traditional agricultural landscape to make the ODE of rural restaurants more humane and naturalistic for elders to rest and enjoy the view. In addition, the group dining with elders also pays high attention to the service, and restaurant managers should pay attention to it in terms of service facilities for the elderly. Another item that stands out is the high preference for good street lighting among the group dining with elders, perhaps for safety reasons, but they have a relatively low preference for spotlights and strip lights. To sum up, there are some differences in consumer preferences between parent–child groups and dining with elder groups. Restaurants aimed at these two groups should be designed and managed with quality and hygiene, green and nature, and consumer safety as the focus of ODE in rural restaurants. In response to the different preferences between different populations suggested by the study, researchers of children's facilities, children's safety, and landscape lighting could also conduct further and more detailed studies in rural areas.

Combined with the results of the three groups, we find that consumers are highly interested in the landscape category. This result can be explained by the fact that consumers have a tendency to seek naturalization of the environment and a higher preference for landscapes with local characteristics, and it also confirms that "naturalness" is an important factor in landscape preference [67,68]. Historical culture and natural resources in the traditional countryside are important pull factors for rural tourism, whether it is at the planning level, design level, or management level, neither the culture nor the natural resources of the traditional countryside should be ignored in the face of its value. The conservation and sustainable use of rural landscape resources through scientific and technological means is essential for the full implementation of the principle of ecological priority. The ODE of rural restaurants can provide a natural, comfortable, and authentic environment for consumers, using the rural landscape environment with local characteristics to attract consumers to achieve the purpose of promoting the environmental protection of rural environmental resources and the sustainable development of the rural catering industry.

Urban and rural area construction and development cannot simply focus on top-down development from the engineering dimension but also need to be linked to social needs. In order to reveal the complexity of the urban and rural construction processes, the participants (subjects of interest) should be included in the scope of investigation, and a more microscopic and detailed observation of the interaction between the participants should be conducted [27,69]. With planning and management based on a human-oriented perspective, the government can reduce costs, improve effectiveness, and enhance efficiency in policy development and project design [70]. Managers can better target restaurant positioning, restaurant themes, and environmental design to improve consumer satisfaction and repurchase willingness, thereby increasing restaurant competitiveness. The research in this paper combines landscape architecture with tourism management, and through social media data analysis, we try to explore refined management of rural restaurants and human-oriented design considerations of ODEs, which can provide a reference for governments and managers. For example, Gibson et al. argue that as cities have gradually brightened up, rural landscape lighting has been lagging behind [71]. The right policies and projects may be able to effectively integrate rural restaurant lighting projects with rural landscape lighting to enhance rural infrastructure. In addition to market and social factors, restaurant managers should also consider the location of their projects in a local context, taking advantage of their location and targeting different customer segments to make a more economical, efficient, and sustainable project. Managers who need to improve the quality of their country's restaurants can also do so by combining the most prominent problems in their restaurants with consumer preferences in order to effectively improve the attractions of their restaurants. In restaurant publicity, restaurant managers can also increase the value of advertising by targeting different groups of people according to the characteristics of the restaurant.

5. Conclusions

Based on the user-generated content of social media platforms, this study explores the classification of ODE of rural restaurants, analyzes consumer preferences for landscape categories and elements, and provides guidance for the development of rural tourism and rural restaurants. The results of this study can provide practical advice to planners and managers at different levels and provide some value to rural tourism development and rural environmental protection. However, this study also has some limitations: (1) The data for the study comes from social media, where most of the people active on social media are young or highly educated, and the data are not universally available. (2) In terms of segmentation, we have only divided the age groups through textual evaluation or the content of the people appearing in the photos, the results of the study can only represent the perceived preferences of consumers with children, consumers accompanying the elderly, and the general public. Further research is needed to know the preferences of specific children or the elderly themselves. (3) The classification in this study is based on an exploration of villages in western China. Villages in different regional and cultural contexts will have different landscape qualities, and future research should be conducted in different regions to test the applicability and generalizability of the landscape element preferences in this study. In addition, after the pandemic, people's changes in the use and perception of green spaces [72], dining habits, and satisfaction are also changing [73]. Perhaps an exploration of the changes in the rural ODEs after the pandemic based on social media data will also reveal new and different findings to complement the study of consumers' preferences and satisfaction in rural ODEs.

To our knowledge, there are few studies on consumer preferences for rural ODEs. Although we only sampled in Chengdu, China, the study is still valuable in several ways. Firstly, from the aspect of refined management and design of urban and rural planning, the study of restaurant management and design is carried out based on the real needs of people, hoping to resonate with more researchers from related fields and to jointly explore the human-oriented considerations and exploration of urban and rural planning. Secondly, the results of the study provide consumer-based recommendations for improving the competitiveness of rural restaurants in terms of design and management. At the same time, we also call on people at all levels to make rational use of the diverse values of rural culture and natural resources in order to truly achieve a win-win situation for the development and conservation of rural areas.

Author Contributions: Conceptualization, M.Y. and J.Q.; methodology, M.Y.; software, W.F.; validation, M.Y. and W.F.; formal analysis, W.F. and S.Z.; investigation, M.Y. and W.F.; resources, M.Y., J.Q. and J.L.; data curation, W.F.; writing—original draft preparation, M.Y. and W.F; writing—review and editing, M.Y. and J.Q.; visualization, W.F. and J.L.; supervision, J.Q.; project administration, M.Y.; funding acquisition, M.Y. and J.Q. All authors have read and agreed to the published version of the manuscript.

Funding: This research was funded by the National Natural Science Foundation of China, grant number 52078423. Sichuan Science and Technology Plan Key R&D Projects, grant number 2020YFS0054. Sichuan Provincial Social Science Key Research Base (Sichuan Cuisine Development Research Center), grant number CC22W32. Sichuan Tourism University "Rural Recreation Tourism and Habitat Enhancement Innovation Team", grant number 21SCTUTP06. and 2021 National Student Innovation and Entrepreneurship Training Program, grant number 202111552069.

Institutional Review Board Statement: The study was conducted according to the guidelines of the Declaration of Helsinki, all the necessary information regarding the study was given. The photos we chose were publicly posted on social media platforms and the study did not expose the users to any harm. Therefore, this experiment was conducted with the approval of the Academic Committee of Southwest Jiaotong University, but no submission for review was required.

Informed Consent Statement: Not applicable.

Data Availability Statement: The data presented in this study are available on request from the corresponding author. The data are not publicly available due to privacy.

Acknowledgments: We thank co-workers from "Ecology and Design Research Studio" for data collection efforts, and the anonymous reviewers who provided invaluable advice on how to improve the manuscript.

Conflicts of Interest: The authors declare no conflict of interest.

References

1. Henderson, J.C. Food tourism reviewed. *Brit. Food J.* **2009**, *111*, 317–326. [CrossRef]
2. Huang, Z.F.; Zhang, Y.G.; Jia, W.T.; Hong, X.T.; Yu, R.Z. The research process and trend of development in the New Era of rural tourism in China. *J. Nat. Resour.* **2021**, *36*, 2615–2633. [CrossRef]
3. He, Y.; Wang, J.; Gao, X.; Wang, Y.; Choi, B.R. Rural tourism: Does it matter for sustainable farmers' income. *Sustain. Sci.* **2021**, *13*, 10440. [CrossRef]
4. Yang, M.; Luo, S. Effects of rural restaurants' outdoor dining environment dimensions on customers' satisfaction: A consumer perspective. *Foods* **2021**, *10*, 2172. [CrossRef] [PubMed]
5. Long, H.; Liu, Y.; Li, X.; Chen, Y. Building new countryside in China: A geographical perspective. *Land Use Policy* **2010**, *27*, 457–470. [CrossRef]
6. Liu, Y.X.; Gao, Y.; Liu, L.L.; Yang, Z.C. Exploration of "people-oriented" village planning and its practice: A case study of Zhunao village, Daxing district, Beijing city. *China Land Sci.* **2020**, *34*, 18–27, 68. [CrossRef]
7. Brouder, P.; Karlsson, S.; Lundmark, L. Hyper-production: A new metric of multifunctionality. *Eur. Countrys.* **2015**, *7*, 134–143. [CrossRef]
8. Torquati, B.; Tempesta, T.; Vecchiato, D.; Venanzi, S.; Paffarini, C. The value of traditional rural landscape and nature protected areas in tourism demand: A study on agritourists' preferences. *Landsc. Online* **2017**, *53*, 1–18. [CrossRef]
9. Devesa, M.; Laguna, M.; Palacios, A. The role of motivation in visitor satisfaction: Empirical evidence in rural tourism. *Tour. Manag.* **2010**, *31*, 547–552. [CrossRef]
10. Cavicchi, A.; Stancova, K.C. Food and gastronomy as elements of regional innovation strategies. In *Spain: European Commission, Joint Research Centre*; Institute for Prospective Technological Studies: Seville, Spain, 2016; pp. 30–34.
11. Findlay, A.M.; Short, D.; Stockdale, A. The labour-market impact of migration to rural areas. *Appl. Geogr.* **2000**, *20*, 333–348. [CrossRef]
12. Lundmark, L. Restructuring and employment change in sparsely populated areas. In *Examples from northern Sweden and Finland*; Gerum, Kulturgeografiska Institutionen, Umeå Universitet: Umeå, Sweden, 2006.
13. Scozzafava, G.; Contini, C.; Romano, C.; Casini, L. Eating out: Which restaurant to choose. *Brit. Food J.* **2017**, *119*, 1870–1883. [CrossRef]
14. Rinaldi, C. Food and gastronomy for sustainable place development: A multidisciplinary analysis of different theoretical approaches. *Sustainability* **2017**, *9*, 1748. [CrossRef]
15. Palmieri, N.; Perito, M.A. Consumers' willingness to consume sustainable and local wine in italy. *Ital. J. Food Sci.* **2020**, *32*, 222–233. [CrossRef]
16. Palmieri, N.; Forleo, M.B. The potential of edible seaweed within the western diet. A segmentation of Italian consumers. *Int. J. Gastron. Food Sci.* **2020**, *20*, 100202. [CrossRef]
17. Liu, Y.; Jang, S.S. Perceptions of Chinese restaurants in the US: What affects customer satisfaction and behavioral intentions. *Int. J. Hosp. Manag.* **2009**, *28*, 338–348. [CrossRef]
18. Auty, S. Consumer choice and segmentation in the restaurant industry. *Serv. Ind. J.* **1992**, *12*, 324–339. [CrossRef]
19. Hul, M.K.; Dube, L.; Chebat, J. The impact of music on consumers' reactions to waiting for services. *J. Retail.* **1997**, *73*, 87–104. [CrossRef]

20. Robson, S.K. Turning the tables: The psychology of design for high-volume restaurants. *Cornell Hotel. Restaur. Adm. Q.* **1999**, *40*, 56–63. [CrossRef]
21. Ryu, K.; Jang, S. DINESCAPE: A scale for customers' perception of dining environments. *J. Foodserv. Bus. Res.* **2008**, *11*, 2–22. [CrossRef]
22. Ryu, K.; Jang, S.S. The effect of environmental perceptions on behavioral intentions through emotions: The case of upscale restaurants. *J. Hosp. Tour. Res.* **2007**, *31*, 56–72. [CrossRef]
23. Horng, J.; Hsu, H. A holistic aesthetic experience model: Creating a harmonious dining environment to increase customers' perceived pleasure. *J. Hosp. Tour. Manag.* **2020**, *45*, 520–534. [CrossRef]
24. Albright, C.L.; Flora, J.A.; Fortmann, S.P. Restaurant menu labeling: Impact of nutrition information on entree sales and patron attitudes. *Health Educ Q.* **1990**, *17*, 157–167. [CrossRef] [PubMed]
25. Bai, L.; Wang, M.; Yang, Y.; Gong, S. Food safety in restaurants: The consumer perspective. *Int. J. Hosp. Manag.* **2019**, *77*, 139–146. [CrossRef]
26. Breuste, J.H. Decision making, planning and design for the conservation of indigenous vegetation within urban development.Landsc. *Urban Plan.* **2004**, *68*, 439–452. [CrossRef]
27. Luque-Ayala, A.; Marvin, S. Developing a critical understanding of smart urbanism? *Urban Stud.* **2015**, *52*, 2105–2116. [CrossRef]
28. Qin, X.; Zhen, F.; Wei, Z. The discussion of urban research in the future: Data driven or human-oriented driven. *Sci. Geogr. Sin.* **2019**, *39*, 31–40.
29. Biltgen, P.; Ryan, S. *Activity-Based Intelligence: Principles and Applications*; Artech House: Boston, MA, USA, 2016.
30. Guan, C.; Song, J.; Keith, M.; Zhang, B.; Akiyama, Y.; Da, L.; Shibasaki, R.; Sato, T. Seasonal variations of park visitor volume and park service area in Tokyo: A mixed-method approach combining big data and field observations. *Urban For. Urban Green.* **2021**, *58*, 126973. [CrossRef]
31. Tieskens, K.F.; Van Zanten, B.T.; Schulp, C.J.; Verburg, P.H. Aesthetic appreciation of the cultural landscape through social media: An analysis of revealed preference in the Dutch river landscape. *Landsc. Urban Plan.* **2018**, *177*, 128–137. [CrossRef]
32. Li, Y.; Xie, L.; Zhang, L.; Huang, L.; Lin, Y.; Su, Y.; AmirReza, S.; He, S.; Zhu, C.; Li, S. Understanding different cultural ecosystem services: An exploration of rural landscape preferences based on geographic and social media data. *J. Environ. Manag.* **2022**, *317*, 115487. [CrossRef] [PubMed]
33. Zhang, X.; Xu, D.; Zhang, N. Research on Landscape Perception and Visual Attributes Based on Social Media Data—A Case Study on Wuhan University. *Appl. Sci.* **2022**, *12*, 8346. [CrossRef]
34. Huang, L. Application of big data in improving landscape plant landscaping method. *J. Phys. Conf. Ser.* **2021**, *1852*, 32024. [CrossRef]
35. Qin, X.; Zhen, F.; Zhu, S.; Xi, G. Spatial pattern of catering industry in Nanjing urban area based on the degree of public praise from internet: A case study of Dianping. *Com. Sci. Geogr.* **2014**, *34*, 810–817. [CrossRef]
36. Jung, H.; Yoon, H.; Song, M. A Study on Dining-Out Trends Using Big Data: Focusing on Changes since COVID-19. *Sustainability* **2021**, *13*, 11480. [CrossRef]
37. Koufie, M.G.E.; Kesa, H. Millennials motivation for sharing restaurant dining experiences on social media. *Afr. J. Hosp. Tour. Leis.* **2020**, *9*, 1–25.
38. Zhu, D.; Li, B. Behavioral science and public policy: Pursuit of policy effectiveness. *Chin. Public Adm.* **2018**, *8*, 59–64. [CrossRef]
39. Kim, W.G.; Li, J.J.; Brymer, R.A. The impact of social media reviews on restaurant performance: The moderating role of excellence certificate. *Int. J. Hosp. Manag.* **2016**, *55*, 41–51. [CrossRef]
40. Introduction to Huaguo Village, Shanquan Town. Available online: http://www.longquanyi.gov.cn/lqyqzfmhwz_gb/c151772/2022/04/08/content_b211846c19334066a99bd05a96579b01.shtml (accessed on 8 April 2022).
41. Lu, L.; Li, H.; Ding, Z.; Guo, Q. An improved target detection method based on multiscale features fusion. *Microw. Opt. Technol. Lett.* **2020**, *62*, 3051–3059. [CrossRef]
42. Taze, D.; Hartley, C.; Morgan, A.W.; Chakrabarty, A.; Mackie, S.L.; Griffin, K.J. Developing consensus in Histopathology: The role of the Delphi method. *Histopathology* **2022**, *81*, 159–167. [CrossRef]
43. Bao, Y.H.; Ren, J. Wetland landscape classification based on the BP neural network in DaLinor lake area. *Procedia Environ. Sci.* **2011**, *10*, 2360–2366. [CrossRef]
44. Mokhtar, M.K.; Mohamed, F.; Sunar, M.S.; Aziz, A.; Sidik, M. Image Features Detection and Tracking for Image Based Target Augmented Reality Application. In Proceedings of the 2019 IEEE Conference on Graphics and Media (GAME), Pulau Pinang, Malaysia, 19–21 November 2019.
45. Raghunandan, A.; Mohana; Raghav, P.; Aradhya, H. Object detection algorithms for video surveillance applications. In Proceedings of the 2018 International Conference on Communication and Signal Processing (ICCSP), Chennai, India, 3–5 April 2018.
46. Guo, R.; Li, S.; Wang, K. Research on YOLOv3 algorithm based on darknet framework. *J. Phys. Conf. Ser.* **2020**, *1629*, 12062. [CrossRef]
47. Koyuncu, H. Determination of positioning accuracies by using fingerprint localisation and artificial neural networks. *Therm. Sci.* **2019**, *23*, 99–111. [CrossRef]

48. Gupta, S.; Gupta, R.; Ojha, M.; Singh, K.P. A comparative analysis of various regularization techniques to solve overfitting problem in artificial neural network. In Proceedings of the International Conference on Recent Developments in Science, Singapore, 22–24 June 2017.
49. Lim, Y.; Weaver, P.A. Customer-based brand equity for a destination: The effect of destination image on preference for products associated with a destination brand. *Int. J. Tour. Res.* **2014**, *16*, 223–231. [CrossRef]
50. Ohe, Y.; Kurihara, S. Evaluating the complementary relationship between local brand farm products and rural tourism: Evidence from Japan. *Tourism Manag.* **2013**, *35*, 278–283. [CrossRef]
51. Whiting, J.W.; Larson, L.R.; Green, G.T.; Kralowec, C. Outdoor recreation motivation and site preferences across diverse racial/ethnic groups: A case study of Georgia state parks. *J. Outdoor Rec. Tour.* **2017**, *18*, 10–21. [CrossRef]
52. Wilson, K.; Ramella, K.; Poulos, A. Building school connectedness through structured recreation during school: A concurrent Mixed-Methods study. *J. Sch. Health* **2022**, *92*, 1013–1021. [CrossRef]
53. Liu, J.; Yang, L.; Xiong, Y.; Yang, Y. Effects of soundscape perception on visiting experience in a renovated historical block. *Build. Environ.* **2019**, *165*, 106375. [CrossRef]
54. Su, M.M.; Dong, Y.; Wall, G.; Sun, Y. A value-based analysis of the tourism use of agricultural heritage systems: Duotian Agrosystem, Jiangsu Province, China. *J. Sustain. Tour.* **2020**, *28*, 2136–2155. [CrossRef]
55. Rossetti, T.A.S.; Lobel, H.; Rocco, V.I.C.; Hurtubia, R. Explaining subjective perceptions of public spaces as a function of the built environment: A massive data approach. *Landsc. Urban Plan.* **2019**, *181*, 169–178. [CrossRef]
56. Zhang, F.; Zhou, B.; Liu, L.; Liu, Y.; Fung, H.H.; Lin, H.; Ratti, C. Measuring human perceptions of a large-scale urban region using machine learning. *Landsc. Urban Plan.* **2018**, *180*, 148–160. [CrossRef]
57. Zhang, Y.; Li, S.; Dong, R.; Deng, H.; Fu, X.; Wang, C.; Yu, T.; Jia, T.; Zhao, J. Quantifying physical and psychological perceptions of urban scenes using deep learning. *Land Use Policy* **2021**, *111*, 105762. [CrossRef]
58. Liu, W.; Li, C.; Tong, Y.; Zhang, J.; Ma, Z. The places children go: Understanding spatial patterns and formation mechanism for children's commercial activity space in changchun city, china. *Sustainability* **2020**, *12*, 1377. [CrossRef]
59. Labrecque, J.A.; Ricard, L. Children's influence on family decision-making: A restaurant study. *J. Bus. Res.* **2001**, *54*, 173–176. [CrossRef]
60. Isele, P.C.; Mussi, A.Q. Inclusive Architecture: Landscape Codesign in Children's Playgrounds. *J. Civ. Eng. Archit.* **2021**, *15*, 429–436. [CrossRef]
61. Sharifi, A.; Khavarian-Garmsir, A.R. The COVID-19 pandemic: Impacts on cities and major lessons for urban planning, design, and management. *Sci. Total Environ.* **2020**, *749*, 142391. [CrossRef]
62. Ulrich, R.S. Human responses to vegetation and landscapes. *Landsc. Urban Plan.* **1986**, *13*, 29–44. [CrossRef]
63. Zube, E.H.; Sell, J.L.; Taylor, J.G. Landscape perception: Research, application and theory. *Landsc. Plan.* **1982**, *9*, 1–33. [CrossRef]
64. Angelaki, S.; Triantafyllidis, G.A.; Besenecker, U. Lighting in Kindergartens: Towards Innovative Design Concepts for Lighting Design in Kindergartens Based on Children's Perception of Space. *Sustainability* **2022**, *14*, 2302. [CrossRef]
65. Yalciner, I.P.; Hasirci, D. Preschool children and sunlight. In *ICERI2018 Proceedings*; IATED: Seville, Spain, 2018.
66. Ganesan, L.; Abu Bakar, A.Z.; Othman, M. A qualitative study on factors influencing older consumer dining out behaviour. In Proceedings of the 3rd UUM International Qualitative Research Conference (QRC), Melaka, Malaysia, 10–12 July 2018.
67. Tveit, M.; Ode, A.S.; Fry, G. Key concepts in a framework for analysing visual landscape character. *Landsc. Res.* **2006**, *31*, 229–255. [CrossRef]
68. Tveit, M.S. Indicators of visual scale as predictors of landscape preference; A comparison between groups. *J. Environ. Manag.* **2009**, *90*, 2882–2888. [CrossRef]
69. Hollands, R.G. *The Routledge Companion to Smart Cities*, 1st ed.; Routledge: London, UK, 2020.
70. The American Presidency Project. Executive Order 13707-Using Behavioral Science Insights to Better Serve the American People. Available online: http://www.presidency.ucsb.edu/ws/index.php?pid=110815 (accessed on 8 September 2022).
71. Gibson, J.; Olivia, S.; Boe-Gibson, G. Night Lights in Economics: Sources and Uses1. *J. Econ. Surv.* **2020**, *34*, 955–980. [CrossRef]
72. Ugolini, F.; Massetti, L.; Calaza-Martínez, P.; Cariñanos, P.; Dobbs, C.; Ostoić, S.K.; Marin, A.M.; Pearlmutter, D.; Saaroni, H.; Šaulienė, I.; et al. Effects of the COVID-19 pandemic on the use and perceptions of urban green space: An international exploratory study. *Urban For. Urban Green.* **2020**, *56*, 126888. [CrossRef] [PubMed]
73. Jia, S. Analyzing restaurant customers' evolution of dining patterns and satisfaction during COVID-19 for sustainable business insights. *Sustainability* **2021**, *9*, 4981. [CrossRef]

MDPI
St. Alban-Anlage 66
4052 Basel
Switzerland
Tel. +41 61 683 77 34
Fax +41 61 302 89 18
www.mdpi.com

International Journal of Environmental Research and Public Health Editorial Office
E-mail: ijerph@mdpi.com
www.mdpi.com/journal/ijerph

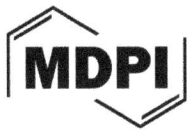

www.ingramcontent.com/pod-product-compliance
Lightning Source LLC
LaVergne TN
LVHW070510100526
838202LV00014B/1828